RUTH STRYKER, R.N., M.A.

Assistant Professor
Long Term Care Administration
Programs in Hospital and Health Care Administration
School of Public Health
University of Minnesota
Minneapolis, Minnesota

1977

W. B. SAUNDERS COMPANY
Philadelphia • London • Toronto

Second Edition

Rehabilitative Aspects of Acute and Chronic Nursing Care

W. B. Saunders Company: West Washington Square
Philadelphia, PA   19105

1 St. Anne's Road
Eastbourne, East Sussex BN21 3UN, England

1 Goldthorne Avenue
Toronto, Ontario M8Z 5T9, Canada

Library of Congress Cataloging in Publication Data

Stryker, Ruth Perin.

Rehabilitative aspects of acute and chronic nursing care.

Includes bibliographies and index.

1. Rehabilitation nursing.   I. Title.

RT120.R4S85 1977   610.73   76-54042

ISBN 0-7216-8637-0

Rehabilitative Aspects of Acute and Chronic Nursing Care   ISBN   0-7216-8637-0

Last digit is the print number: 9   8   7   6   5   4   3   2   1

To
MRS. BEVERLY FAHLAND,
the rehabilitation nurse from whom
so many of us have learned.

PREFACE TO
THE SECOND EDITION

When the word "rehabilitation" is used, beware of any assumption about its meaning. It may refer to a house, a neighborhood, a criminal, the disabled, someone culturally disadvantaged, the mentally ill, the chemically dependent or a cancer victim. If rehabilitation means the restoration or reorganization of a lost or underdeveloped function or ability, one can rule out the house and neighborhood, but one must still ask (1) who is being rehabilitated and (2) what is the condition requiring rehabilitation? In other words, a book on rehabilitation must focus on a specific population and identify that population for its readers.

The aim of this book is to provide the nurse with greater understanding and skill in working with persons having neuromusculoskeletal problems. Also, it primarily addresses itself to adult and elderly populations. In most instances, the concepts and skills described are applicable to a variety of conditions. It is hoped that the reader will be able to transfer knowledge appropriately when a specific disease is not mentioned. For instance, the one-handed dressing technique can be utilized by a person with hemiplegia, upper extremity amputation or a fractured arm. Range of motion exercises can be used by and for the elderly and patients with stroke, spinal cord injury, arthritis and some neurological conditions, as well as post fracture and post surgery. A new chapter, Maintaining Sexuality, which emphasizes spinal cord injury and the aged, is also applicable to a majority of patients seen on many medical and surgical units.

While a problem-oriented approach to nursing is desirable in most instances, specific disease-oriented concerns obviously do exist. For this reason, six supplementary texts are suggested. There are obviously others and many are listed at the end of each chapter. The following six basic texts are recommended:

Carini, Esta, and Owens, Guy: *Neurological and Neurosurgical Nursing.* St. Louis, C.V. Mosby Co., 1973.

Downey, John A., and Low, Niels L. (Eds.): *The Child with Disabling Illness: Principles of Rehabilitation.* Philadelphia, W. B. Saunders Co., 1974.

Ehrlich, George E. (Ed.): *Total Management of the Arthritic Patient.* Philadelphia, J. B. Lippincott Co., 1973.

Ford, J.R.: *Physical Management for the Quadriplegic Patient*. Philadelphia, F.A. Davis Co., 1975.

Larson, Carroll, and Gould, Marjorie: *Orthopedic Nursing*. St. Louis, C.V. Mosby Co., 1974.

Licht, Sidney (Ed.): *Stroke and Its Rehabilitation*. Baltimore, Waverly Press, 1975.

I have also tried to integrate a broader range of problems, especially those of the elderly, into each chapter. This will be particularly noticed in Chapter 3 – An Overview of Rehabilitation Nursing, Chapter 4 – Psychological Reactions to Disability, and Chapter 6 – Planning Patient Care. Chapter 19 – The Elderly in the Community – is a new addition to the book. While all chapters have been revised, expanded and updated, there are major changes in Chapter 4 – Psychological Reactions to Disability, Chapter 6 – Planning Patient Care, Chapter 7 – Communicating with Patients with Communication Problems, Chapter 8 – Assisting Patients with Bowel and Bladder Problems, Chapter 11 – Planning for Discharge and Chapter 12 – Positioning and Skin Care. The book was designed for students and practitioners, but it can also be used as a faculty reference and may sometimes be useful to selected patients and families.

A patient's optimum rehabilitation potential can be permanently reduced by poor nursing care at any point in the health care system, whether that be the emergency room, an intensive care unit, a medical-surgical station, a chronic care section, a nursing home, a clinic or the home. Therefore, although obviously every nurse cannot become a rehabilitation expert, basic rehabilitation concepts and skills are necessary to knowledgeable nursing care in all settings.

RUTH STRYKER, R.N., M.A.

ACKNOWLEDGMENTS

Content for a book arises from the melding of the author's life experience and study of a particular area of interest. In this instance, my association with the University of Minnesota and Sister Kenny Institute has added very special insights and knowledge to former experiences in other work settings. These opportunities to study rehabilitation, to know patients and to teach students have guided the design and content of the book.

Many persons have assisted immeasurably with the book, especially the first edition. For this edition, I am particularly grateful to Thomas P. Anderson, M.D., Associate Professor, Department of Physical Medicine and Rehabilitation, University of Minnesota, for his review of Chapter 9, Maintaining Sexuality, and to Beverly Fahland, R. N., recently retired as instructor at Sister Kenny Institute. Mrs. Fahland's expertise and critical eye once again influenced the accuracy and depth of content of the book, particularly in the area of skills and equipment. Also, Mary Albury, artist at Biomedical Graphics Communications Department, University of Minnesota, has clarified many of the techniques by the addition of her new illustrations.

Last, but certainly not least, special gratitude goes to my husband, Ken, who had to share the first year and a half of our marriage with the writing of this book.

PREFACE TO
THE FIRST EDITION

Rehabilitation has all too frequently been thought of as a specialty. What is even more unfortunate is that it has also been thought of as something that follows acute and convalescent care. It is true that preventive and maintenance measures are an integral part of restorative care of the chronically ill and disabled, but such measures undertaken during acute care can both shorten and enhance restorative care. Because these facets of care are so often overlooked, this book has been particularly designed to help nurses implement rehabilitative steps in acute and long-term care, regardless of the physical setting.

We are here primarily concerned with physical rehabilitation. The psychosocial aspects of physical disability are considered because of their close relationship with physical care, but it should be made clear that we are not dealing with psychiatric rehabilitation.

Since the principles, philosophy, techniques, devices and psychosocial concepts of rehabilitation are applicable to patients with a great variety of conditions, specific disabilities are not discussed in detail. The types of conditions under consideration, however, are mainly neuromuscular-skeletal disorders.

It is not so much what disease the patient has as how it affects him that the nurse must consider. Her responsibility is to know how to help the patient deal with his problems. For example, a nursing problem may not be a matter of whether the patient has arthritis or hemiplegia, but of how to handle a painful extremity *versus* a paralyzed one. Even if two patients have arthritis, the degree of pain and deformity, prognosis, intelligence, interests and social and economic factors may vary greatly. Therefore, the emphasis of this book is on knowledge that can be abstracted and integrated, and on tools that can be adapted to many situations.

It is the author's hope that nurses reading this book will be stimulated to incorporate appropriate preventive, maintenance and restorative measures in their patient care regardless of the setting in which they practice nursing.

RUTH STRYKER, R.N., M.A.

CONTENTS

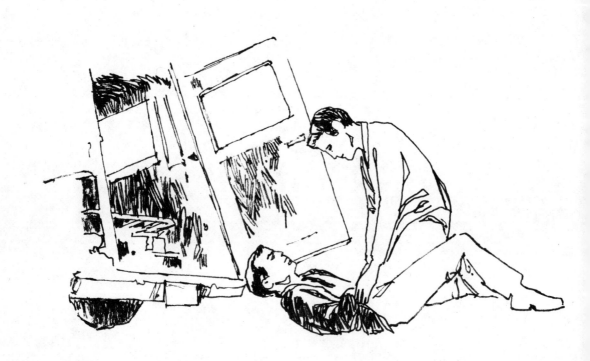

Unit I
INTRODUCTION

Chapter 1

THE HISTORY OF REHABILITATION—IS IT JUST BEGINNING?

The history of rehabilitation reflects mankind's persistent discomfort, apathy and insensitivity toward disadvantaged persons, whether they be old, poor, mentally impaired or physically disabled. Throughout history such persons have been ridiculed, persecuted or totally ignored. Primitive man abandoned the disabled and old with the philosophy that only the fit should survive. In many cultures such as nomadic tribes, only the fit could survive. It took many centuries before even a minimally humane attitude was exhibited.

The history of rehabilitation of the physically disabled and the aged is intimately tied to the development of medicine—physical medicine in particular—and the growth of a social consciousness and sense of responsibility. As one traces the history of treatment methods as well as the attitudes of people toward persons with deformities and disabilities, one sees that it has taken centuries to achieve today's standards. Yet with all of our enlightenment, we continue to demonstrate both apathy and anxiety about these individuals. We do this by segregating them from the rest of society, ignoring building codes, and by providing inadequate funds to care for them. Let us hope that during the last quarter of the 20th century, greater numbers of disabled and aged persons will be living more satisfying lives.

HIGHLIGHTS OF THE PAST

Hippocrates, Father of Medicine, born 460 B.C., described many deformities and said in his book, *On Surgery,* "It should be kept in mind that exercise strengthens and inactivity wastes." This is a basic principle underlying physical medicine and rehabilitation and sometimes not used even today! The Roman physician Galen (A.D. 130–200) first described the muscles and bones of the body. While some of his errors were perpetuated for centuries, his contributions relate directly to physical rehabilitation.

Various forms of treatment and assistive devices were recorded very early. Early treatment methods such as heliotherapy have been used since the days of mythology when the sun was worshiped as a god for its healing power. Artificial limbs are recorded at about the same time as Hippocrates, while the first known crutch was recorded on an Egyptian tomb dated 2380 B.C. The Greek gymnasts were the first to teach massage. In the time of Jesus, electrotherapy first happened, apparently quite accidentally. A man named Anthero was walking on the beach and stepped on a Torpedo (an electrified fish). This reportedly rid him of the gout instantaneously. These fish were used later for the treatment of headaches.

Next came the Dark Ages, a period known for its lack of progress in both scientific and social advancement. During this time, the handicapped were treated with cruelty or indifference and in some cases, they were both laughed at and persecuted.

During the 14th century, gunpowder was invented and the cannon was first used. This single invention resulted in new kinds of war injuries which required a new medical approach. Care of men with cannonball wounds stimulated an interest in rehabilitation. For the first time, there were many persons who were maimed and disabled from a cause other than an accident of birth. Unfortunately, even during the 20th century it has taken a war to stimulate interest in rehabilitation.

While a few religious orders had shown concern for the disabled, society at large first began to accept its responsibility in England in 1601, the year the Poor Relief Act was passed. This law did three main things: (1) it outlawed begging, which had previously been sanctioned as legitimate, (2) it classified dependent people and (3) it provided an attempt at assisting both the poor and the disabled. Our present welfare system, a legacy of the 1601 English Poor Laws, is still wrestling with some of these same issues.

In the 18th century, two seemingly unrelated threads of history occurred. The British physician John Hunter described what has become the basis of muscle re-education and focused on the important relationship of patient-will and range of motion. At the end of this century, Phillippe Pinel liberated the insane at the Asylum De Bicêtre. This was not only the beginning of psychiatric rehabilitation, but it was also the first time that occupational and recreational therapy were used as treatment methods. At last, both physical and psychological care had begun.

THE 20TH CENTURY

During the last decade of the 19th century and the first decade of the 20th century, major steps in laying the groundwork for modern rehabilitation took place. This was first exhibited in an interest in training crippled children. Nursing literature shows evidence of convalescent nursing care and the need for occupational therapy. The term occupational therapy referred to use of idle time and was not used in our modern sense. It was also during this period that the first medical social service department was started at Bellevue Hospital in New York. Two other dimensions were added—home care and education. The first visiting nursing service was begun by Lillian Wald and the first professorship of physical therapy in the United States was held by R. Tait McKenzie at the University of Pennsylvania beginning in 1911.

Once again a war influenced the field of rehabilitation. At the time of World War I, the term "rehabilitation" began to be used instead of such terms as "physical reconstruction" and "reclaiming the cripple." In addition, the Red Cross Institute for Disabled Men opened to provide injured soldiers with an opportunity for vocational training. The unfortunate part of this program was that medical rehabilitation was unsuccessful. The death rate of those with spinal cord injuries was very high, and for some patients the life expectancy was only about one year. Therefore, because total rehabilitation was not always possible, its importance was minimized.

A need for the dissemination of information resulted in the first issue of the Archives of Physical Medicine and Rehabilitation in 1919. This magazine has since become the official journal of the American Congress of Rehabilitation Medicine formed in 1923 to provide a forum for communication among the many disciplines concerned with rehabilitation medicine. Its membership includes all of the professions on a so-called "rehabilitation team."

A desire to set standards and requirements for the practice of rehabilitation medicine culminated in the founding of the American Academy of Physical Medicine and Rehabilitation (originally the Society of Physical Therapy Physicians) in 1938. Their initial objective was accomplished in 1947 when the American Board of Physical Medicine and Rehabilitation was established. Requirements for certification require a three-year residency or a specific equivalent. Only certified physicians are eligible for membership in the Academy. Physicians practicing this specialty are called physiatrists.

In 1941, Dr. Frank H. Krusen wrote *Physical Medicine,* the first inclusive textbook on treatment methods. Not only was this book the first comprehensive textbook on this subject, but it also presented collected data which related treatments to outcomes. His scientific approach was a major step. Dr. Krusen, sometimes referred to as the "father of physical medicine," spent a major part of his life at the Mayo Clinic and at Temple University. The Krusen Rehabilitation Center and the Krusen Research and Engineering Center, located at Temple University, are reminders of his enormous contribution to the field.

During World War II, the possibilities of rehabilitation were shown dramatically under the direction of Colonel Howard A. Rusk, Chief of the Army Air Force's Convalescent Training Program. He was able to demonstrate how rehabilitation could improve the lives of men who had been hospitalized since World War I. In some instances, men were discharged after 20 years of hospitalization. Dr. Rusk later became the director of the Institute of Physical Medicine and Rehabilitation at the New York University Medical Center. His contributions and writings are well known to both professionals and laymen.

After World War II, there continued to be much interest in all phases of rehabilitation. Along with industrial growth came an increased number of industrial injuries. More automobiles brought still more injuries. This brought further need of rehabilitation. Legislation during this period, such as the Vocational Rehabilitation Act of 1943 and its amendments of 1954, broadened the scope of both vocational and medical rehabilitation services to disabled citizens. It also made funds available for professional training and research.

Since then, giant strides in technology have occurred and again there is greater emphasis on rehabilitation, not only of industrial, auto, Korean and Viet Nam war injury victims but of all persons with chronic illness, including the aged. Medicare legislation instituted in the 1960's has further stimulated the demand for rehabilitation. Further demands can be expected as insurance mechanisms for catastrophic and chronic illness are developed. Extended care facilities, nursing homes, rehabilitation units and home care programs have adopted more advanced techniques. The influence of rehabilitation is really just beginning.

Nurses concerned with quality of rehabilitation nursing had been meeting informally all over the United States for many years. Feeling an increased need to share their knowledge and experience, they formed the Association of Rehabilitation Nurses (ARN) in 1974. The first annual conference of this organization was held in Minneapolis in 1975. At this first meeting, plans for a long-term care section were under way, indicating the intense interest in the aged.

INTEGRATING REHABILITATION CARE INTO HEALTH EDUCATION

One aspect of the history of rehabilitation has been its slow incorporation into educational programs. This has created a lag in knowledge, education, and practice. That there are great variances in medical programs is shown by a study done by the Commission on Education in Physical Medicine and Rehabilitation. This group surveyed the incorporation of physical medicine and rehabilitation into undergraduate medical education. This was first done in 1929 and by 1965, 80 of the 87 medical colleges in the United States had some type of program in their curriculum. Of these, 59 were directed by physiatrists (a physician specializing in physical medicine and rehabilitation) and 21 were directed by non-physiatrists. Physiatry is the branch of medicine dealing with the diagnosis and treatment of disease and injury by physical agents (such as manipulation, massage, heat, water, exercise and so forth) and with the physical, psychological, social and vocational restoration of the seriously disabled or chronically ill person.

While the physiatrists and non-physiatrists had similar views and problems related to the school and teaching, the physiatrist directed programs reported that it takes 100 clock hours to reach their objectives, while the non-physiatrist directed programs average about 15 hours to reach their objectives. It therefore becomes obvious that in the field of medical education, there is a wide variance in exposure to the philosophy, techniques and treatment programs of physical medicine and rehabilitation.

While there has been no similar study of nursing education, graduates of baccalaureate, master's, associate degree, and diploma programs report a wide variance in their exposure to rehabilitation nursing. Many report that their rehabilitation education consisted merely of a tour through a rehabilitation center and learning range of motion and other techniques traditionally associated with rehabilitation nursing. It is for this reason that short courses in long-term care continue to be both necessary and popular even if some course content is a review for a few students. A majority of nurses attending such courses find much new material. This indicates a need for greater emphasis on rehabilitation in the total nursing curriculum. As long as we continue to have this lag in the basic education of both doctors and nurses, patients will suffer from lack of the optimum care possible.

THE FUTURE

PREVALENCE OF CHRONIC ILLNESS

During the early 1900's, mortality rates seemed to measure our state of ill-health quite adequately. This was because most diseases resulted in death, and our life expectancy was only 47 years of age, so that not many of us lived long enough to develop a chronic disease. Today, however, we have a significant number of serious but non-fatal diseases. To assess the extent of chronic disease is very difficult.

Chronic illness may be a slow, insidious process with mild or unnoticed beginnings. Some persons may be more aware of their symptoms than others. In addition, precision of diagnosis varies and a chronic disease may go unnoticed in some instances. Because most chronic illnesses and disabilities are not reportable, accurate statistics on the incidence and prevalence of chronic illness in the United States are very difficult to obtain and depend on extensive efforts to collect and interpret accurate data. The National Health Interview Surveys and the National Center for Health Statistics suggest the following figures:

Arteriosclerosis and Related Conditions: 25 per cent of all adults have definite or suspected heart disease. In addition to being a prevalent chronic disease, cardiovascular disease is the number 1 killer, causing over 1,000,000 deaths each year.

Cancer: It is estimated that more than 1,000,000 persons were under treatment for cancer in 1975, and the incidence is rising. One out of 4 persons will have cancer, and 1 out of 3 will be saved. Cancer is the number 2 killer in the United States today.

Arthritis: About 20.2 million, or 1 out of 10, persons have some form of arthritis. While this condition is rarely fatal, it is the leading cause of limited activity.

Mental Retardation: There are approximately 6,000,000 retarded persons, some of whom are able to live in the community or in a sheltered living arrangement. About 126,000 are born annually—one every five minutes.

Visual Impairment: There are about 9,596,000 visually impaired persons in the United States, of whom 1,306,000 have severe impairment and 475,000 are legally blind. In the elderly population, visual problems are very prevalent. Seventy-three per cent of those visually impaired by cataract are over 65 years of age. Fifty-nine per cent of those visually impaired by glaucoma are over 65.

Hearing Impairment: It is estimated that 1 out of 10 persons has at least some hearing difficulty. Over 236,000 are totally deaf, and the condition increases with age. Twenty-eight per cent of those 65 to 74 years of age have impaired hearing, and 48 per cent of those 75 to 79 years of age have diminished hearing. Hearing impairment among nursing home residents is reportedly 5 times greater than in the general population.

Cerebral Palsy: There are probably 750,000 persons with varying degrees of severity of cerebral palsy, and 15,000 infants are born with this condition annually.

Multiple Sclerosis and Related Demyelinating Diseases: There are 500,000 persons with some kind of demyelinating disease, and half of these persons have multiple sclerosis.

Muscular Dystrophy: The estimate for this condition is 200,000.

Parkinson's Disease: It is estimated that between one and one and one-half million persons have some degree of parkinsonism, with 50,000 new cases each year.

Paraplegia and Quadriplegia: The Paraplegia Foundation estimates that there are between 125,000 and 200,000 persons with this condition in the United States, with 12,000 new cases annually.

Other figures would lead us to believe that 87 per cent of all chronic illness is due to a disabling disease while 13 per cent is due to accidents and injuries. The U. S. National Health Survey estimates that one-half of our civilian non-institutionalized population suffers from a chronic physical or mental condition. One out of every 12 persons reported partial or total limitation in their major activity. As might be expected, this was in a greater proportion among the aged and the less educated, the non-white and rural groups.

In addition to the population of persons with specific chronic diseases, an increasing sector of our population is growing old. This group of persons have chronic disabling conditions that limit their mobility, usually in addition to one or more actual diseases. There are currently more than 22,000,000 persons over 65 years of age. This comprises about 11 per cent of our population, compared to only 4 per cent in 1900 when the life expectancy was 47 years of age. Life expectancy today is 71 years of age. By the year 2000, there will be an estimated 30 million persons over 65. This will naturally add to the incidence of chronic disease, since anyone who lives to this age will be likely to have a multiplicity of chronic diseases.

NEW DEVELOPMENTS

Besides breakthroughs in the control of cardiovascular disease, cancer and other diseases, other frontiers are being developed. The classical goal of rehabilitation — to optimize remaining body function — may soon be expanded to include augmenting by electrical means body function beyond what nature provided or left remaining. This exciting new development comes from the emerging field of neuromodulation, the term used to describe the effects of electrical stimulation of the nervous system. While neuroaugmentive devices and neuroaugmentive surgery are still new, future developments promise improved lives for many severely disabled persons.

Basically, neuromodulation is accomplished by implanting an electrode into an affected area, which is then activated by an external transmitter operated by the person. Currently research is being conducted in pain control, auditory and visual augmentation, and control of epilepsy, cerebral palsy, spasticity and other conditions. Thus far, the numbers of persons who have benefited from neuroaugmentive devices are small, but disabled persons should be assessed for possible help from this area every year or two so that they may take advantage of any new breakthroughs or refinements of devices and surgical techniques.

POTENTIAL FOR REHABILITATION PRACTICE

In Volume II of the report of the Commission on Chronic Illness, the shortage of personnel in the field of rehabilitation is noted and attributed partly to the following: (1) rejection of the aged and disabled by both the public and professional persons, (2) the belief so widely held among health professions that long-term care is uninteresting and not very productive, (3) facilities for care of the chronically ill need to be more community-oriented, (4) good medical care of chronic illness is difficult to purchase economically. These facts were published in 1959 and are still true today!

Even with our increased knowledge, our better education and our expansion of facilities and financial support, it is estimated there are still hundreds of thousands of persons who are being deprived of adequate rehabilitation programs. This is due in part to cost, in part to lack of education in basic health programs and in part to inertia on the part of both communities and professionals.

We have made strides in the fields of rehabilitation, physical medicine and community responsibility for the poor, the aged and the disabled. However, what we know how to do does not match what we are presently doing. Since a major objective is to add quality to the life of any person who has a chronic disease or disability regardless of age, it is heartening that some health workers are accomplishing results once considered impossible. Several institutions are discharging chronically ill and even some of their terminally ill patients. Senile persons are becoming oriented. Many severely handicapped people not only are earning a living but are also raising families and contributing immensely to their communities. As we expand our education in this field, as new drugs and surgical procedures are developed, as more effective technological equipment becomes available, as less social isolation occurs and as greater financial support becomes available, the full extent of future historical steps will unfold. In the meantime, today's more creative patient care is tomorrow's history. The impact of rehabilitation programs is just beginning.

REFERENCES

Commission on Chronic Illness: *Chronic Illness in the United States.* Vols. II, III and IV. Cambridge, Harvard University Press, 1959.

Erhardt, Carl, and Berlin, Joyce, (Eds.): *Mortality and Morbidity in the United States.* Cambridge, Harvard University Press, 1974.

Indeck, W., and Printy, A.: A skin application of electrical impulses for the relief of pain. *Minnesota Medicine, 58*:305, April, 1975.

Keith, Robert Allen: Physical Rehabilitation: Is it ready for the revolution? *Rehabilitation Literature, 30*:170, 1969.

Krusen, Frank H.: *Physical Medicine.* Philadelphia, W. B. Saunders Company, 1941.

Loetterle, B. C., et al.: Cerebellar stimulation: pacing the brain. *American Journal of Nursing, 75*:958, June, 1975.

Morrissey, Alice B.: *Rehabilitation Nursing.* New York, G. P. Putnam's Sons, 1951.

National Health Education Committee: *The Killers and Cripplers: Facts on the Major Diseases in the United States Today.* New York, David McKay Co., 1976.

National Center for Health Statistics: Selected reports from the *Health Interview Survey, Series 10, Vital and Health Statistics,* 1975.

Shanas, E., et al.: *Old People in Three Industrial Societies.* New York, Atherton, 1968.

Spangler, D. P.: *Service Needs of Paraplegics and Quadriplegics.* National Paraplegia Foundation, 1965, pp. 5, 10, 12.

A Study of Undergraduate Teaching Programs in Rehabilitation Medicine in American Medical Colleges. Minneapolis, Commission on Education in Physical Medicine, 1966.

Working With Older People. Volume II: *Biological, Psychological and Sociological Aspects of Aging.* U.S. Department of Health, Education and Welfare, P.H.S. Publication 1495, Superintendent of Documents, U.S. Government Printing Office, Washington, D.C. 20402, April, 1970.

Chapter 2

THE CONCEPTS OF
REHABILITATION

In order to help the reader acquire a broad knowledge of the concepts and meanings of rehabilitation, this chapter examines some of the major definitions. Rehabilitation has been defined by many different disciplines: pioneers in physical medicine, psychologists, vocational counselors and other professionals who have worked in the field. As a result, each one speaks from a somewhat different perspective and provides us with a fresh distinction or new insight. Each definition was no doubt developed because someone thought someone else's statement was inadequate or incomplete!

An examination of some of the major descriptions of rehabilitation will of course lead to my own definition. Interestingly, it is virtually impossible to find a definition of rehabilitation nursing in the literature! It is hoped that this approach will enable the reader to view rehabilitation as a broad underlying part of total patient care in any setting, as well as lay a foundation for future chapters.

REHABILITATION — A PHASE OF HEALTH CARE?

Unfortunately, the rehabilitation potential for a particular patient often is unknown, forgotten, thought to be unimportant, ignored or left until it is too late. There are many reasons why health professionals allow this to happen, some known and some unknown.

One reason for the deficit of rehabilitative care is the way we learn about it. If we learn about rehabilitation at all in our basic education, it is often referred to as the "third phase of medical care." This phrase itself suggests that rehabilitation is separate from acute and convalescent care. It tends to isolate the area of rehabilitation and implies that it follows after everything else is done. Unfortunately, that is what happens all too often in common practice. How often have you seen rehabilitation integrated into an acute care plan?

This kind of thinking deprives a patient of several vital aspects of rehabilitation. First, it deprives the patient of most of the important preventive aspects of care, such as prevention of further injury, contractures, decubitus ulcers, other physical deterioration and unnecessary loss of morale. Second, it inhibits making a maximum effort to maintain existing abilities. Third, it prevents patients from visualizing a future that may be relatively satisfying and, fourth, it does not help families to prepare themselves and their environment for necessary changes.

Perhaps the most unfortunate result of such failures is that a professional person with limited knowledge of rehabilitation develops an attitude of hopelessness stemming from ignorance rather than knowledge. This person unknowingly deprives the patient of proper assistance. Lack of help quite naturally indicates to most patients that no help is possible and that the situation is hopeless. Since the health professional, doctor, nurse or other therapist is looked to as an authority, it is imperative that he or she have at least a nodding acquaintance with what can be done and where to send a patient for help.

Isolation of rehabilitation practice has another negative effect: it implies that it is a specialty that must be learned. Only if one works at a rehabilitation center, where severely disabled persons are cared for, is it necessary to learn more specialized knowledge. When a nurse cares for a very narrow and specific patient population, she has an opportunity to become an expert in a specialty.

Rehabilitation nursing and psychiatric nursing can be compared. The principles of psychiatric nursing are not only used in a mental health center: they are used in any setting. The same is true for rehabilitation nursing. A rehabilitation *attitude* along with certain knowledge and skills must be basic to all phases of patient care, whether one works in a hospital for acute diseases, in a nursing home or in the patient's own home. Rehabilitation must be infused into general care, and the maintenance and preventive aspects of rehabilitation must be ongoing throughout a patient's life. It is a part of health care, not a phase of it. It is with this thought in mind that we examine our definitions.

DEFINITIONS OF REHABILITATION

People who work in the field of rehabilitation must come to terms with a very special world of reality. They do not cure, they cannot fully restore and they often do not see every patient goal attained. They do, however, frequently achieve "almost miracles." They are able to do this because they are convinced that "Rehabilitation is basically an optimistic process which concedes that despite continuing and even catastrophic disability, a better way of life for the patient is possible." This basic philosophy, stated by Dr. Paul M. Ellwood, balances the reality of a tragedy with the reality of an adaptive life and sets the stage for the following definitions.

The definition given by the National Council on Rehabilitation is as follows: "Rehabilitation means the restoration of the individual to the fullest physical, mental, social, vocational and economic capacity of which he is capable." The word *rehabilitation* is used when a person has lost functional ability because of accident or disease. The word *habilitation* is used when a person has a congenital deficiency. Habilitation can be defined as stated above by merely substituting the word "development" for "restoration."

This definition is obviously very broad in its approach and encompasses five major facets of a person's life. Many patients will not have a disability severe enough to require rehabilitation in all five areas, but others may require intensive help in each category. For example, it is quite conceivable that a school teacher who becomes a paraplegic can go back to teaching, even if it is in a different setting. In this case, the vocational problem is relatively minor. Another paraplegic might have been a bellhop and would obviously have to change his means of livelihood. The vocational emphasis in these two rehabilitation programs would be quite different. It should be noted that in addition to stressing the different facets of rehabilitation, this definition emphasizes the all-important aspect of restoration but omits the vital concept of prevention.

One of the most important concepts of rehabilitation, that one be restored to the fullest ability of which one is capable, is included in the Council's statement. Lacking the benefits of a good rehabilitation program, many people are living at a level less than that of which they are capable. This may mean physically, socially or one of the other major areas.

Another definition of rehabilitation is given by Dr. Frank Krusen, a pioneer physiatrist. His definition is as follows: "Rehabilitation is a creative procedure which includes the cooperative efforts of various medical specialists and their associates in other health fields to improve the mental, physical, social and vocational aptitudes of persons who are handicapped, with the objective of preserving their ability to live happily and productively on the same level and with the same opportunities as their neighbors."

This definition adds a very important component that is not mentioned in the previous statement—the matter of creativity. After one has worked with handicapped people over a period of time, one finds that there is no one answer that is applicable to all patients. While there are many devices that can be adapted and used by many patients, each individual must ultimately create his own environment and ways of coping with it. Individual ingenuity is often remarkable. A very good example is the Hoyer Lift. This important piece of equipment was developed by Ted Hoyer, a quadriplegic pastor, because of his own personal needs. This invention not only was useful to him but has also become an essential piece of equipment to many other handicapped people, both at home and in institutions.

The second important concept expressed in Dr. Krusen's definition is that of the health team. No one profession can provide a total rehabilitation program. In order to provide an intensive program, a variety of health professionals need to be available. This may include doctors, nurses, physical therapists, occupational therapists, social workers, psychologists, speech therapists, recreational therapists, vocational counselors, teachers, dieticians, and other persons such as orthotists and prosthetists. However, no team, regardless of its composition, can be truly successful unless both the patient and his family have an opportunity to participate fully.

The Community Health Service of San Francisco defines rehabilitation as "the process of decreasing dependence of the handicapped or disabled person by developing to the greatest extent possible, the abilities needed for adequate functioning in his individual situation." This statement stresses the all important factor of minimal dependence. In order to have self-respect, ego satisfaction and a sense of contributory living, it is vital that a disabled person develop as much independence as possible. Also, this definition stresses abilities rather than disabilities. To focus on an ability instead of a disability is to reorient treatment goals from the present to the future.

Helen J. Yesner, a social worker, defines rehabilitation as "a treatment process designed to help physically handicapped individuals to make maximal use of residual capacities and to enable them to obtain optimal satisfaction and usefulness in terms of themselves, their families, and their community." This useful statement makes it very clear that one is referring to residual capacities and the maximal use of these capacities. In other words, rehabilitation is a realistic approach to reduced physical abilities. This definition also articulates the very important relationship of patients to their families and their communities. In other words, families and communities can affect eventual treatment outcomes as much as, if not more than, health care professionals.

Dr. Wilbert Fordyce, a psychologist, says that rehabilitation is "concerned typically with people who have disabilities with enduring and pervasive effects. The essence of the rehabilitation process is recognition that what has happened to the patient affects and will continue to affect many aspects of his life extending beyond the limits of bodily function." Dr. Fordyce makes it eminently clear that there are permanent effects, which are not just physical, that will affect the patient's life. This is important because many professionals find it more comfortable to relate mainly to the physical problem while overlooking or de-emphasizing the other areas needing attention.

Dr. Sedgwick Mead defines rehabilitation as "a transient episode during which a human being with a physical-psychological impairment is given the opportunity to realize in himself latent potentialities for improved independence of action and of personal care." Dr. Mead adds the important factor that is somewhat implied in Dr. Krusen's use of the word "creative." The individual will find latent potentialities in himself that would never have been developed had it not been for the disability. This will help him in becoming independent not only in his physical actions but also in his decision making about his own life. Another feature of this definition is one that health workers too frequently forget — the rehabilitation process is merely a transient episode in this person's life. This transient episode, of course, seemingly can be successful in an institution yet have little influence on the person after he goes home. Unless there is adequate follow-up to see that the rehabilitation process has become a part of the person's life, the success of a rehabilitation program is unknown. Later chapters discuss discharge planning and the importance of making this transient episode useful to the patient on a very permanent basis.

Dr. Howard Rusk says: "Rehabilitation is a program designed to enable the individual who is physically disabled, chronically ill or convalescing to live and to work to the utmost of his capacity. It is an integral part of clinical, non-institutional and community responsibility in meeting the problems of chronic illness." (cited by Terry, p. 13). This definition suggests that convalescing people may require rehabilitation and that it may not necessarily occur in an institution. It may take place within a community, in the home or on an outpatient basis rather than at a rehabilitation center. It is very probable that a greater number of community oriented rehabilitation programs may develop in the future.

Miss Mary Switzer, longtime director of the Vocational Rehabilitation administration, which later became the Social and Rehabilitation Service, describes rehabilitation as a bridge for the patient, "spanning the gap between uselessness and usefulness, between hopelessness and hopefulness, between despair and happiness" (cited by Terry, p. 13). She also points out the supportive role of the health worker by emphasizing the very important psychological goals of persons with a physical disability.

None of these definitions is seen from a nurse's viewpoint. This author sees an urgent need to encourage rehabilitation to become part of general nursing care and to emphasize the relationship between preventive and restorative care. Our definition of rehabilitation is as follows: Rehabilitation is a creative process that begins with immediate preventive care in the first stage of an accident or illness. It is continued through the restorative phase of care and involves adaptation of the whole being to a new life.

SUMMARY

Reviewing various definitions of rehabilitation highlights key facets of the process. It is obvious that one is dealing with the physical, psychological, social, economic and vocational components of a person's life. In order for rehabilitation to be effective, it must begin as early as possible. Rehabilitation is a creative process that allows maximal use of existing abilities, emphasizes independence vs. dependence and requires an attitude of realistic optimism. The patient and his family are essential members of a team of health workers that will make it possible for rehabilitation to have a permanent effect on the patient's life after the actual medical program has ended.

REFERENCES

Community Health Services, Community Health Council of the United Community Fund of San Francisco: *Report on Rehabilitation of Chronically Ill and Disabled Persons in San Francisco.* April, 1960, p. 4.

Holley, Lydia: The physical therapist: who, what and how? *American Journal of Nursing, 70*:1521, July, 1970.

Krusen, Frank H., Kottke, Frederic V., and Ellwood, Paul M. (Eds.): *Handbook of Physical Medicine and Rehabilitation,* 2nd Ed. Philadelphia, W. B. Saunders Company, 1971.

Licht, Sidney: *Rehabilitation and Medicine.* Baltimore, Waverly Press Inc., 1968.

Riffler, K.: Rehabilitation: the evolution of a social concept. *Nursing Clinics of North America, 8*:665, December, 1973.

Spencer, William A.: A new use for the rehabilitation process—Introspection. *Archives of Physical Medicine and Rehabilitation, 51*:187, 1970.

Terry, Florence J., et al.: *Principles and Technics of Rehabilitation Nursing,* 2nd Ed. St. Louis, The C. V. Mosby Co., 1961.

Yesner, Helen J.: Psychosocial diagnosis and social services—One aspect of the rehabilitation process. *In* Krusen, F., et al. (Eds.): *Handbook of Physical Medicine and Rehabilitation,* 2nd Ed. Philadelphia, W. B. Saunders Company, 1971, p. 196.

Chapter 3

AN OVERVIEW OF
REHABILITATION NURSING

In order for patients to receive the greatest benefit from a rehabilitation program, it is imperative that nurses perceive rehabilitation as a process that begins when a patient first suffers from acute disease, trauma or the early symptoms of a progressively debilitating disease. Over 50 per cent of the patients in most acute-care general hospitals have one or more chronic diseases, and about 25 per cent of these are over 65 years old. Each nursing department certainly needs this kind of information in order to plan staff development programs and staffing patterns.

The elements of rehabilitation nursing need to be viewed as a part of basic nursing rather than as a specialty. Those who work at rehabilitation centers where patients are severely disabled naturally require additional knowledge in this field of nursing. However, this is a matter of degree and depth of knowledge rather than one of learning a completely new body of knowledge. Both early care during the acute phase of a condition and continued care after a rehabilitation program are essential to the patient's ultimate and continued adjustment. With this in mind, it becomes evident that at least some degree of knowledge of rehabilitation nursing is required by all nurses. The nurse who is convinced of this need will translate her knowledge into actions that go beyond the mere feeding and turning of patients.

BASIC AIMS OF REHABILITATION

The entire health care team is concerned with the two basic aims of rehabilitation, namely, prevention and restoration. It might be argued that the nurse has a greater role in the area of prevention than any other member of the health care team. This will become more apparent in later chapters dealing with specific nursing measures and responsibilities. For the present, it will be useful to understand the nurse's overall function in these two areas.

PREVENTION

Prevention must be future-minded, whether it concerns (a) maintaining function in order to prevent deterioration of an unaffected organ or part or (b) preventing further injury to an affected organ or part. Prevention must be a continuous aspect of care throughout the life of any patient with a chronic condition.

One should note that the prevention of deterioration of the body is the basis of physical fitness programs for all of us. This concept of maintaining bodily functions and abilities is vital in the rehabilitation process. Unfortunately, preventive measures are unspectacular unless they are omitted, and the rewards for their use are almost always unseen. For instance, a pressure sore is both visible and dramatic, but the lack of one is not. Hypostatic pneumonia in someone with a fractured hip, hip flexion contracture of the amputee, a pressure sore from a cast or leg brace and confusion from lack of mental activity serve as more specific examples of things that can be prevented with proper care. The absence of these and similar complications attests to good rehabilitation nursing practices.

Prevention of further injury or additional disability of the affected organ or body part is the other area of concern. For example, when there is an automobile accident, the ambulance driver is probably the first person to handle the patient. The way he moves and lifts the person from the street into the ambulance can prevent further injury. The emergency room nurse can also prevent further impairment by her knowledge of body mechanics, body alignment and first aid. If we visit the patient throughout his hospital stay, we will see measures taken to prevent contractures, food drop, pressure sores, dependency and so forth. In the case of a nursing home patient, both physical and mental changes can be reduced. Maintaining existing abilities by preventing additional injury or deterioration of seemingly uninvolved parts requires special nursing knowledge and skills. It is the nurse who can and must see that fewer and fewer patients endure treatment or, what is worse, hospitalization or institutionalization for preventable conditions. Far too many patients must suffer prolonged or postponed rehabilitation programs because of the need to correct or minimize a problem that never should have been allowed to occur.

RESTORATION

The second aim of rehabilitation is to restore as much function as possible to the injured or diseased part. This is the area of rehabilitation in which the nurse working in a rehabilitation center will have a greater depth of knowledge than the nurse in a nursing home, extended care facility, public health agency or general medical surgical area of a hospital. However, some nurses in these other areas require the same degree of specialized knowledge as those in the rehabilitation center.

The nurse works with the health team to help the patient to regain strength, to restore speech, to walk, to re-learn activities of daily living and to gain new ways to handle bowel and bladder problems. While prevention of further impairment and maintenance of existing ability continue throughout a patient's rehabilitation program (and lifetime), restoration takes precedence at this time. It is the area of restoration that is often responsible for the tendency to isolate rehabilitation as a specialty. It is hoped that there will be a greater awareness of the interrelatedness of these different areas in the total process of rehabilitation, a great many of which occur simultaneously rather than separately. The result of this awareness will be a higher level of total patient care.

Even where nurses have acquired a greater degree of rehabilitation knowledge, we find varying degrees of activity in the area of restoration. A nurse may have attained increased knowledge and insight through self-study, inservice education, seminars or short courses, or by attending a formal postgraduate program at a college or university. While many nursing skills contribute to physical restoration, other skills contribute to restoration of the psychosocial area.

ROLE OF THE REHABILITATION NURSE

WHERE WILL SHE PRACTICE?

At least some rehabilitation knowledge is required whether the nurse works in the emergency room, the intensive care unit, the extended care facility, the medical service, the geriatric service, the surgical service or the psychiatric service. Prevention of further impairments and maintenance of existing abilities are particularly vital, no matter where the patient is. We often forget about the physical disabilities that accompany mental diseases. If a person with schizophrenia is allowed to sit in a chair all day, he can develop hip flexion contractures just as easily as someone who is allowed to remain in Fowler's position too long. Problems with ambulation are often severe in mental hospitals. Conversely, we frequently do not use appropriate psychiatric knowledge in our care of patients with physical problems.

In other words, basic rehabilitation knowledge can be used whether the patient has hemophilia, cancer, arthritis, multiple sclerosis, mental illness or cerebral palsy; whether he has had a stroke, a spinal cord injury or a burn. It is up to the nurse to apply the appropriate concepts and techniques to the patients under her care.

KNOWLEDGE, SKILLS AND ATTITUDES

Certain knowledge, skills and attitudes, while pertinent to many areas of nursing, are required in greater depth by the nurse who works with patients having a chronic illness or in a rehabilitation program. First of all, the nurse needs a good understanding of the psychological effects of long-term illness in order to respond appropriately to patient needs during the various stages of adjustment to a disability. Also, she needs to increase her knowledge of anatomy, physiology and pathophysiology, especially of the nervous system, the musculoskeletal system and the urinary system. She also needs to know something about kinesiology — the science of body movement. She will have to be able to communicate with persons who have difficulty in expressing themselves and understanding others. She will need to know how to plan ways in which a patient can achieve bowel and bladder control.

The nurse must also be aware of the interrelatedness of psychosocial and economic problems. What radical changes are occurring to the family as a result of the disease? Is this the breadwinner who has been struck down by some accident or illness? Is this the housewife who must be replaced in the family? Is it a child? What social and vocational obstacles lie ahead? How do individual perceptions of the condition affect planning? What environmental alterations will be needed? Lastly, she must know and use community resources. In the community, the public health nurse will both find rehabilitation candidates and follow those who have completed a program. Public health nursing follow-up is a key factor in maintaining rehabilitation gains in many instances.

In addition to specialized knowledge, the rehabilitation nurse needs to be expert in certain skills. While these skills are used in hospitals treating acute disease, a greater number of variations are required when dealing with the disabled. Each of these skills will be discussed in later chapters.

Position changes are essential to maintain body alignment, to prevent skeletal deformities and to prevent pressure sores. If a patient comes to a long-term care facility with a contracture or one or more pressure sores, nursing ingenuity will be vital.

Another necessary skill is the performance of transfer techniques. How has the patient been taught to transfer himself? What kind of technique does he use? What kind of equipment does he use? What kind of wheelchair does he have? Can he transfer independently? How much assistance if any, is needed? Can these techniques be used at home?

Skill in performing range of motion exercises will be required. Passive, active assistive and active range of motion exercises vary with the age and condition of the patient. Range of motion exercises will be applied to the disabled part as well as the non-disabled parts to prevent additional problems resulting from disuse.

Finally, the rehabilitation nurse needs to possess special attitudes. All of us have observed the difference in temperament between the operating room nurse and those in slower moving areas of the hospital. Operating room problems are immediate, often a matter of life and death, and the pace is quick. Rehabilitation problems are long-term, a matter of future adjustment, and the pace is slow by comparison. It is important that we know ourselves as well as what will be required of us personally when we select a field of work. Consequently we can suggest that the nurse who prefers quick results work where the pace is more compatible with her temperament.

The rehabilitation nurse needs to be slightly slow-geared. She must have patience and understanding in order to be sensitive to her patient and to adjust her actions accordingly. At certain times the patient may need a lot of encouragement, at other times pressure is required and on occasion a person may need to be slowed down in his efforts.

The nurse must encourage the patient and praise him not only for achievement but also for effort. The latter is important since results may not be evident for weeks or even months.

Patients need time to perform their tasks, not only when they are first learning but also, perhaps, permanently. No one learns to perform an act from observation. Practice is essential. No one learns to play the piano by watching somebody else play it. This is equally true in relearning or learning new ways to eat, dress, walk, and so forth. We want to allow the patient time. This means allowing ourselves time to let patients do things for themselves.

Some nurses find it difficult to refrain from assisting patients during periods of learning. The helping role of the nurse in rehabilitation differs from that in acute care. The emphasis is not to help the patient but to help him to help himself. When a nurse first works with patients who have a disability or a chronic disease, she must be especially cognizant of the ultimate goal—patients must become independent of the nurse in every way allowed by the disability.

In many respects the functions of the rehabilitation nurse are similar to those of nurses in other settings. However, there are certain areas of priority and emphasis to which a rehabilitation nurse must address herself.

The nurse will encourage progress from simple to complex procedures; she will proceed from providing much assistance to providing as little as necessary;

and she will help the patient to make the adjustment from hospital living to home living. She will need to be constantly vigilant for the many small things that can make the difference between dependent and independent living. She will be aware of the needs that lie ahead, so that returning home presents the least number of unexpected obstacles.

PLANNING PATIENT CARE

This role includes the integration of objective data from the patient's history and physical examination, careful observation of the patient, application of nursing knowledge and, finally, patient participation. These tools and data will help the nurse to assess patient problems more accurately and, ultimately, to assist him to a greater degree. The areas of concern include the physical, psychological, social and environmental spheres of the patient's life. Patient care planning will be discussed in greater detail in the next chapter.

IMPLEMENTING PREVENTIVE NURSING MEASURES

Some nurses have a somewhat narrow awareness of what nursing care encompasses. A most unfortunate practice is to limit the activities of the nurse to those ordered by a physician. This is only one function—the dependent (on the physician) function of the nurse. Even more regrettable, and frequently disastrous, is that the nurse sometimes waits for the physician to order nursing care!

The use of footboards, bedboards, turning schedules, positioning techniques, range of motion exercises (in most cases), transfer belts, comfort measures and so forth should be initiated by the nurse, not the physician. Her assessment of patient needs takes place over a 24-hour period and is more current than that of any other health professional, including the physician. Therefore, our aim must be to enhance patient care through the initiation of independent nursing measures.

A broadened scope of independent nursing practice has been encouraged and developed in a variety of ways. At the Rehabilitation Institute in Chicago, every full-time registered nurse is a nurse therapist. Nurse specialists holding Master's degrees are available for consultation and teaching. At the time of admission, each patient is assigned to a nurse therapist who is responsible for that individual's plan of care throughout his or her stay. The nurse also continues to work with the family, the patient and other team members after discharge whenever possible. Nurse therapists use their independent judgment in making decisions relating to assessment, evaluation, care plans, adapting equipment, teaching in the areas of diet, fluids, bowel and bladder control, pain control, rest, and sleep. Essential to the success of the nurse therapist is the concept that the patient has a responsibility to coach the care givers on his needs. In other words, the patient is expected to identify and communicate needs that require attention.

Primary nursing is another way of better utilizing the skills of the nurse. Briefly, in primary nursing, the nurse who plans the patient's care also gives the care. Each nurse carries a case load of four to six patients, reports to other care givers when not on duty, communicates directly with the physician and other departments and is held accountable for her patient load. Again, patient participation is not only desired, it is encouraged and expected. Marram's *Primary Nursing* describes this concept and system in detail.

The Loeb Center in New York pioneered in the concept of nursing as a therapy that can both upgrade care and actually shorten hospitalization time. All of these ways of expanding the role of the nurse have several things in common: greater utilization of the nurse's higher professional skills and knowledge (with less time on administration of care), clearly identified accountability for one to one care, increased participation by the patient as a member of the health team, and allowing patients to identify with one person for their overall care.

The nursing home is a growing area of practice. In a few homes where a highly skilled multiprofessional staff exists, patients who were originally admitted as lifetime residents are frequently discharged! This becomes a problem of readjustment for both patients and families, who often experienced great conflict about the initial decision to enter a nursing home. Discharge from a nursing home may imply a poor initial decision, poor home care, a lack of community resources or good rehabilitation nursing care in the home. As all personnel begin to study the results of good geriatric care, they will find more ways of bringing new and unexpected results.

COORDINATION OF A MULTIDISCIPLINARY APPROACH

Coordination is a key role of the nurse who cares for patients receiving attention from a variety of health workers. This does not refer to the administrative function of coordinating appointments, requests and other activities. It refers to the coordination of the learnings from various therapies into the patient's activities throughout his day.

For example, if a patient spends 30 minutes with the speech therapist two or three times a week, he will need to use what he learns between appointments. In order to do this, the nurse must know what the speech therapist would like the patient to practice. Such information must be incorporated in the plan of care. This same concept of coordination holds true of other departments such as physical therapy and occupational therapy. If a patient learns a transfer method at 10:00 A.M. and is allowed to transfer carelessly the other $23\frac{1}{2}$ hours of the day, his learning will obviously be slow and difficult. In addition, he will become discouraged, and it will negatively affect his motivation for further learning.

In order to coordinate patient learnings, the nurse must have open channels of communication between departments. This is sometimes done informally at lunch, during coffee or through telephone calls. However, such informal methods do not guarantee a systematic information flow for each patient. Most rehabilitation centers find that interdisciplinary patient conferences provide an excellent avenue for sharing information. Such meetings are mutually helpful because therapists become more aware of problems encountered outside the confines of their treatment areas. Ultimately, of course, the patient benefits from a treatment team whose members view his problems together. In this way, no therapy works in isolation.

TEACHING

A major role of the rehabilitation nurse is that of patient and family teaching. The patient usually has much to learn. He may need to learn new ways of performing activities of daily living (ADL's) such as dressing, bathing, eating and toileting. He may need to learn to walk again, to use a wheelchair or a variety of other new living adaptations.

In order to accomplish the goal of successful patient and family teaching, the nurse must know as much about learning as she does about teaching. The teaching and learning processes are discussed in Chapter 9.

SUPPORT

The nurse has her more traditional role in the area of support. It is in this role that she uses her communication skills—listening, in particular. She will need to help both patients and families to visualize a new life, altered though it may be. Her assistance in interpreting the differences between short-term and long-term goals will prevent misunderstanding at various stages of a rehabilitation program. Listening, realistic encouragement, helping to clarify misunderstanding, and acceptance of patient feelings will provide support for the patient and his family at a time when both confusion and fear are most acute.

PERSONAL QUALITIES

In addition to the overall knowledge, skills and attitudes just described, there are certain personal qualities that a rehabilitation nurse must either have or develop. These qualities come from the subjective experience and observation of this author. However, this chapter would not be complete without them.

The first point is that objectivity is not appropriate to rehabilitation nursing. Roget's College Thesaurus defines objective as "not subjective, unemotional, unprejudiced, unbiased, impersonal. See indifference." How can it be possible to maintain indifference as one comes to know a person—the fears, weaknesses, strengths and problems of an individual? We cannot help but come to like, dislike, admire, or perhaps pity a person with whom we work over a period of months or years. We cannot help but have human subjective responses. Certainly the nurse cannot spend her energies being overwhelmed by another's misfortunes, because it would incapacitate her ability to give nursing care. Nor can she let her nurturing qualities involve her in unhealthy personal relationships.

What quality can strike a balance between the chill of objectivity and the dangers of overinvolvement? *Responsiveness* would seem to be a desirable answer. Responsiveness implies receptivity to both the feelings and the needs of others. It requires a person who is capable of recognizing and accepting feelings of self and who is able to channel those feelings into therapeutic directions. By concentrating attentively to another's broad needs, more appropriate immediate responses can be given. Admittedly, this a delicate balance, but it can be achieved through greater awareness and more thoughtful consideration.

A second essential quality relates to the need of patients to be in earlier contact with nurses who have expertise in rehabilitation. This requires a degree of *assertiveness*. Nurses must describe their potential contributions and expertise both to medical surgical colleagues and to physicians. Early intervention by a rehabilitation nurse can expedite a person's rehabilitation program. What can be done in the beginning? What adaptive devices are available? What early goals can be achieved? What resources are available? All too frequently a patient with a disability is surrounded by a conspiracy of silence caused by personnel who are ignorant of what can be done and a fear of an unfavorable outcome. Nurses today are discussing assertiveness in many areas of practice. Nowhere would this quality benefit patients more than in the field of rehabilitation.

As a final point, *imaginativeness* is an essential quality of the rehabilitation nurse. This requires that she practice viewing the world around each patient with new eyes. Because patients do have certain needs in common, such as care plans, teaching self care, range of motion and so forth, the release of new ideas for individualized environments is inhibited. The necessary routinization of certain aspects of care also curtails our ability to see more creative solutions to patient problems. Admittedly, this is the most difficult quality to develop; a few comments may be useful, however. First, maintaining an awareness of the need for greater imaginativeness will at least keep us from forgetting about it. Second, rehabilitation people tend to contradict themselves philosophically; that is, we talk about an emphasis on ability rather than disability and in the same breath teach personnel problem-solving techniques and problem-oriented charting, which has the negative effect of emphasizing problems. To counteract this, it would seem profitable to also view patients from an ability-oriented perspective. A greater emphasis on abilities is a more positive approach and is more likely to release a flow of ideas and thus increase our chances of giving more imaginative care.

SUMMARY

The nurse's role in rehabilitation has been discussed. The aims of rehabilitation, the necessary knowledge, skills, attitudes and personal qualities and the major functions of the nurse have been introduced.

REFERENCES

Alfano, Genrose J.: The Loeb Center for Nursing and Rehabilitation. *Nursing Clinics of North America, 4*:487, 1969.

Allgire, Mildred J., and Denney, Ruth R.: *Nurses Can Give and Teach Rehabilitation.* New York, Springer Publishing Co., 1960.

Anderson, Helen C.: *Newton's Geriatric Nursing.* 5th Ed. St. Louis, C. V. Mosby Co., 1971, Chapter 12.

Anderson, N.: Rehabilitation nursing practice. *Nursing Clinics of North America, 6*:303, June, 1971.

Bergstrom, Doris: Rehabilitation nursing. *In* Licht, Sidney (Ed.): *Rehabilitation and Medicine.* New Haven, Elizabeth Licht, Publisher, 1968, Chapter 4.

Bonner, Charles D.: *The Team Approach to Hemiplegia.* Springfield, Illinois, Charles C Thomas, 1969.

Brown, Esther Lucile: *Nursing Reconsidered: A Study of Change.* Philadelphia. J. B. Lippincott Co., 1970.

Chafee, C. E.: Rehabilitation needs of nursing home patients: A report of a survey. *Nursing Research, 17*:477, 1968.

Clipper, Margaret: Nursing care of the stroke patient. *In* Licht, Sidney (Ed.): *Stroke and Its Rehabilitation.* Baltimore, Waverly Press, 1975, Chapter 8.

Gebbie, K., and Lavin, M.: Classifying nursing diagnoses. *American Journal of Nursing, 74*:250, February, 1974.

Guidelines for the Practice of Nursing on the Rehabilitation Team. American Nurses' Association, 10 Columbus Circle, New York, New York 10019, 1965.

Hirschberg, Gerald G., Lewis, Leon, and Vaughan, Patricia: *Rehabilitation: A Manual for the Care of the Disabled and Elderly.* Philadelphia, J. B. Lippincott Co., 1976.

Johnson, E. E., et al.: Self-medication for a rehabilitation ward. *Archives of Physical Medicine and Rehabilitation, 51*:300, 1970.

Klumb, K. Bernice: What is rehabilitation nursing? *California Health, 16*:4, 1958.

Kos, Barbara: The nurse's role in rehabilitation of the myocardial infarct patient. *Nursing Clinics of North America, 4*:593, 1969.

Long, Janet: *Caring for and Caring About Elderly People — A Guide to the Rehabilitative Approach.* Philadelphia, J. B. Lippincott Co., 1972.

Marram, Gwen D., et al.: *Primary Nursing.* St. Louis, C. V. Mosby Co., 1974.

Martin, Nancy, King, Rosemarie, and Suchinski, Joyce: The nurse therapist in a rehabilitation setting. *American Journal of Nursing, 70*:1694, 1970.

Meocita, Sister Mary: Rehabilitation — Bridge to a useful and happy life. *Nursing Outlook, 10*:581, 1962.

Poole, Pamela E.: Nurse, please show me that you care. *Canadian Nurse, 66*:25, 1970.

Rusk, H. A.: Rehabilitation belongs in the general hospital. *American Journal of Nursing, 62*:62, 1962.

Rusk, H. A.: *Rehabilitation Medicine.* 3rd Ed. St. Louis, C. V. Mosby Co., 1971, Chapter 13.

Schwartz, Doris: Incident from a family study. *American Journal of Nursing, 65*:89, 1965.

Steen, Joyce: Liaison nurse: ombudsman for the chronically ill. *American Journal of Nursing, 73*:2102, 1973.

Stryker, Ruth Perin: *Back to Nursing.* 2nd Ed. Philadelphia, W. B. Saunders Company, 1971.

Stryker, Ruth Perin: Every nurse a rehabilitation nurse. *Nursing, 2*:13, 1972.

Tryon, Phyllis A., and Leonard, Robert C.: Giving the patient an active role. *In* Skipper, J. K., and Leonard, R. C. (Eds.): *Social Interaction and Patient Care.* Philadelphia, J. B. Lippincott Co., 1965.

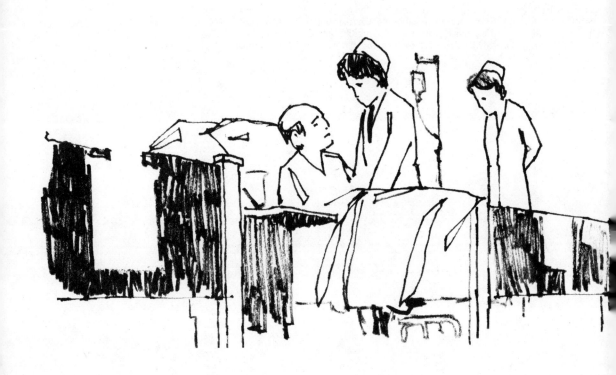

Unit II
NURSING CARE

Chapter 4

PSYCHOLOGICAL REACTIONS TO PHYSICAL DISABILITY

A successful physical rehabilitation program ultimately depends on psychological adaptations. If these adaptations do not occur, the ultimate goals of rehabilitation cannot occur. Many non-productive disabled persons represent failures in the psychosocial aspects of rehabilitation rather than in the physical aspects. When a patient needs psychotherapy, it may be that he will not be ready for an intensive physical rehabilitation program until he reaches a certain level of understanding and acceptance of himself. This chapter can only highlight various psychological factors in chronic disease and disability, as the topic is vast and complex. For a deeper understanding of psychological reactions to physical disability, the reader is referred to the sources listed at the end of this chapter.

FACTORS DETERMINING PATIENT RESPONSES

INTRINSIC FACTORS AFFECTING RESPONSES

Age of Onset

One of the most important factors that affect a person's adjustment to physical impairment is age of onset. For example, a person with a congenital disability will have problems related to growth and development, to play and to school. This person will have to find ways, not *new* ways, of self care. While such a person may have to adjust to a body image that differs from others, he or she is not adapting to an *altered* body image. However, if the disability occurs during adolescence, reactions will be very different. At this stage of development, physical strength, physical beauty and physical activity are considered extremely important. There are rather special adjustments to be made for this particular age group, not only because of their primary concerns but also because of yet undeveloped personality facets.

If a disability occurs in adulthood, the reaction and response will be still different. A sense of loss, much like grief, is experienced. This relates to the loss of not only a physical function but also a way of life. Adult fears primarily revolve around sexual function, bowel and bladder continence, economic capability and social acceptance.

Disability occurring in an elderly person may be more expected but is no less distressing. While mild disability occurs to almost all older persons, it is unfortunate that patient's families and society are less willing to expend time, money and energy rehabilitating the elderly than they are for other age groups. The chapter on the elderly will deal with this age group in more detail.

Type of Onset

Psychological reaction to a disability can be quite different in the case of a disease that has an acute or traumatic onset compared with that of a slowly progressive disease. With acute disease or trauma, the disability becomes stabilized, and one's future can be dealt with on this basis. There is a final limitation to the amount of disability, and the patient, once over the initial shock, can work toward an adjustment, knowing what he or she can and cannot do. The psychological impact in an acute onset is usually greater in persons disabled by an accident than in those disabled by a disease. This is because of the factors in accidents that may later contribute to guilt, anger, depression and other negative emotions.

In the case of a person who has a progressively deteriorating disease, or one with remissions and exacerbations, such as arthritis or multiple sclerosis, the person's physical and psychological adjustment will fluctuate according to the stage of the disease. A patient may try to prepare for the changes that come with exacerbations, but changes in the degree of disability from one month to another are relatively unknown, causing uncertainty and anxiety.

Prognosis

The outcome of a disability is strongly influenced by the condition itself—that is, whether the condition will stabilize, whether there will be remissions or whether there will be gradual and continual deterioration. In many instances a depressing prognosis may cause both health personnel and patients to feel that all forms of rehabilitation are futile. This position is not justifiable. Just because the outcome of a particular disease is death or progressive disability, there is no reason why life should not be as independent and as worthwhile as possible. This is when the preventive and maintenance aspects of rehabilitation become primary.

The element of prognosis is rich in opportunity for misunderstandings. How does the person perceive the prognosis of the condition? Does his view of its implications differ from that of the family or the personnel giving care? Does he expect that a permanent injury will be more handicapping than it actually will be? It is important to explore such possibilities through the course of treatment.

Previous Personality

Naturally a severe disability affects a person's personality and behavior. However, one of the myths of traumatic illness is that a disability actually causes a personality problem. This is rarely true. A good example is the case of a paraplegic teenager who is disobedient, is careless with cigarettes, wheels his wheelchair down a ramp backwards and does other reckless tricks. This behavior is not caused by his disability. If you know that this young man was trying to dive flat into three feet of water when he sustained his injury, you realize his psychological problems preceded the injury, not vice versa.

Except for some accidents, there may be little or no relationship between personality and the cause of the disability. An individual's personality, however, does seriously affect his ultimate success in adapting to a new life. In all instances of disabling accident or disease, there are initial emotional reactions that will vary greatly from person to person. These will be discussed later in this chapter. In essence, it is vital to remember that the patient's previous personality signals (1) what kind of help will be needed, (2) what kind of help is likely to be accepted and (3) how the ultimate adaptation will occur.

Intelligence

While intelligence is a factor in predicting what the patient will be able to learn, drive and motivation often compensate to some extent for ability. By the same token, ability may not be evidenced without some motivation. Many questions must be asked. Does the person have the ability *and* interest to become a teacher, a social worker, a psychologist? Is a trade more appropriate? What is the person's basic ability in terms of choosing future schooling? The latter will have a great deal to do with intelligence. Recently, in one of the rooms at the Sister Kenny Institute there were two patients, one who had had a diving accident and one who had had a motorcycle accident. Both were paraplegics; one had an I.Q. of 142, while the other had an I.Q. of 80. General intelligence will certainly make the educational goals of these men different.

Aptitude and Interest

A patient may have certain interests that can be built on and used as a new life style is developed. For example, the boy with the I.Q. of 142 has a choice of many professional occupations, such as law, social work, teaching and counseling, but he may be interested in only two of the four possibilities, or none. It is important that psychometric tests be used to help identify interests and aptitudes that will aid in selecting appropriate fields of endeavor. The classic example of new directions is the artistic aptitude that is so often uncovered after a patient becomes disabled. The International Art Show (of disabled artists) exhibits many fine pieces of artwork done by such persons. Genuine artistic talent is often exhibited by persons who must paint with a non-dominant hand, with a foot or with the mouth. With disability, new interests and abilities are frequently discovered and developed.

Degree of Physical Dependency

Dependency may be due to lack of will, lack of proper rehabilitation or extensive physical disability. The amount of physical independence achievable is determined by the degree of dependency caused by the physical disability. The role of rehabilitation is to minimize the physical dependency as much as possible by reaching new ways of performing various activities, by identifying adaptive devices that make activities possible, by using a proper prosthesis and by adjusting the environment. When there is much physical dependency, psychological adjustment becomes more difficult.

The degree or intensity of disability need not be overriding, however. It may be helpful to distinguish between disability and handicap. *Disability* is the degree of impairment that can be objectively described, while *handicap* refers to a person's total adjustment. The degree of disability does not determine the amount of handicap. This author knows a quadriplegic who is married, manages his own business and travels all over the world. He has a severe disability, but he is minimally handicapped. I also know a paraplegic who is unmarried, does not work and stays home to be cared for by an attendant. He is severely handicapped with a lesser disability. Psychological assistance should be sought whenever the handicap is greater than the disability warrants.

EXTERNAL FACTORS DETERMINING ADJUSTMENT

Psychological Environment

While every person is ultimately responsible for his or her own adjustment, the adjustment is often adversely affected by other persons in the environment. These include family, friends and health personnel. Family relationships and roles may be altered by chronic illness. An important family member may reject the person. Friends may stand back. An attendant may desire that a patient be dependent. In brief, a patient will be influenced by the role expectations of those around him. Therefore, it is essential that families, friends and personnel adopt healthy expectations for the patient and help him to achieve them.

Physical Environment

Whether a patient can go to the bathroom or not may simply depend on his ability to open the bathroom door. Whether or not a patient can go to a movie may be determined by the number of steps at the entrance. Whether a person can take a particular job may depend on the physical arrangement of the building—the number of steps, the entry, whether there is parking available, whether the bathrooms can accommodate a wheelchair or whether there are elevators. The removal of environmental barriers can ensure a fuller social life, education and employment for disabled persons.

Economic Conditions

The economic condition of a patient is very important to ultimate adjustment. Can he afford to buy proper equipment? Can he afford to adapt his house? Can he afford the new education? Can he afford an attendant if one is needed? Can he support a family if he is the breadwinner? Can a housekeeper be employed if the disabled person is either the homemaker or a child? Ultimate adjustment is strongly influenced by financial conditions, although assistance may only be required initially.

Society has a financial obligation in this essential aspect of the patient's adjustment. We cannot refuse to help the athlete who entertained us, the veteran who fought for us, the innocent victim of a chance birth defect. When services are provided and used, they usually repay society as well as assist the person needing the assistance.

Social Expectations

It is often difficult to assess what the patient expects of himself and what his friends expect him to be able to do. Social expectations, either his or his friends', can determine whether he goes out to dinner, whether he goes to a movie, whether he plays bridge or whether he participates in activities that sometimes are seemingly impossible, such as hunting. In reality, these things are usually feasible. Travel is more difficult with a disability, but it is not impossible. There are motels, hotels and restaurants that present no barriers for the disabled. Most airlines will accept persons with disabilities, but they must be notified ahead of time if a wheelchair is used. All of these activities are vital to the person's social well-being, but he must first realize that normal social encounters are possible. Friends must learn to expect the disabled person to work, socialize and travel. If he is excluded from these areas, his life will obviously be more circumscribed and less satisfying.

Community Resources

Every state and local community varies in terms of resources available to the disabled patient. Some states have no or only one rehabilitation center. There is variation especially in the resources available for certain diseases or types of disabilities. Is this a young child who needs a special school? Is this a young person who needs not only a physical rehabilitation program but also counseling and vocational guidance? If a person lives in a small community, will he need to be moved for a temporary period to a community where agency resources are available?

Once an appropriate agency has been located, the next step is to have a counselor who has the skills and the personality that will be helpful to this particular patient. In many places the psychology department and the social service department have personnel who are especially effective with certain age groups or certain conditions. Often the young adult or the older teenager more effectively relates to a young counselor. A counselor who is a mother or father image may or may not be detrimental. A very young professional "whippersnapper" can irritate an older person just by virtue of his young age. Aside from age differences, one should be especially conscious of the relationship, the understanding and the support given by important persons in any agency. It is sometimes helpful to reassign personnel. This does not have to be unpleasant, since people who work with people will usually recognize their limitations and individual reactions. Families should be encouraged to be open about such problems.

It is very important for some member of the health team, usually the social worker, to coordinate referrals, so that the patient does not have to endlessly find his way from one resource to another, one by one. This is discussed in more detail in chapter 11.

RESPONSES OF PATIENTS TO ILLNESS

Esther Lucile Brown refers to patients as "people in trouble." Even if one merely goes to a hospital for diagnostic tests, there is a loss of identity and role activity, whether it be that of worker, friend or family member. There is a loss of home, sometimes compensated for by the presence of familiar objects. There is a loss of friends except during visiting hours. Also, patients invariably lose strength as a result of bedrest, painful treatments and uncomfortable diagnostic procedures. These occur to both the acutely and the chronically ill person whenever institutionalization is necessary. But the person with a chronic disability has an additional loss—the permanent loss of a function.

The patient with a condition that will create a permanent disability has a multifaceted adjustment ahead. While the basic problem is physical, more important problems relate to his or her future. Financial needs, vocational needs, housing requirements, transportation availability and psychosocial adjustment all take precedence at one time or another.

MEANINGS OF ILLNESS

Our Western culture places high value on beauty, good physical condition, youth, perfection and physical ability. This emphasis pervades our entertainment and leisure activities as we pursue sports, exercise and do-it-yourself activities. When someone is born with or develops a physical disability, feelings of bewilderment, frustration, distress and shame often dominate until new understanding and deeper values develop.

The concept of body image can best be understood in the context of child development. We learn to master our bodies during the preschool years: grasp, walking, talking, bowel and bladder control and coordination are usually achieved by the age of 3. With each accomplishment, we experience a feeling of success and competence. Throughout adulthood, most of us continue to develop physical abilities, such as piano playing, playing tennis or driving a car. If, however, something happens to our bodies, whether it be paralysis, amputation, a heart condition or disfigurement from arthritis, we feel ashamed and even guilty. We are embarrassed because a lifetime of indoctrination to the values of physical perfection is challenged. Suddenly, whether our problem is visible or not, we feel incompetent, unattractive and unable to hold up our end of things.

This cultural facet of illness, especially chronic illness because it does not go away, is further complicated by each person's background and individual personality. Each person will attach a particular meaning to illness. This may be conscious or unconscious. All too frequently persons view illness or disability as punishment for past sins or evil desires. Certain religious beliefs strengthen this kind of thought and feeling. Such individuals may actually take comfort in their illness and believe they do not deserve to get well. In other words, the illness atones for their sins. These beliefs will obviously have to be dealt with before successful treatment outcomes can be expected.

Another response that can adversely affect a treatment outcome occurs in the kind of person who finds a disability a release from an intolerable situation. This usually revolves around a family problem such as a bad marriage or caring for a burdensome family member.

Other persons who receive secondary gains from a disability might be accident victims who want to continue to receive disability payment and dependent persons who welcome the opportunity to have a more concrete reason for dependence. A disability may also satisfy a masochistic need for punishment.

CHANGE—ADAPTATION TO A CHRONIC DISABLING DISEASE

Peter Marris, in his book *Loss and Change,* explores the concept of grieving as applied to many situations of change. He found that even when people wanted a change, as in accepting a sought-after job, their reactions expressed an internal conflict much like grief. In fact, he defines grieving as the psychological adjustment to loss (not necessarily death).

This is best explained when one understands that, as Marris states, "the fundamental crisis of bereavement arises not from the loss of others, but from the loss of self." He goes on to explain that the intensity of grief is related to the degree of disruption and the intensity of involvement. His conclusions lend insight into the patient confronted with drastic change of the body and its function and the ways his life must be altered in order to function anew.

Marris believes that the principle of adaptation involves bereavement: "Life becomes meaningless. The context of purposes and attachments to which events are referred for their interpretation has been so badly disrupted by the loss that it at first seems irreparable." This is what happens to the disabled person initially. His or her sense of identity is shattered but not yet altered. The meaning of life has yet to be "reshaped," "retrieved" and "reformulated."

Management of change does not occur until after mourning has taken place. This process is considered a psychological necessity, not weakness or self indulgence. Change "depends on the articulation of conflicting impulses." This is a key concept for rehabilitation personnel to understand. They must be able to listen to patients and allow them to go about their psychological repair.

PHASES OF ADAPTATION

Persons faced with a loss of major body functions and/or parts will proceed through a series of phases much like those experienced in mourning. The duration of each phase may differ, and a person may skip a phase or plateau altogether. It is the job of the staff to understand that it is important for patients to feel comfortable in expressing their anger, anguish, depression and other feelings at each phase in order for progress to occur.

The initial reaction to a disability, especially if it is the result of trauma, is *shock*. This may be manifested by withdrawal or anxiety. The person is fearful not only about the specific loss but also about his or her total life's orientation.

At the same time, *dependency* occurs and is considered healthy. Initially, when the patient is experiencing the impact of the loss with its shattering effect on the ego, it will require time to begin to gather new resources and to reinforce old ones. Depression, anger and varying degrees of dependency are expected during this early period. As the patient begins to realize that life simply cannot continue as it was, he will gradually begin to formulate a new self-image.

During the period of shock and mourning, the patient has many fears. How will he take care of himself? Will he be able to care for his family? Will he be a sexually adequate marital partner? Will it be possible to have bladder and bowel control? For the physically active person who discharged feelings through athletics, what other healthy outlets are there? These questions, unanswerable at this time, are overwhelming.

The second stage is that of *denial*. This serves the purpose of giving the patient time to gather new strength to deal with the task of coping with his disability. Staff must be careful not to confront patients with too much reality too soon. Usually, the staff will notice the patient gradually accepting the situation with little help required on their part.

A third stage, that of *turbulence,* occurs in varying degrees, especially with younger persons. The turbulent stage may be marked by depression, overt hostility and manipulativeness. Staff must be particularly firm and consistent during this period, which is usually a particularly trying one.

The fourth stage, that of *working through* the many new insights and roles, is the longest. The process of change may begin when the patient realizes he has always judged himself by so-called normal standards, which are more conventional than realistic. It causes a person pain and a feeling of inferiority when he cannot do what is considered "normal," or when he looks "different."

Therefore, in adapting to a disability, the patient must begin to enlarge his or her scope of values. What seemed important yesterday may become unimportant today. New values with deeper meanings will emerge. Most persons with a severe disability say that they eventually become a far better person as a result of the kind of soul searching and analysis required for living with that disability.

As the person identifies and re-examines the "normal" values held by society, he will be able to subordinate the ideal of perfect physique as deeper and more enduring values emerge. For instance, if the patient can no longer walk except on leg braces, he must realize that this is not the only thing that matters in life. Another part of the adjustment process is the containment of the effects of the disability. In other words, the disability need not affect all situations. If it is a physical disability or one that alters the appearance, it does not have to affect every situation of one's life. As these ideas begin to be appreciated, the patient can begin to have greater self-acceptance and acceptance of others.

Goals often must be changed so that the patient can experience realistic successes. A goal of walking without a limp becomes doing things in spite of a limp. Throughout this process, one becomes less comparison-minded, more cooperative rather than competitive. As independence and personal responsibility begin to increase, a new self-image develops. The final adjustment relates to the person's self-conduct and his concept of the disability.

Not everyone can work through these problems successfully. Personnel should be aware of any patient who does not seem to experience at least some anguish, anxiety and depression, since these feelings are a part of the healing process, the first step to an acceptance of disability. If the patient does not have some of these initial reactions, he may be denying that his life has changed substantially. Psychologists are in agreement that the patient must be given time for such feelings to occur before the process of adaptation begins.

Jerome Siller says that the goal of rehabilitation is to promote ego integrity and a feeling of self-worth. He goes on to explain that these things cannot be hurried or rushed. Too rapid an approach to rehabilitation may hinder rehabilitation. As the patient is assimilating the disability and recovering from a period of disorganization, grief, fear of death and anxiety about an inability to cope with the future, he will also begin to devaluate himself less. He will come to realize that disability and lack of worth are not synonymous.

ACCEPTANCE OF DISABILITY

As times goes on, the patient gradually comes to "accept" his loss. Acceptance is a term that is used both frequently and thoughtlessly. People accept things in many ways. One might cope with a disability and yet have unrealistic goals. Another might accept the diagnosis but deny the implications of the disability.

Some experts feel that a goal of the patient's total acceptance of his disability is unrealistic. Because there is some truth to this, many persons prefer to use the term "assimilate a disability." As the patient begins to work through his initial shock, depression, fear and anger, he begins to develop an inner acceptance and to move toward social integration. He realizes that his total life style, while responsive to the reality of his problem, does allow for personal gratification. He begins to experience satisfaction from what he can do, rather than defeat from what he cannot do. Acceptance means giving into the treatment, but it does not mean constricting one's interests or remaining unnecessarily dependent.

This stage arrives after months for some, after years for others, and for a few never. Progression and regression are likely to occur and some patients reach a stage of adaptation which becomes a plateau. Each person must be allowed to move forward in his own way, not ours.

Just prior to discharge, the patient may have a sudden rush of fear that may be manifested by symptoms similar to those of the turbulence phase. This is due to the fear of leaving the safety of the hospital on a permanent basis. Trial visits at home can minimize this reaction, but they may not eliminate it.

The final adaptation takes place at home and may be observed by few health workers. Only the occasional follow-up visit to the home, doctor's office or clinic permits us to know how the person is doing in the community. Dr. Carl Herman says: "His reaction depends to large degree on the confidence and self esteem he has developed during his rehabilitation program and to an equal degree on the receptivity and acceptance of his family, employer and society." This combination of successes is the ideal adaptation to disability and is the goal of rehabilitation. The patient will have become a person with new requirements and deprivations, new privileges and expectations, and new rewards and opportunities.

RESPONSES OF HEALTH PERSONNEL

PERSONAL RESPONSES

There has been social prejudice against the disabled throughout the history of mankind. It is important that we occasionally remind ourselves of this, for undoubtedly none of us (including the disabled) has entirely escaped the influence of our cultural prejudice. The Greeks viewed the physically impaired as inferior. The early Hebrews attributed these conditions to punishment by God. While we know better and think more scientifically today, some of our behavior does not reflect the knowledge we have acquired. Rearing of handicapped children is usually not "integrated." The "charity" aspect of certain fund drives and the pity that is stimulated by them reflects some of our historical attitudes. Even in a rehabilitation center, we are often seen trying to place middle class values on patients from a lower socioeconomic sector of society.

In the health care setting, personnel may manifest their discomfort in the presence of a disabled patient in a variety of ways that can range from overt hostility to avoidance. The health worker (physician, nurse, physical therapist, etc.) who is struggling with his own feelings or conflicts involving dependency on a parent or spouse will not be able to tolerate working with the disabled if he views them as primarily dependent. The "rescue fantasies" of some physicians are seriously challenged by chronic incurable disease. The need to conquer illness cannot be met when caring for a person with arthritis. Some personnel may sense a partial death in disability or displace parental conflicts on patients. Persons who have an unconscious need to dominate or be dominated do not make good rehabilitation workers.

Personnel who work with long-term patients should examine themselves for such qualities. Each person needs to become aware of his own attitudes. For example, fear of dependency, often exhibited by overindependence, could adversely affect a patient at a dependent stage. This type of staff member may label the patient "a baby," accuse him of refusing rehabilitation or subtly treat him disparagingly. This kind of behavior prevents any therapeutic communication between staff and patient and may delay or hinder the patient's own adjustment.

In Siller's studies of people who lived and socialized with the handicapped, some of the following reactions were identified. There was a feeling of guilt for being able-bodied. Many developed a fear of becoming disabled themselves. Others experienced a sense of uneasiness and uncertainty about how to deal with the disabled. They feared saying or doing something that would be wrong or embarrassing. The problem of social embarrassment and social ostracism was more serious with certain types of conditions. Some felt an aversion or revulsion toward a particular disability. People were afraid of staring, or of not staring. Disabled persons will almost certainly encounter some of these reactions and attitudes, and it is therefore important that they be given the opportunity to develop healthy relationships.

People who work with rehabilitation patients are liable to have similar feelings. Therefore, they will need to identify and explore their own reactions. By doing so, personnel can resolve negative feelings, so that they will not adversely affect the patient during crucial periods of learning and adjustment. In some instances, a health worker may frankly realize that she or he should not be assigned to a particular patient and will request a transfer. Such decisions show consideration of the patient.

Before discussing more positive aspects of personnel behavior, a brief overview of the difficult patient—that is, the patient who becomes difficult as a result of poor attitudes on the part of health workers—may be helpful. Donald Peterson succinctly defines a difficult patient as "one whose needs are not met—emotional or physical or both." He goes on to describe the kinds of nurses who can cause this: the nurse who is dissatisfied with nursing or her job, the nurse who accepted the teaching that she should be objective and not sympathetic, the one who speaks about the patient rather than to him in his presence, the one who plans care in a conference where the patient cannot hear or refute information that is discussed. When a patient becomes a problem because of indifferent treatment by difficult personnel, reassignment to a caring person will make the patient no longer troublesome. The nurse's task in rehabilitation is complex because she must deal with regression, masochism, dependency and transference. She must therefore be able to distinguish between difficult behavior that is caused or intensified by persons in the environment and that which is caused by the patient's stress while coping with a personal crisis.

THERAPEUTIC RESPONSES

The patient's job is to get well. The role of the professional person is to assist him in doing so. As the patient begins to convalesce, he is sometimes likened to an adolescent. Leaving a protective world causes great ambivalence between the need for dependency and the need for independence. At this point in the patient's life, the professional needs to stimulate independence, to show confidence in a successful outcome and to make clear that the ultimate rewards of independence are gratifying and fulfilling.

One of the ways in which health personnel can help the patient during acute stress is to help him cope with simple tasks. If the patient can experience some early successes, it will assist him in rebuilding his self-image. In fact, physical rehabilitation of function is sometimes thought of as a series of strategies to assist rehabilitation in the other areas. It is also important to involve members of the patient's family. If they are stable, they can be of immense assistance.

Throughout the stages between acute distress and ultimate adjustment to the disability, all health personnel, especially the nurse and the physician, need to observe the patient's reactions. They must listen to the patient and accept what he has to say. Words that are too cheery are inappropriate in the early stages of illness. In fact, this kind of attitude may simply add irritation to an already overwhelming number of emotions. Personnel working with the disabled might well confront their *own* inevitable disability, prepare for it and learn "acceptance" in themselves, so that they can pass on positive attitudes to their patients.

The nurse must adapt her approach to different patients, and often to the same patient. She must be sensitive to the times when she can move ahead and recognize when the person needs to be left alone. Frequent self-reflection will be helpful. Does she find herself imposing her values on the patient? What motivates her actions—her patient's needs or her own? Is she so emotionally involved with a patient that she feels no one else can care for him? Is she so overwhelmed by the disability that she is unable to assist her patient? Does she remind herself that *she* is not responsible for her patient's disability? Does she try to smooth over disturbed behavior or does she try to find out its cause?

This chapter cannot deal with all the various responses that will assist the patient to a healthier condition. However, the nurse is encouraged to study basic communication with patients so that she can listen better, answer questions better and better sense patients' problems and feelings. The nurse should make a point of studying blocks to communication and various ways of helping patients to express their feelings. This is the key to assisting any patient in any illness. For the nurse working with long-term care patients this is crucial, because she is with them during a prolonged period of varying degrees of stress.

Patient Participation

The patient who is given the opportunity to become a co-manager of his or her care develops and maintains self-esteem. After the acute phase of care during the very first few weeks following the initial disability, patient participation becomes a key to vital psychological adjustment. It may even motivate early participation in plans for the future. Since motivation comes from within, it is the job of the health professional to find out what interests will be stimulating to the patient. What is it that he or she would really like to learn and do? The more a plan is based on input from patients, the more helpful the health counseling will be.

In addition to positive interpersonal relations and therapeutic communications, the nurse must be aware of the problems of learning, not merely in relation to teaching new skills but also in relation to learning new behaviors. Wilbert Fordyce believes that change in behavior is best achieved by applying appropriate learning principles. He directs his efforts "toward applying appropriate learning principles directly to the behavior to be changed rather than trying to change inferred underlying attitude on feeling states." In other words, rather than trying to change the underlying attitude or feeling states so that new behaviors may occur, he aims to change the behavior "with the expectation that adjustments in underlying feelings and attitudes . . . will follow."

The nurse will more than likely participate in operant conditioning programs for patients in a rehabilitation setting. The nurse is urged to study this subject in greater depth. A good beginning would be to see Chapter 6 by Wilbert Fordyce in the *Handbook of Physical Medicine and Rehabilitation* by Krusen et al.

Briefly, however, the crucial element of operant conditioning is manipulation of behavior to achieve certain goals. In starting an operant-based management program, the patient must be told about the goals of the program. This will avoid the issues that are often raised about the ethics of operant conditioning.

Operant conditioning operates as follows. First, behaviors to be increased or decreased are identified. Next, potential reinforcers are identified. These must be readily available, since a reinforcer must be delivered as soon as possible after a behavior that is supposed to be influenced. The nurse must be alert to an individual's response, as a particular consequence may be a reinforcer to one person and a punisher to another. For example, if a patient refuses physical therapy, frequent rests or a cigarette may become the planned reinforcer after periods of participation. As behaviors change in the desired direction, the problem then becomes that of maintaining the change after discharge from the hospital. This is done by providing reinforcers through work and social and leisure activities.

SUMMARY

The ultimate adjustment to a disability will depend upon both the individual's internal factors and external factors in the environment. Some of the feelings experienced by persons with a disability have been discussed to give health personnel who must deal with such feelings a better understanding of their sources and characteristics. With a greater knowledge of communication and some insight into one's own reactions to disability, nurses will be able to provide more meaningful psychological support to patients.

REFERENCES

Aiken, L., and Aiken, J.: A systematic approach to the evaluation of interpersonal relationships. *American Journal of Nursing, 73*:863, May, 1973.

Armacost, Betty, et al.: A group of "problem" patients. *American Journal of Nursing, 74*:289–292, February, 1974.

Buscaglia, Leo: *The Disabled and Their Parents: A Counseling Challenge.* Thorofare, New Jersey, Charles B. Slack, 1975.

Brown, Esther Lucile: *Newer Dimensions of Patient Care,* Parts 1, 2 and 3. New York, Russell Sage Foundation, 1965.

Campbell, Ann: Outreach, new dimensions in rehabilitative services for the physically and socially handicapped. *Rehabilitation Literature, 31*:162, 1970.

Carlson, Carolyn E.: *Behavioral Concepts in Nursing Intervention.* Philadelphia, J. B. Lippincott Co., 1970.

Christopherson, Victor A., et al.: *Rehabilitation Nursing Perspective and Applications.* New York, McGraw-Hill Book Co., 1974.

Fordyce, Wilbert E.: Psychological assessment and management. Chapter 6 *in* Krusen, Frank H., et al.: *Handbook of Physical Medicine and Rehabilitation.* 2nd Ed. Philadelphia, W. B. Saunders Co., 1971.

Gellman, William: Roots of prejudice against the handicapped. *Journal of Rehabilitation, 25*:4–6, January–February, 1959.

Goldin, G. J., et al.: *Dependency and Its Implications for Rehabilitation*. Toronto, Lexington Books, 1972.

Grayson, Morris: *Psychiatric Aspects of Rehabilitation*. New York, The Institute of Physical Medicine and Rehabilitation, New York Medical Center, 1952.

Herman, Carl D.: Psychiatric rehabilitation of the physically disabled. Chapter 38 *in* Krusen, Frank H., et al.: *Handbook of Physical Medicine and Rehabilitation*. 2nd Ed. Philadelphia, W. B. Saunders Co., 1971.

Kalish, Richard: *The Dependencies of Old People*. Ann Arbor, Institute of Gerontology, 1969.

Lederer, Henry D.: How the sick view their world. *In* Skipper, James K., and Leonard, Robert C. (Eds.): *Social Interaction in Patient Care*. Philadelphia, J. B. Lippincott Co., 1965, p. 155.

Litman, Theodor: Physical rehabilitation: a social psychological approach. *In* Jaco, E. Gartly (Ed.): *Patients, Physicians and Illness*. New York, Free Press, 1972.

Lyon, Glee Gamble: Stimulation through remotivation. *American Journal of Nursing*, 71:982–986, May, 1971.

McCollum, Audrey T.: *Coping with Prolonged Health Impairment in Your Child*. Boston, Little, Brown and Co., 1975.

Marris, Peter: *Loss and Change*. New York, Pantheon Books, 1974.

Orade, Donnal, and Waite, Nancy: Group psychotherapy with stroke patients during the immediate recovery phase. *American Journal of Orthopsychiatry*, 44:386–389, April, 1974.

Peterson, Donald: Developing the difficult patient. *American Journal of Nursing*, 67:522–525, March, 1967.

Safilios-Rothschild, Constantina: *The Sociology and Social Psychology of Disability and Rehabilitation*. New York, Random House, 1970.

Siller, Jerome: *Attitudes of the Nondisabled Toward the Physically Disabled*. New York, New York University, School of Education, May, 1967.

Siller, Jerome: *Structure of Attitudes Toward the Physically Disabled*. New York, New York University, School of Education, November, 1967.

Siller, Jerome: Psychological situation of the disabled with spinal cord injuries. *Rehabilitation Literature*, 30:290, 1969.

Skipper, J. K., and Leonard, R. C. (Eds.): *Social Interaction and Patient Care*. Philadelphia, J. B. Lippincott Co., 1965.

Smith, Dorothy W.: Patienthood and its threat to privacy. *American Journal of Nursing, 39*:509, 1969.

Strauss, Anselm: *Chronic Illness and the Quality of Life*. St. Louis, C. V. Mosby Co., 1975.

Tarver, Joyce, and Turner, A. Jack: Teaching behavior modification to patients' families. *American Journal of Nursing, 74*:282–283, February, 1974.

Weiss, James (Ed.): *Nurses, Patients, and Social Systems*. Columbia, Missouri, University of Missouri Press, 1968.

Wright, Beatrice A.: *Physical Disability: A Psychological Approach*. New York, Harper and Row, 1960.

Chapter 5

REDUCING THE HAZARDS OF BED REST

In 1863, The British physician John Hilton wrote a book reporting rest of body systems through the prescription of bed rest. This concept has often been misinterpreted as a recommendation for rest of the whole person rather than of one system or part. Since that time, people have often been put to bed and forgotten. This unfortunate practice has caused many problems in nursing homes, has unnecessarily reduced the strength of patients hospitalized by acute disease and has caused physical deconditioning and deterioration that could well have been prevented.

Since bed rest is so commonly used, it is surprising that there have been few controlled studies of its results. Given a specific condition among a group of patients, do those who rest get well faster than those who are ambulatory? Several such studies have been done, and the results may be surprising. Browse cites in one study by J. A. Wier in 1957 where 200 patients with the diagnosis of tuberculosis were on drug therapy: 100 patients were ambulatory, and the other 100 were placed on bed rest. The result was that both groups of patients had the same rate of recovery as measured by chest x-ray findings. Similar recovery rates of ambulatory and bedfast patients have also been found in studies of persons with gastric ulcers and respiratory infections. At present a great deal of information comes from the aerospace program, because astronauts undergo physiological changes in a weightless atmosphere similar to those undergone by patients placed on bed rest.

In our daily practice it is important that we use the knowledge that is presently available. We need to understand the problems caused by immobility or bed rest, and to know what action we can take to minimize them. Many of these precautions are nursing measures and can be independently initiated by the nurse. A majority of patients in almost all settings can benefit if this basic knowledge is applied.

PURPOSES OF RESTRICTED MOTION

There are three main causes of restricted motion, or patient inactivity. First, anyone who has a spinal cord injury or a brain injury will obviously have limited motion due to paralysis. Second, someone who has pain from arthritis, from an injury or from surgery will naturally move less in order to reduce the amount of pain. Third, weakness caused by aging, neuromotor diseases or nutritional problems will cause reduced activity. The patient will automatically decrease his activity in these instances.

There are, of course, specific reasons for using bed rest. Let us examine them. A physician prescribes bed rest for the following *therapeutic* purposes. First, bed rest usually relieves pain whether it is the result of surgery, sprains, trauma or disease. Second, bed rest may be required to immobilize a wound, such as a fracture or a cataract. Third, bed rest may be prescribed to limit exercise and activity, as in the case of a patient who has suffered a myocardial infarction. In certain conditions, self-discipline or the use of a chair may be just as adequate as, and less damaging than, bed rest. Fourth, bed rest may be prescribed to provide support when there is too little strength to fight the pull of gravity, as in the case of a weak and debilitated patient. However, in these cases a vicious circle can result, since prolonged rest can in turn cause a greater degree of weakness. Reduced activity rather than bed rest should be considered as soon as possible for these patients. Fifth, bed rest increases cardiac output and venous return, as in the case of shock when patients are placed in the supine position. Sixth, bed rest might be prescribed to reduce the effects of gravity in such conditions as edema, varicosities or venous ulcers. A reduction of the effect of gravity is also desirable in such conditions as a protruding hernia or a prolapsed rectum. On the other hand, gravity is desired when tipping is required to relieve copious secretions of the lungs.

It is important to understand not only the purposes of inactivity and bed rest, but also the adverse effects of bed rest. When a patient is in bed, the nurse must know why. Thus, if one part of the body must be rested, the rest of the body need not become totally inactive also. The nurse must note what immobilizing factors exist in a particular situation and what the patient's response to those factors are and relate this information to the disorder under treatment. She then seeks to prevent immobilization whenever possible, or to reduce its effect and to help the patient cope with unavoidable immobility. The knowledge and skill of the nurse can enhance the therapeutic effects and reduce the adverse effects of bed rest.

THE ADVERSE EFFECTS OF BED REST

In 1947 Doctor R. A. Asher, a British physician, wrote an article entitled "The Dangers of Going to Bed." In it he describes what an "overdose" of bed rest can do: "Look at a patient lying long in bed. What a pathetic picture he makes! The blood clotting in his veins, the lime draining from his bones, the scybala stacking up in his colon, the flesh rotting from his seat, the urine leaking from his distended bladder and the spirit evaporating from his soul." If one re-reads his statement, one becomes aware that he has taken each system of the body and dramatically stated what occurs during prolonged inactivity.

The basis of an organ's functional ability is use. Rest or restricted motion constitutes a period of non-use and results in a loss of ability of that organ. This means that when bed rest (as opposed to rest of an affected part) is prescribed, deterioration of healthy parts of the body also occurs. This implies a need for gradual activation after rest, as well as necessary precautions during the period of rest. A brief discussion of each system will help to explain these points.

EFFECT ON THE CARDIOVASCULAR SYSTEM

The cardiovascular system is affected by bed rest in four ways: (1) increased work load of the heart, (2) orthostatic hypotension, (3) reduction of cardiac reserve and (4) possible increase in thrombus formation. In a study by Coe, it was demonstrated that the heart must work 30 per cent harder in the supine position than the sitting position. The pulse drops from about 89 to 60 and the blood pressure remains about the same. The supine position alters the distribution of blood in the body. Since hydrostatic pressure equalizes when the patient is supine, approximately 11 per cent of the blood leaves the legs and most of this goes to the thorax. This means that the blood volume of the heart increases, which in turn causes greater work for the heart with each contraction.

The workload of the heart can also be increased by the Valsalva maneuver, described as follows. When someone holds his breath, the chest is held fixed, air is pushed against the closed glottis and intrathoracic pressure increases. When the person then breathes, there is a sudden increase in venous return to the heart, causing tachycardia. This occurs when a person turns in bed (10 to 20 times an hour), gets on and off a bedpan and strains at the stool. It is because of this that a heart patient should be taught to breathe through his mouth when turning in bed. This is why a commode is recommended for these patients, and it is part of the rationale for chair rest versus bed rest.

Bed rest reduces the effects of gravity and results in generalized vasodilatation accompanied by increased venous return, cardiac output and blood volume. When patients who have been lying in bed for any length of time first sit up, the decreased efficiency of their orthostatic neurovascular reflexes causes their skin to become clammy and pale, and they may feel weak or faint. Their blood pressure drops (orthostatic hypotension) when they become erect.

In a study conducted by Taylor, healthy young men were put to bed for 21 days. At the end of this time they were given work requiring moderate exertion. It was found that their heart rates on the average had increased about 40 beats per minute, compared to their heart rates during similar exertion before the period of bed rest. It took 5 to 10 weeks for their heart rates during work to return to the rates prior to the period of rest. It is to be noted that this occurred in healthy young men. Is it any wonder that it takes persons who have been ill much longer to regain function and strength?

These responses to bed rest give us physiological reasons for certain nursing measures. We elevate the head of a cardiac patient in order to prevent increased work by the heart. Passive and active range of motion exercises and any possible self-care promote return flow of blood to the heart. Isometric exercises, while not recommended for cardiac patients, might be prescribed by a physician in other conditions. We get a postoperative patient up slowly, check his pulse and help him to adapt from the horizontal to the vertical position. Besides frequent changes of position, we may use a tilt table and ask patients to dangle if they have been in bed for a long time.

There is some disagreement in the literature as to the relationship of bed rest and thrombus formation. Browse states that there is no documented evidence of formation of thrombi due to stasis alone. He says, however, that stasis (the result of decreased muscular contractions, which promote venous return from the extremities) accompanied by hypercoagulability and any damage to the intima of the blood vessel can cause thrombi. Preventive and therapeutic medical and nursing measures usually include the following: early ambulation for postpartum and postoperative patients, prescription of anticoagulant therapy based on prothrombin times and the administration of anticoagulants on time. It is important for the nurse to position the patient's legs to prevent any damage to the intima of the vein. For example, if the patient is in a lateral recumbent position with his upper calf on his lower tibia, the nurse must be very careful that the knee does not press on the popliteal vein. This is especially vital if the patient is unconscious or paralyzed.

EFFECT ON THE RESPIRATORY SYSTEM

Bed rest affects the respiratory system by (1) interfering with chest expansion, (2) reducing the movement of secretions and (3) causing deficient ventilation. In most instances a healthy person can compensate for respiratory problems by moving about in bed and coughing. However, if a patient is sedated, weak, paralyzed or unconscious, it is essential for the nurse to take measures that will counteract any ill effects on the respiratory system. When a patient is in the supine postion, he has decreased respiratory movement due to pressure of the bed against the rib cage. In fact, one investigator found that it takes twice the effort to breathe in a supine position as it does in an upright position.

Certain drugs or a tight abdominal binder can also reduce chest expansion. In addition, stasis and pooling of secretions may cause bronchitis or hypostatic pneumonia. Eventually, there is less aeration in already collapsed alveoli, resulting in the production of a greater amount of carbon dioxide. In 1951, Monroe studied geriatric patients who had been diagnosed as having pulmonary emphysema. Autopsies, however, revealed no evidence of emphysema. He concluded that the shortness of breath had been due to lack of fitness. Inadequate oxygenation of the geriatric patient will affect cardiac and brain function as well as respiratory function.

Nursing measures are especially important for the paralyzed, the postoperative or the weak patient. First of all, the nurse must make sure that the patient does deep breathing at intervals throughout the day and night. Whenever possible the patient should sit up in a chair to increase ease of respiration and to stimulate greater depth of respiration. It is important to have the patient cough in order to loosen secretions. Turning the patient will help prevent pooling of secretions on one side. The frequency of deep breathing, turning and coughing varies from 2-hour to 4-hour intervals and, depending on the patient, may be required around the clock. If the patient is able the nurse can teach him to do this for himself. In addition, careful observations — depth of respirations, their type and regularity, the effort required, the presence of secretions, the patient's color — are essential. In general, the nurse needs to initiate preventive measures earlier to counteract the effects of inactivity on the respiratory system in most patients.

EFFECT ON THE URINARY TRACT

It is estimated that between 15 per cent and 30 per cent of patients who require prolonged bed rest develop stones. Urine output increases, as does the concentration of urinary calcium, which trebles in two weeks of rest and is even greater if there is also bone disease or paralysis. The amount of calcium, the volume of urine and the pH and concentration of citric acid determine the solubility of calcium. During rest, the level of citric acid stays the same while that of calcium increases. As a result, calcium is less soluble, and urinary stones develop.

Certain nursing measures will reduce the effect of bed rest on the urinary tract. First of all, the force of gravity should be encouraged by having the patient sit up when he voids. This prevents the renal pelvis from becoming distended as a result of urine stasis in the calyces of the kidney. It is also important to turn the patient at frequent intervals. Forcing fluids is helpful. Some physicians reduce the amount of calcium in the diet, especially if the patient has a spinal cord injury or a bone disease.

EFFECT ON THE MUSCULOSKELETAL SYSTEM

Bed rest has adverse affects on both bone and muscle tissue. Bones demineralize and muscles change in strength, size, general appearance, chemistry and function.

When activity is reduced, bone strength is reduced because of the loss of bone matrix and calcium. Calcium lost in this process results in the development of calculi of the urinary tract. Patients also become fracture prone, and osteoporosis becomes imminent. Daily weight bearing is practiced to reduce the likelihood of these potential problems.

It is estimated that muscle weakness and atrophy begin from the third to the seventh day in bed. Most affected are the anti-gravity muscles of the limbs used for standing and walking. In lower extremity fractures, preventive measures to both the fractured limb and the non-fractured limb can shorten the period of recovery considerably.

In addition, the patient has an obvious loss of mobility. When there is regular motion of bones, joints and muscles, loose connective tissue is present. When there is greatly reduced or no motion, connective tissue becomes dense—a condition known as fibrosis. This can cause a loss of motion within only a few days, which in turn results in contractures. Contractures occur very quickly in stroke victims. About 60 per cent develop a shoulder contracture, and 30 per cent develop an ankle contracture. An amputee may develop a contracture on the operative side within a few days. Incidentally, it takes weeks and sometimes months to reverse fibrosis, and the condition can become permanent if allowed to go on for too long a time. This is the basic reason for doing range of motion exercises of every joint that does not require immobilization, and for positioning body parts in proper alignment. This kind of nursing intervention can be thought of as preventive and maintenance. See Chapter 14, Range of Motion Exercises, for details.

Perkins described the length of time needed to regain range of motion following shoulder dislocation with varying periods of immobilization. The findings were as follows:

LENGTH OF IMMOBILIZATION	RECOVERY OF RANGE OF MOTION
0 days	18 days
7 days	52 days
14 days	121 days
21 days	300 days

Another effect of immobilization on the musculoskeletal system is the loss of muscle strength and endurance. The strength of a muscle is the maximum tension that the muscle can exert, and if a patient is unconscious he may lose as much as 3 per cent of his muscle strength every day. It is also estimated that an arm in a cast loses over 3 per cent of its strength each day. When a muscle reconditioning program begins, it will take a longer time to regain strength than it did to lose it. Weakness and disuse atrophy can be reduced somewhat by certain nursing measures. Three times a day the patient can be asked to give two or three strong contractions of such muscles as the biceps, the quadriceps and the abdominal and gluteal muscles.

EFFECT ON THE SKIN

Since a decubitus ulcer can develop in 24 hours, constant nursing vigilance is essential. Unfortunately, many nurses do not think about decubitus ulcers until they occur, at which time their interest is focused on treatment. It is estimated that 95 per cent of all decubitus ulcers are preventable, which only contributes to a sense of guilt whenever an ulcer develops. It is important that the nurse understand that she has no reason to feel guilty if she has taken all ordinary preventive measures. Certainly, in the very debilitated and undernourished it is almost impossible to prevent the development of some decubitus ulcers.

Decubitus ulcers tend to occur over bony prominences (see Fig. 13–2). Pressure on the tissue causes reduced circulation in that tissue and, ultimately, tissue death. Since decubitus ulcers can occur within 24 hours, all preventive measures should be started at the time of admission of any patient who has limited motion whether due to disease, injury or paralysis. Throughout any period of immobilization, constant vigilance by the nurse is essential.

Nursing measures include (1) maintaining skin cleanliness, (2) maintaining adequate circulation by turning at frequent intervals and by protecting bony prominences and (3) preventing pressure from external sources such as clothing, casts, braces or adaptive devices.

Whenever a patient is turned, the nurse should inspect the skin to see if there is redness. If so, gentle massage is indicated. If the redness does not readily disappear, the turning schedule should be shortened. In other words, one should base the frequency of a turning schedule on skin inspection, allowing only quickly transient redness to occur.

There are many pieces of equipment that are helpful in aiding the prevention of decubitus ulcers. However, the nurse must not expect equipment such as alternating pressure mattresses, lamb's wool, foam rubber or turning frames to do her nursing care for her. These are aids to nursing care. They are helpful, but they cannot replace observation, good positioning and turning. See Chapter 13, Positioning Methods and Skin Care, for more detailed nursing care.

EFFECTS ON THE ALIMENTARY TRACT

According to some authors, there is no clinical evidence that gut motility or biochemical processes are changed when the patient is on bed rest. Studies of children who swallowed foreign objects indicate that for both the ambulatory child and the child on bed rest, objects are passed through the alimentary tract and eliminated in the stool at the same rate. Inactivity has two effects on the colon, however. First, gravity inhibits the feces from passing through the ascending colon, so that transit in this segment is faster in a supine position. Also with the patient supine, the rectum is more likely to fill gradually rather then suddenly from the sigmoid colon. The principal problems of elimination, usually constipation, seem to be related to a change in diet and a reduced amount of activity. In addition, weakened muscle tone or a disease involving the gastrointestinal tract will obviously alter elimination habits.

For these reasons, nursing measures must be related to the patient's former habits and to the patient's activity and general physical condition. This is why bowel programs of inactive persons can be based on a frequency of every other day or only three times a week. This is usually adequate for older people. The problem lies not just in teaching the nurse that a daily bowel movement may not be essential but also in teaching patients that this is not necessarily healthy especially if regular laxatives are required to achieve it.

Nursing measures include an awareness that in a multiple-bed room, a patient suppresses the sensation to evacuate and sometimes does not feel it at all. Therefore, every effort to provide privacy is vital. A commode or bathroom is always preferable to a bedpan. Lying on the right side will encourage emptying of the stomach. The diet must have adequate protein and enough bulk and liquids to encourage elimination.

Lastly, it is important for the nurse to know that diarrhea may be a sign of fecal impaction. She should also check for impaction if there has been no bowel movement after approximately three days or if stools have been hard and inadequate. See Chapter 8, Assisting Patients with Bowel and Bladder Problems, for more detailed nursing care.

EFFECT ON THE INTELLECT AND EMOTION

Bed rest does not alter a person's personality, but it may bring out a latent psychosis or neurosis. More commonly, bed rest is simply depressing and anxiety producing. In addition, it is a psychological axiom that when a physician prescribes rest, the patient considers his condition more serious than if the physician had not prescribed rest.

Once the patient is in bed, he experiences feelings of helplessness, of inadequacy and of dependency on those around him. These feelings can cause withdrawal or rebellion against the doctor's orders. One of the more serious problems relates to the loss of role activity, whether that be son, daughter, mother, father or spouse. In addition, isolation from friends and familiar surroundings, a private room or an area where there is little stimulation causes intellectual and sensory deprivation. Several studies have indicated that a perfectly normal person who is completely isolated for as little as 24 hours may begin to hallucinate.

Lack of occupation leaves time for both introspection and concentration on illness. This can increase both the physical and psychological stress of the illness. This becomes a vicious circle, and it becomes harder and harder to interest the patient in other activities.

The effect of isolation has been studied at terminal care centers, where it has been shown that patients who have good psychological support, an active milieu and adequate stimuli improve to the point where they can be discharged. Cambridge Rehabilitation Center in Massachusetts, once a terminal care hospital, now discharges 300 geriatric patients a year. The Masonic Hospital for cancer patients at the University of Minnesota discharges far more patients than they first anticipated when they built their hospital.

Nursing measures to counteract ill effects of bed rest and inactivity are infinite in variety. One of them is helping the patient to identify and fulfill his needs. This may include his seeing visitors, reading, having a library cart come to the room, or watching television. It may include his working on hobbies, trying new activities, or carrying out some part of his regular occupation. All of these measures are vital in helping the patient maintain his sense of self-esteem, his sense of identity and his sense of worth. Since institutionalization can cause a loss of these vital psychological supports, we must, as nurses, do everything we can to counteract them.

THE KEY TO NURSING ACTION

The key to nursing action is to find a balance between therapeutic rest and therapeutic activities. In other words, the nurse must first of all know why the patient is to have bed rest, identify which system or part requires rest and then plan for this to be accomplished. In addition, she must be aware of the need to protect the affected areas and to maintain the abilities of unaffected parts in order to prevent complicating problems. By doing this she provides a balance between rest and activity, so that maximal physical and psychological energy can be directed toward recovery. Frequently, however, the strain of doing nothing causes fatigue, mild aches and tenseness. For example, it may very well be better to have a patient feed himself if he is overly upset about being fed by someone else.

Whenever possible, the patient needs to participate in his care plan. This does not mean asking the acutely ill patient to make decisions. There are times when the nurse must make the decisions, but for the most part the patient needs to be consulted and to have an opportunity to participate in his own care. The nurse can assist him in dividing his day between reading, television, visitors, hobbies and rest. She can subsequently plan and prepare for more activity as he progresses.

SUMMARY

The nurse must use the tools of her trade to promote rest for the healing of the immobilized part or organ, and to prevent further impairment of that injured part. She must help to maintain the function of parts and organs that do not require immobilization and provide both the physical and psychological environment that will make these goals most possible.

REFERENCES

Asher, R. A. J.: Dangers of going to bed. *British Medical Journal, 2*:967, 1947.
Bonner, Charles D.: Rehabilitation instead of bed rest? *Geriatrics, 24*:109, 1969.
Brower, Phyllis, and Hicks, Dorothy: Maintaining muscle function in patients on bed rest. *American Journal of Nursing, 72*:1250–1253, July, 1972.
Browse, Norman, L.: *The Physiology and Pathology of Bed Rest.* Springfield, Illinois, Charles C Thomas, 1965.
Carnevali, Doris, and Bruechner, Susan: Immobilization—reassessment of a concept. *American Journal of Nursing, 70*:1502, 1970.
Coe, W. S.: Cardiac work and the chair treatment of acute coronary thrombosis. *Annals of International Medicine, 40*:42, 1954.

Conrad, Linda: The Valsalva maneuver: a clinical inquiry. *American Journal of Nursing, 71*:553, 1971.

Dietrick, J. E., Whedon, G. D., and Shorr, E.: Effects of immobilization upon various metabolic and physiologic functions of normal men. *American Journal of Medicine, 4*:3, 1948.

Dock, W.: The undesirable effects of bed rest. *Surgical Clinics of North America, 25*:437, 1945.

Downs, Florence: Bed rest and sensory disturbances. *American Journal of Nursing, 74*:434–438, March, 1974.

Goldstrom, Deborah: Cardiac rest: bed or chair? *American Journal of Nursing, 72*:1812–1816, October, 1972.

Hettinger, Theodor: *Physiology of Strength.* Springfield, Illinois, Charles C Thomas, 1961.

Jackson, C. Wesley, and Ellis, Rosemary: Sensory deprivation as a field of study. *Nursing Research, 20*:46, 1971.

Jones, J. A.: Deprivation and existence or stimulation and life: our choice for the elderly. *Journal of Gerontological Nursing, 2*:17, March/April, 1976.

Kelly, Mary M.: Exercises for bedfast patients. *American Journal of Nursing, 66*:2209, 1966.

Kottke, F. J.: Deterioration of the bedfast patient. *Public Health Reports, 80*:437, 1965.

Kottke, F. J.: Preventing deterioration in the bedfast patient. *R.N.,* February, 1967, p. 71.

Lavin, Mary Ann: Bed exercises for acute cardiac patients. *American Journal of Nursing, 73*:1226–1227, July, 1973.

Madden, Barbara, and Affeldt, John E.: To prevent helplessness and deformities. *American Journal of Nursing, 62*:59, 1962.

Mead, S.: A century of the abuse of rest. *Journal of the American Medical Association, 182*:344, 1962.

Mills, John A., et al.: Value of bed rest in patients with rheumatoid arthritis. *The New England Journal of Medicine, 284*:453, 1971.

Muller, E. A.: Influence of training and of inactivity on muscle strength. *Archives of Physical Medicine, 51*:449–462, August, 1970.

Olson, Edith V., et al.: The hazards of immobility. *American Journal of Nursing, 67*:780, 1967.

Perkins, G.: Rest and movement. *Journal of Bone and Joint Surgery, 35B*:526, 1953.

Taylor, H. L., et al.: Effects of bedrest on cardiovascular function and work performance. *Journal of Applied Physiology, 2*:223, 1949.

Thomson, Linda: Sensory deprivation: a personal experience. *American Journal of Nursing, 73*:266, February, 1973.

Wylie, Charles M.: The value of early rehabilitation in stroke. *Geriatrics, 25*:107, 1970.

Zubek, J. P. (Ed.): *Sensory Deprivation: Fifteen Years of Research.* New York, Appleton-Century-Crofts, 1969.

Chapter 6

PLANNING PATIENT CARE

Everybody talks about nursing care plans, but the vast majority of patients enter and leave an institution having had a Kardex card which noted only medical treatments, examinations and medications. A written plan for nursing care is all too often a nonexistent entity. Even when care plans are required by law, as in the case of the nursing home, they are more concerned with transmittal of information than with testing and validating nursing care.

What goes wrong? Most nurses agree with the concept that a care plan is important. Why, then, do we have so little practical appreciation of a plan, as evidenced by its absence or inadequacy in so many instances? The reasons are not entirely clear. The nurse may have been inadequately taught, had inadequate supervised practice, had little experience or she may see it as unimportant. We may not know where to find out how to prepare a good plan. We may not know how to interview or assess needs. We may be afraid of the kind of patient involvement required to make an effective plan. Or we may find the incessant demand to meet all patient needs so overwhelming a goal that we give up and do very little.

If one looks honestly at the nursing factor, it is quite evident that we will be unable to meet all of the needs of our patients. Thinking that we can is not only unrealistic but self-defeating. I know a paraplegic person who says that 10 per cent of his rehabilitation (just a beginning) occurred in the rehabilitation center and 90 per cent occurred after discharge. This kind of statement should help to keep us humble and put our contributions in proper perspective. However, we *are* able to select needs with which we can work and with which we have learned to deal effectively. This in itself can reduce patient discomfort and tension and can enhance future adjustment. This 10 per cent can be the foundation for the other 90 per cent, and we sell ourselves short by not realizing what an immense contribution the nursing component can make to patient care.

Lack of time is not a justifiable answer because a plan does not have to be written like a thesis. With practice, developing a care plan is far less time consuming than it first appears. It takes a lot more time to learn a transfer procedure than it does to transfer a patient, because the learning stage and the practice stage take time. The same thing is true of learning to do care plans. It is most unfortunate that nurses think it takes the same amount of time to develop a nursing care plan in the work situation as it does in the classroom.

This chapter is written with the conviction that nursing care plans make an important difference in the quality of nursing care. This conviction is the result of working at institutions where some patients have plans and others do not. It is also the result of interviewing patients who have had plans and others who have not. This, along with the findings of countless authors as well as personal experience, brings a sense of urgency to the proper content and use of care plans.

In order to make a nursing care plan work, there needs to be some system or a form to assist the nurse in organizing her information. Administrative staff spend a great deal of time and effort on developing forms. While this is helpful, it sometimes diverts time and energy that should be spent addressing the conceptual issues and content of nursing therapy.

Most forms are developed for particular situations, and it is likely that one form will not be suitable for all types of patients. While all forms will have both strengths and weaknesses, these are far less important than the strengths and weaknesses of what the nurse sees and does for her patient.

It is desirable to have one nurse primarily responsible for the care plan of each patient. She may have several patients, and other members of the staff will be encouraged to contribute to the plan through discussions and conferences. This enables the patient to identify with a particular nurse and places direct responsibility on one person rather than on many team members. When nursing tasks are assigned to various levels of personnel, total care becomes fragmented, and some aspects of care are overlooked because it is assumed that "someone else is doing the job."

Developing a plan, implementing it and evaluating it can make nursing a most challenging and stimulating profession because it constantly presents new facets for exploration. Without such plans, nursing becomes ritualistic, with constant repetition of procedures and techniques offering little challenge to the nurse and giving small comfort to the patient.

One aspect of care planning is often hotly debated; that is, should it be called a nursing care plan or a patient care plan? Here, we are talking about nursing care of a particular patient. The term patient care plan assumes an interdisciplinary role, which is somewhat presumptuous unless, of course, all disciplines actually do record and participate in the plan. We are also talking about something other than care given by a physician, a physical therapist or an occupational therapist. We are discussing care given by a nurse. This is the rationale for using the term, nursing care plan, in this chapter.

While this chapter deals with nursing care plans in general, nursing care of patients who have chronic diseases with life adaptation problems will be used as examples. The Commission on Chronic Illness defines chronic disease as comprising all impairments or deviations from normal which have one or more of the following characteristics: they are permanent; they leave residual disabilities; they are caused by nonreversible pathologic alteration; they require special training of the patient for rehabilitation; and they may be expected to require long periods of supervision, observation or care. The greatest health problem for such a patient is the adaptation of his life rather than an actual threat to his life.

Patient needs go unmet for a variety of reasons, but lack of information, inaccurately identified needs, inadequate evaluation and lack of patient participation are primary causes. The nurse must seek facts and relate them to needs. The patient may not have participated in his care plan. He may even have a feeling that his life is being manipulated by so-called experts. Such problems can be avoided if the nurse knows that patient needs cannot be known without continuous communication with the recipient of that care. Without this information, nursing practice becomes limited in effectiveness. She should be specific in planning how she involves her patient. Does she invite responses concerning care from the patient and family? Is this done by direct question, observation, informal conversation, planned teaching times and conferences with other persons on the health team?

OBTAINING INITIAL INFORMATION

Initial nursing care can actually be given without knowing the medical diagnosis or any traditional kinds of information. Ultimately, of course, nursing measures are based on the condition of the patient, observations by the nurse, scientific knowledge of the various facets of illness and a particular condition, and patient and family interactions.

A patient interview form is a useful tool at the time of admission (Fig. 6–1). It is sometimes called a nursing history. It may simply be used as a check-list, or the nurse may actually record on the sheet. It should not become a part of the chart as it is likely to become a dormant piece of paper which in no way contributes to planning the patient's care. Therefore, such a sheet is best used as a worksheet or a checklist to initiate a care plan.

There are other matters which can be considered in an admission interview, depending on the information received from an individual patient. The example is given merely to suggest initial information which can be used to explore problems and needs in order to lay the foundation for nursing care. Routine

---

ADMISSION INTERVIEW WORKSHEET

Patient Name_____Date_____

1. Have you ever been hospitalized before? If so, describe.

2. What is your goal for this hospitalization?

3. What problems including your present illness restrict your activities?

4. Do you have any difficulty sleeping? If so, what do you find helpful?

5. Are you on any medications or a special diet?

6. Do you have any food or drug allergies?

7. Do you have any eating problems? Handling utensils? Dentures?

8. Do you have any visual or hearing deficits? Glasses? Hearing aids?

9. Do you have any trouble with elimination of urine? Have you used a catheter?

10. When and how often do you have a bowel movement? Do you use a laxative regularly?

11. What family do you have?

12. Do you wish to restrict any visitors or phone calls?

13. Do you have any questions you would like answered now?

14. Is there anything else we should know in order to give you better care?

Figure 6–1 Admission Interview Worksheet form.

kinds of information such as vital signs, height and weight may or may not be included.

It should be noted that some questions might not be pertinent to all patients. Most of them, however, can be modified for any patient who is able to be interviewed. This information along with information from the patient's chart, including the face sheet, which describes the patient's religion and occupation, begins a plan of care. If the patient is in a multiple-bed room, it is important to provide him with as much privacy as possible during his interview. While the nurse is interviewing the patient, she will naturally observe general appearance, facial expression and speech. She will try to assess the level of anxiety the patient is experiencing and observe his general behavior.

This time can also be used to give initial information concerning use of the electric bed, signal cord, radio, telephone, intercom and so forth. It is important to introduce him to other patients in his room. Naturally he should be told who will be taking care of him. Personnel can then introduce themselves as they come on duty.

Another essential source of information and assistance is the family. In addition, consultations, the referral sheet (if there is one), lab data and x-ray reports can provide guides to nursing measures. Besides knowledge of sciences from the nurse's basic education, other resources must be sought, such as reference readings concerning a particular condition as well as conversations with the attending physician and other health personnel caring for the patient.

THE PROBLEM-SOLVING APPROACH

Since nursing care is so frequently based on assumptions and intuition rather than scientific facts, it is no wonder that the profession is seeking a more precise method to determine nursing care. We too often draw our conclusions without having enough facts. Even when we gather facts, our perceptions sometimes prevent us from using them to the patient's advantage.

Patient assessment must be based on the biological, psychological and social history of the individual. In this way, one's view of the patient does not stress one particular facet of the illness or the illness itself. Rather, it stresses the various effects that the illness has upon the individual. Throughout a patient's illness it is hoped that the nurse and other members of the health care team can help the patient to maximize his potential during each phase of illness. The nurse has a role to conserve the patient's strength and to support him especially during periods of increased stress. This will naturally vary from time to time throughout an illness or a hospitalization. She will capitalize on his functional abilities and his wellness rather than on his disabilities and his disease.

Many times we do not understand a patient because of a problem within ourselves. For instance, we may have a predisposition about certain persons or situations and draw a conclusion from our own predisposition rather than from the situation. A second problem is that we may form a snap judgment based on a first impression which has lasted without further evidence. Third, we may be so preoccupied with our own problems and tasks that we do not hear what the patient is saying. Fourth, while it is difficult for us to admit it, we may not be free of prejudice. An example might be the person who thinks that poor people are shiftless. Anyone who has known poor people knows that there are shiftless poor people and that there are extremely self-determined and responsible poor people. Projection is another cause of lack of understanding. In this case, we attribute our motives to others when in reality they may be having entirely different needs, reactions and desires.

As the nurse combines a greater awareness of her own reactions with increased response to actual rather than perceived patient motives, she will begin to encourage greater patient participation and to call upon a wider variety of resources. She will begin to feel less need to control each situation and ultimately will be able to plan care with the patient, the family and her co-workers without feeling insecure.

Basically, the nursing care plan is developed by using the scientific method of problem solving. Adapted to care plans, this includes five basic steps.

1. Collection of data.
2. Identification of problems.
3. Hypothesis or tentative approach to the problem.
4. Evaluation of the effectiveness of the plan.
5. Readjustment of the plan and continuation of evaluation.

This is how a nursing care plan is developed although each step may not always be consciously considered. Knowledge of care and practice helps to make this process a habit.

It is important for the nurse to realize that some problems should also be worked on by other members of the health team. When the problem-oriented medical record is used in rehabilitation, this becomes apparent. In the problem-oriented medical record, many members of the health team record their findings on the *same* sheet. There is not a special sheet for each therapy, a special sheet on which the doctor records and so forth. A list of problems for a given patient is placed on the front of the chart. Each problem is dated at the time it is entered and again when it becomes inactive. In this way, patient outcomes are readily apparent. As an example, a list of active problems for a particular patient might include foot drop on right, bowel plan being re-evaluated, infection of bladder. The entire health team would then address themselves to these problems.

Should a new problem develop, this would be added and become activated. As a problem such as the bladder infection disappears, it becomes inactive. In this way, the focus of all members of the health team is on the patient's problem rather than on what each discipline is doing for the patient. For further information on the problem-oriented medical record, the reader is referred to the references at the end of this chapter.

In brief, the nurse uses the problem-solving approach to prepare a nursing care plan in the following manner:

• First she gathers her information (data) from the various sources previously described.

• Second, she reviews the data in order to identify specific patient problems. How the problem is stated is important. It is well to remember prevention at this juncture. For instance, in some conditions, a hip flexion contracture could develop. At the moment there may be no problem, but a worthy objective might be to prevent the problem of hip flexion contracture.

• Third, a planned approach is stated in terms of a nursing action. In this case, range of motion and positioning would be two nursing actions associated with the objective of preventing a contracture.

• Fourth, the patient's response to the nursing action must be observed. If the patient develops a hip flexion contracture in spite of the measures taken, different approaches are necessary. If not, it can be considered a successful approach to a given objective.

• Fifth, readjust the plan according to the patient response and evaluate the new approach in terms of patient outcomes and/or responses.

THE PLAN

FACTORS TO BE CONSIDERED

Physician's orders are a part of the total plan. However, medications, treatments, parenteral fluids, preparation for examinations and so forth become only one factor in the patient's plan. These activities are dependent upon the doctor and not initiated by the nurse.

This chapter is concerned with care that is initiated by the nurse. In some instances, it may be initiated in consultation with other members of the health team. Certainly hygienic factors such as the bath, oral hygiene, shaving and nail care are nursing functions. The environment is in part a nursing responsibility. This would include heat control, noise, care of patient property and furniture arranged so that it is convenient to the patient rather than conforming to the arrangement in other rooms.

The nurse must assess and describe in the care plan what assistance the patient requires with meals, ambulation, dressing, communication and so forth. Safety factors must be included in the plan. For long-term care patients, attention to sensory deficits which could harm or injure the patient is vital.

The nurse must plan for maintaining an open airway, maintaining proper body alignment, preventing circulatory constriction, preventing cross infection and providing relief of pain. She needs to include elements which relate to elimination, such as proper care of the catheter, privacy for a bowel program and an adequate amount of fluid. She must include psychological support and arrange for spiritual counseling if such is desired. Patient and family teaching are integrated in the plan throughout a program of rehabilitation, since their participation is always necessary.

As the person leaves the care of one health agency or institution and goes to another, a nursing summary must go with the patient to assure the continuation of individualized care. Such a referral, of course, presupposes that a good care plan exists and that it would be useful to the family, the nursing home or the public health nurse assuming responsibility for care.

PRESCRIBING NURSING CARE

June Rothberg defines nursing therapy as "knowledgeable intervention in the form of nursing activities." In order to do this, the nurse must know the needs and goals of individual patients and be able to select appropriate methods of assisting the patient. This is based on knowledge of the patient's physical, psychological and physiological problems as well as those which he might experience socially, economically and environmentally. She defines a nursing diagnosis as "evaluation by nurses of those factors affecting the patient which will influence his recovery." The fact that nursing care can influence a patient's status either positively or negatively makes meaningful plans mandatory.

While terms and forms vary, the process of stating patient objectives and nursing approaches and then relating them to patient responses is basic to planning care. This process is both dynamic and current if it is monitored and modified according to patient responses. This also keeps the plan future-oriented, which is vital in order to include the preventive and learning aspects of the rehabilitation process.

Little and Carnevali suggest a planning system that uses the letters POAR. This provides the nurse with a framework in which to conceptualize her plan. P stands for problem, O for objective, A for approach, and R for response. Whether one chooses this approach or whether one merely prefers to state objectives, approaches and responses is a matter of individual taste. The mechanics of preparing a plan become less important as the nurse improves the content of her plans.

One of the reasons most nursing care plans cannot be utilized in the way they should be is that the information is incomplete and is therefore not useful; it does not assist the nurse, the student, the aide or the orderly coming on duty. Frequently the care plan merely describes problems. To state that a patient is confused is only partial information. This information would be part of our data gathering process but does not assist the nurse to take care of that patient. Everyone may know that the patient is confused, but what approach is helpful? Does it help orient him if he is spoken to? Does it help him if he is out of bed and walking? Does he respond to relatives? In other words, what approaches would help the nurse to give care? These are the things that the nurse wants to see on her plan.

In reality, it is the approach to the problem that is most essential to the written plan of care. We may gather important data and set objectives, but our approach must vary with new information that is received after we observe the patient's response to the approach. This is especially important in assisting non-professionals to give care.

Figure 6–2 is the nursing care plan developed for a young quadriplegic girl and Figure 6–3 is a plan for an elderly hemiplegic woman. You will note that if you came on duty at 8:00 A.M. and had never worked at this particular facility before, you would be able to take care of these patients with relative ease. In addition, the patients would not be subjected to care by a nurse who did not understand their problems or the kinds of goals they are working toward.

The nurse must make realistic goals and set priorities. She will be unable to meet the total needs of every patient, but she can work on a particular need each day. Sometimes a priority is obvious, such as keeping a patient's airway open in the Intensive Care Unit. Two weeks later the priority for the same patient may be seeing that the patient gets up in a chair and walks down the hall twice a day. The sample plans allow the nurse to identify temporary goals and special areas of emphasis.

All goals of nursing care plans should be stated in terms of patient objectives, nursing approaches and patient responses. It is in this way that the patient actually becomes a co-manager of his own care.

ITEMS FOR SPECIAL ATTENTION AND ASSESSMENT IN CHRONIC DISEASE

If the nurse thinks of a disease as having multiple causations and multiple effects, she is in a far better position to understand and assist her patients. Keeping this concept in mind is especially important when treating persons who are

NURSING CARE PLAN

ADMISSION DATE: _9-22-77_   DIAGNOSIS: _Quadriplegia - C6_   TOLERANCE: _low to moderate_

ALLERGIES: _none_

INDEPENDENCE CODE: INDEPENDENT – I   DEPENDENT –(D)   DIET: _reg._   WEIGHT: _108_

SUPERVISE – S   ASSIST – A   _(dislikes milk_   HOME BATH FACILITIES: _combination_

& bread)   _bath-shower unit_

A.D.L.'s		CODE
BED ACTIVITIES: _wears cervical collar_		D
Coming to sitting position: _may elevate bed to 45° for meals_		D
Turning: _q 2 h c̄ 2 people - support neck_		
BED POSITIONING: Supine: _2_ hrs. Prone: _2_ hrs. Side Lying: _2_ hrs.		
Special Positioning:		
TRANSFERS: _3 man lift_ Bed: Toilet: Tub: Car:		D
UPPER DRESSING: _To wear street clothes - needs total assistance for upper and lower dressing_		D
LOWER DRESSING: _Ace wrap both legs toe to groin - off at h.s._		D
FEET: _Wears tennis shoes c̄ socks_		D
BLADDER PROGRAM: _Foley catheter - instill Renacidin sol. and clamp for 10 minutes b.i.d._		D
BOWEL PROGRAM: Frequency _god p̄ breakfast Position on left side - use chux_		
Suppository: _Dulcolax x_		
Stimulation: _Digital q 15" X 2_		D

A.D.L.'s		CODE
DAILY HYGIENE: Bed: ✓ W/C:		D
BATHING: Invalift: _____ Bed: ✓ Tub: _____ Shower: _____		D
Face-Hair-Arms: _Can wash and dry face if cloth is placed over face for her._		A
Trunk-Perineum: _Keep perineal area clean & dry Kenalog cream to red areas p̄ bathing_		D
Lower Extremities:		
FEEDING: _Let her set the pace. Keep atmosphere relaxed and conversation going. She tends to eat better when distracted. Encourage her to eat finger foods c̄ minimal assistance._		
PSYCHODYNAMICS: _Family - likes to make daily phone call to mother after A.M. PT. Enjoys visits by younger brother & sister_		
Special Interests: _School - just began classes here. Discusses assignments with other students. Social - Shows great interest in boys._		
General Attitudes and Motivation _Does not yet grasp the reality and permanence of her injury. Very enthusiastic about therapies - wants to know why and how of everything. Watches progress of others c̄ similar problems with great interest._		

TEMPORARY GOALS AND SPECIAL AREAS OF EMPHASIS:
1) _Provide discussion times for family - both c̄ & s̄ Jane._
2) _Have family observe P.R.O.M., positioning, O.T. & P.T. appointments whenever possible._
3) _Explain reasons for nursing measures._
4) _Discuss what she will be able to do after she has attained 90% tolerance on tilt table & greater arm strength._
5) _Begin to have Jane a partner in her care by having her hang onto siderails when turning & for back care. Make her responsible for asking for position changes when in W.C._

Figure 6–2 Nursing care plan for 15-year-old quadriplegic.

MEDICATIONS

START DATE		STOP DATE
9/23	Valium 5 mgm h.s.	
9/23	Dimetapp cap ↑ qd	
9/23	Choloral Hydrate 500 mgm hs prn	
9/23	Aspirin gr. X q4h prn	

TREATMENTS

Hot Packs: ————

R.O.M.: *Passive - q8h to all extremities*

NAME: *Jane Doe*

APPLIANCES: *Keep cervical collar on to prevent neck flexion*

Wheelchair Type: *Full reclining, junior chair c̄ vertical projections on handrims, elevating leg rests, removable arm rests*

Time Up: *2 - 3 hours tid*

DISCHARGE PLANNING:

Family Instruction: *Include family in that listed below. Family seeing social worker regularly to help them to deal with their feelings and to help them to help Jane.*

Has been out for overnight: Yes_____ No ✓

Public Health Referral completed: Yes_____ No ✓

Instruction Completed: *No - instruction just beginning*

Instruction Remaining:
1) *Rom - started*
2) *ADL's - started*
3) *Positioning and skin care - started*
4) *Wheelchair handling - started*
5) *Transfers - share with P.T. - start in abt 2 weeks.*

Equipment Needed and Ordered:
1) *Her own wheelchair*
2) *Her own bed at home*
3) *Tenodesis splints*
4) *Adaptive devices for eating, personal hygiene and dressing.*
5. *Begin to discuss possible adjustments in physical layout in the home.*

AGE: *15*   ROOM: *317*   DOCTOR: *Schmidt*   HOSP. NO.: *3001*

Figure 6–2 *Continued.*

NAME: Bertha Dow AGE: 72 M.D.: T. Jones ADM.: Readmitted from son's home where she lived briefly after her husband's death. Contractures and bed sores present on re-admission.
DIAGNOSIS: CVA—rt. hemiplegia

Problem	Patient Care Goal	Next Evaluation	Approach	Responsibility
A. Seizures	Safety and prevention	June 12	A. Observe; daily Dilantin	Nursing and M.D.
B. Aphasia	Communicate wishes	q month—July 1	B. Use gestures and short sentences; repeat	All
C. Contracture—rt. leg	Improve ambulation	q month—July 1	C. P.R.O.M. tid; ambulate in walker tid	P.T. and Nursing
D. Decubitus ulcer—rt. ankle	Heal ulcer	q week—Mondays	D. Turn; use padded ankle support at night; see Karkex for bid treatment	Nursing
E. Incontinent	Void in B.R. as much as possible	qo Monday	E. Take to B.R. after meals and at midnight; cleanse skin well when incontinent	Nursing
F. Poor ability to transfer	More stable and more participation	q month—July 1	F. Use transfer belt and assist P.T. teaching	P.T. and Nursing
G. Difficult swallowing	Proper nutrition and less fear of choking	q month—July 1	G. Frequent small feedings; small bites and soft foods	Nursing and Diet.
H. Loose dentures; sore gums	Greater comfort	Dental evaluation next week	H. Oral hygiene after meals with gentle but firm brushing	Nursing, M.D. and Dentist
I. Grief over recent death of husband	Expression of grief	q month—July 1	I. Allow expression of grief and support Pastor visits twice weekly	All
J. Social needs	Increase interest in surroundings	q month—July 1	J. Attends remotivation group twice a week Daughters visit daily—are supportive Encourage any interest in visiting with other residents Visit with her and try to engage in communications as much as possible	All

Figure 6–3 Nursing Care Plan for a 72-year-old right hemiplegic.

aged or who have a chronic disease, since these patients usually have multiple problems. Therefore, the nurse working with the aged, the disabled, or the chronically ill must be especially cognizant of the triad effect of the disease on the mind, the body and the emotions.

In dealing with these categories of patients, the nurse must find out to what extent the patient is independent in his activities. This is sometimes called the self-care status. In Figure 6–2, you will note that a code is used: I stands for independent, S for supervise, D for dependent and A for assist. The use of a code enables personnel to glance quickly at the care plan to find out in what areas the patient is independent and in what areas assistance or supervision is needed. Important areas for assessment of the chronically ill would include the following:

1. *Bed Activities*. Can the patient move from side to side? Can he turn over? Can he come to a sitting position by himself?

2. *Positioning*. Does the patient need to be in the supine, prone or sidelying positions? How long and at what hours? Aside from turning schedules, what skin problems exist?

3. *Range of Motion (ROM)*. What extremities require ROM? What special precautions are required? What joint might be prone to contracture?

4. *Transfers*. Can the patient go from bed to wheelchair, toilet, tub, car? Does he stand or sit to transfer?

5. *Dressing*. Can he dress the upper part of his body? Can he dress the lower part of his body? Can he manage after the toilet? What kind of shoes and stockings does he use? Is he using a brace? Can he put on his own brace? Does he have Ace bandages?

6. *Bladder Program*. Does the patient have a Foley catheter, a leg bag? What is the schedule for irrigation of the catheter or general voiding?

7. *Bowel Program*. What schedule is planned? Are medications and suppositories used? Are diet and fluid intake adequate?

8. *Daily Hygiene*. Can he bathe himself? Can he brush his teeth or care for his dentures? What about general grooming?

9. *Locomotion*. Wheelchair? Ambulation? Gait? Can he use stairs?

10. *Feeding*. Does he need help? Dentures? Adaptive equipment? Special diet? Is the amount of food increased when physical therapy is strenuous?

11. *Vision*. Does he have impaired vision? A field cut? Wear glasses? Is he susceptible to glare? Does he have adequate light for reading?

12. *Hearing*. Is hearing impaired? Does he wear an aid? Does he lip read? Can he hear better from one side than the other? Is it a problem of comprehension rather than hearing?

13. *Speech*. Have you learned the meaning of seemingly incomprehensible words? Can he write? Does he understand when spoken to? Does he understand writing? Can he do arithmetic?

14. *Mental Ability*. Is he alert? Forgetful? Does he have periods of confusion? Comatose? What about his learning? Does he learn quickly? Does he require repetitive teaching? Is demonstration vital? Is he unable to learn?

15. *Psychological Approach to Patient*. Does the patient need encouraging? Does he need restricting? Does he follow through with learned activities? What are some of his goals that might give us clues in caring for him?

16. *Social Interactions*. Does he enjoy being with others? Do friends and family visit? Does he prefer solitary activities, and if so, which ones?

17. *Discharge Planning*. This is a large area and of course the final goal of the entire hospitalization. What family instructions have been given? Has the pa-

tient gone home overnight? Has he gone to the independent area of the institution where he takes care of himself as practice for the home situation? Has the public health referral been made? Have the patient and family instructions been completed? What instructions need repetition? What equipment will be needed and ordered? Has the house been rearranged so that he can live with maximum ease? (Chapter 11 will discuss this in greater detail).

This list is not meant to be complete, but it suggests the major areas of consideration for patients in a rehabilitation program. It should be noted that many patients in acute-care hospitals and nursing homes are never referred to a rehabilitation setting but nonetheless have problems that fall into the categories described above. Nurses in all settings need to assess the same conditions.

SUMMARY

A nursing care plan is essential to effective nursing care. Effective nursing care, in turn, is based on gathering information about the patient from many sources, including the patient and his family. Once information is gathered and patient objectives are established, nursing approaches are selected. The nurse evaluates her approach on the basis of the patient's response. New goals and approaches are identified with the help of the patient on a continuous basis. Special areas of concern for planning care of a patient with a chronic illness must be included.

REFERENCES

Anderson, Eleanor, M., and Irving, J.: Uninterrupted care for long-term patients. *Public Health Reports, 80*:271, 1965.

Berni, R., and Readey, H.: *Problem-Oriented Medical Record Implementation: Allied Health Peer Review.* St. Louis, C. V. Mosby Co., 1974.

Bloom, Judith, et al.: Problem-oriented charting. *American Journal of Nursing, 71*:2144, 1971.

Bowar-Ferres, Susan: Loeb Center and its philosophy of nursing. *American Journal of Nursing, 75*:810, May, 1975.

Commission on Chronic Disease: *Prevention of Chronic Disease.* Cambridge, Massachusetts, Harvard University Press, 1957, p. 4.

Dinsdale, Sidney M., et al.: The problem-oriented medical record in rehabilitation. *Archives of Physical Medicine and Rehabilitation, 51*:488, 1970.

Garant, Carol: A basis for care. *American Journal of Nursing, 72*:699, 1972.

Hamilton, Constance B., et al.: The nurse's active role in assessment. *Nursing Clinics of North America, 4*:249, 1969.

Hurst, J. W., and Walker, H. K.: *The Problem-Oriented System.* New York, MedCom Press, 1972.

Lazarus, Andrea H.: These are the pitfalls for the nurse: predisposition, preoccupation, prejudice. *Modern Nursing Home, 24*:41, 1970.

van Leeuwen, Elaine: Assessing the family's nursing needs. *Minnesota Nursing Accent, 39*:23, 1967.

Little, Dolores E., and Carnevali, Doris L.: *Nursing Care Planning.* 2nd Ed. Philadelphia, J. B. Lippincott Co., 1976.

McCain, R. Faye: Nursing by assessment—not intuition. *American Journal of Nursing, 65*:82, 1965.

Marriner, Ann: *The Nursing Process: A Scientific Approach.* St. Louis, C. V. Mosby Co., 1975.

Martin, Nancy, King, Rosemarie, and Suchinski, Joyce: The nurse therapist in a rehabilitation setting. *American Journal of Nursing, 70*:1694, 1970.

Mesolella, Daphne W.: Teachers—You are trespassing! *The Canadian Nurse, 66*:21, 1970.

National League for Nursing: *The Problem-Oriented Approach.* New York, NLN, 1974.

Neelon, F., and Ellis, G.: *Syllabus of Problem-Oriented Care.* Boston, Little, Brown and Co., 1975.

Palisin, Helen E.: Nursing care plans are a snare and a delusion. *American Journal of Nursing, 71*:63, 1971.

Rothberg, June S.: Why nursing diagnosis? *American Journal of Nursing, 67*:1041, 1967.

Schwartz, Doris R.: Toward more precise evaluation of patient's needs. *Nursing Outlook, 13*:42, 1965.

Smith, Dorothy M.: A clinical nursing tool. *American Journal of Nursing, 68*:2384, 1968.

Smith, Dorothy M.: Fostering clinical expertness in nursing practice. *Supervisor Nurse, 1*:21, 1970.

Smith, Dorothy M.: Myth and method in nursing practice. *American Journal of Nursing, 64*:68, 1964.

Tayrien, Dorothy, and Lipchak, Amelia: The single-problem approach. *American Journal of Nursing, 67*:2523, 1967.

Wagner, Berniece M.: Care plans, right, reasonable and readable. *American Journal of Nursing, 69*:986, 1969.

Wandelt, Mabel: *Quality Patient Care Scale.* New York, Appleton-Century-Crofts, 1974.

Wang, Brayton: Health maintenance for chronically ill. *The Nursing Clinics of North America, 5*:199, 1970.

Woody, Mary, and Mallison, Mary: The problem-oriented system. *American Journal of Nursing, 73*:1168, 1973.

Woolley, F. R., et al.: *Problem-Oriented Nursing.* New York, Springer Publishing Co., 1974.

Zimmerman, Donna S., and Gohrke, Carol: The goal-directed approach: it does work. *American Journal of Nursing, 70*:306, 1970.

Chapter 7

COMMUNICATING WITH PATIENTS WITH COMMUNICATION PROBLEMS

The purpose of this chapter is to describe measures that can assist the nurse in communicating with persons who have a visual, hearing, speech or language deficit. As the number of persons with chronic illness increases, the number of persons with these problems is also increasing. The diabetic may have reduced vision. The person with a fractured hip may be hard-of-hearing. The brain damaged person is likely to have a speech problem. Since the primary goal of this chapter is to help the nurse find better ways of communicating with such patients, there will be no attempt to describe the many conditions and treatments involved.

Sensory deprivation can be the result of many different problems. Knowledge of the environment can be altered by a reduction of any of the senses (vision, hearing, smell, touch, taste), a distortion in the perception of position, space or kinesthesia or difficulty in the selection and organization of impressions. A combination of biological and psychological factors may be responsible. While this discussion only relates to ways of communicating with patients who have problems with language, speech, hearing and vision, the nurse must keep in mind that her patient may also be experiencing other kinds of sensory deprivation.

COMMUNICATING WITH PERSONS WITH IMPAIRED HEARING

BACKGROUND REMARKS

Audiology may be defined as the science of hearing. Briefly, normal hearing begins when sound stimulates pulsations of pressure in the air around us. These pulsations enter the outer ear and initiate a motion of the drum membrane, which in turn induces the ossicles (the malleus, incus and stapes) to move the fluid in the cochlea. It is here that mechanical energy is transmitted into electrical energy. The sensory hair cells in the cochlea convert mechanical energy into neural impulses which are then transmitted to the brain via the auditory nerve.

Those of us with normal hearing only experience hearing difficulties when sound is either too far away or when there is interference from other sounds, such as from a T.V., dishwasher or siren.

Those with a hearing impairment will have one of two kinds of hearing loss: *conductive* or *sensorineural*. In some persons, both types of loss may occur. Conductive losses are caused by errors in, disease of or injury to the outer or middle ear. They are more amenable to treatment than are sensorineural losses, which are caused by problems of the inner ear. Persons with a conductive loss do not have problems with word discrimination and are therefore assisted if persons around them speak louder. Good results can often be obtained through surgery or amplification or both. Sensorineural losses, on the other hand, are rarely reversible, and any improvement is due to training and the person's ability to adapt.

Unfortunately, hearing loss in the aged (presbycusis) is a sensorineural disorder. Losses are in the high-frequency range and are manifested in poor word discrimination. Therefore, amplification is of limited value.

It is imperative that a proper diagnosis be made before any treatment or training is suggested. First, an otolaryngologist must evaluate the cause of the hearing loss and treat any problem that is correctable. If the loss is sensorineural, the person will be referred to an audiologist who will evaluate hearing function, assess the possible benefit from a hearing aid or training and counsel both the person and the family. The hearing aid dealer will then work with the person in finding the aid that is most beneficial. Present amplification methods do not reproduce normal hearing, so the selection of a hearing aid is usually a matter of individual preference for a particular sound.

ASSISTING THE PERSON TO HEAR

Sound is one of the key ways we communicate not only with other persons but with our environment. A person with impaired hearing has altered perceptions of sound. This may even affect personal safety. A loud noise, a fire alarm or an oncoming car may not be heard until it is too late. In addition, impaired hearing affects interpersonal relations. People who are hard-of-hearing often become very self-conscious about the fact that they do not hear well. This is because they may appear to be stupid, slow-witted, indifferent and inattentive. This in turn can cause varying degrees of depression. In some cases, paranoid tendencies occur when hard-of-hearing persons feel that they are being talked about when they see but do not hear conversations going on around them.

Persons with a hearing loss also have apprehension about understanding others and being able to be understood. Such tension is not only exhausting and unpleasant, but it can result in physical problems too. The patient frequently isolates himself, although some tend to monopolize conversations. Others may show irritation and hostility and be hypersensitive in their reactions to other people. Family problems and friendship problems arise when these characteristics occur.

The nurse needs to be aware of ways to identify a person who is having a hearing problem. The person will be unable to hear his own speech, so the volume of his voice may be too loud or especially soft. Besides a change in tone or volume, speech may be unclear because of less attention to enunciation. The person may not hear the telephone or doorbell. He may seem slow to understand or stupid. In some cases the person leans forward, straining to hear, or comes a little closer to hear or turns one side toward you. They may frequently ask for clarification of what you've said, ignore what was said or respond inappropriately.

When you are speaking to the person who is hard-of-hearing, it is important not to do the wrong thing. Some persons need a somewhat increased volume, while others can hear sounds, but they are not clear. It is not helpful to shout, to speak very slowly or to use exaggerated motions of your mouth, especially if the patient does any lip reading. Incidentally, many hard-of-hearing persons teach themselves some lip reading although they may not always be conscious of this. Do not cover your mouth, smoke, talk with a full mouth or chew gum when speaking. This is even more important for nurses working with patients who lip read. In addition, it is vital not to drop your voice at the end of a sentence.

The best way to speak to someone who is hard-of-hearing is to stand directly in front of him and speak slightly louder and more slowly and distinctly than normal, without exaggerating any of these three qualities. You may have to draw the attention of the person when you are about to speak. Touch is both useful and important psychologically. It is helpful to use familar words, and if there seems to be misunderstanding you might use shorter words or rephrase the statement. Sometimes hearing acuity seems to fluctuate; this may explain the frequent statement, "He can hear when he wants to hear." It is very important for the nurse to avoid showing impatience, as these persons already feel impatient about their hearing ability. Such reactions on the part of others increase the patient's sense of frustration and tend to increase his desire for withdrawal and social isolation.

If a person lip reads, an adequate light on your face is essential when you are talking to the patient. This is particularly important for the night nurse to remember. If communication with someone who has a hearing deficit is especially difficult, paper and pencil communication may be necessary.

If a person has a hearing aid, he needs to be told that sounds will not be identical to those he heard before the use of the aid. It takes time to get used to the new sounds. Background music, conversations of crowds and other sounds are also amplified. These situations are therefore avoided whenever possible. Extraneous sounds can be equally distracting to the person who has a hearing impairment but does not use a hearing aid. When a patient claims his aid no longer helps him, the nurse should check several things. Is there wax on the ear mold, on the receiver or in the ear itself? Are the batteries dead? Are all connections tight? (See Figure 7–1 for one of many types of hearing aids.)

The case can be cleaned with alcohol or acetone, and the mold itself can be washed with warm soapy water. A pipe cleaner can be run through the mold to keep it open and to remove any wax. If the patient complains of a squealing sound, check to see if the ear mold is inserted and secured properly. If further problems arise, the volume should be checked. If this is not satisfactory, the

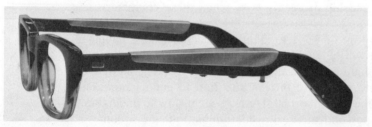

Figure 7–1 Eyeglass hearing aid with controls on bow. (Courtesy Maico Hearing Instruments, Minneapolis, Minnesota.)

transmitter should be checked by the hearing aid company. A supply of batteries should always be available and kept in a cool place. In nursing homes, one person may be assigned to check hearing aids and batteries once a month to make sure that they are functioning properly.

The nurse can help the patient to locate resources. The person may need information on hearing aids, may need to learn to lip read (more accurately called speech reading) or may need to learn sign (hand) language. Organizations that will provide helpful information on resources are the Alexander Graham Bell Association for the Deaf, 1537–35th Street, N.W., Washington, D.C. 20007, and the American Speech and Hearing Association, 9030 Old Georgetown Road, Washington, D.C. 20014. The references at the end of the chapter provide suggestions in more specific areas of assistance.

In summary, the nurse's responsibility is to see that the patient receives an adequate medical evaluation, that he is referred to appropriate resources, that his hearing equipment is in proper order and that every effort is made to help him hear. This will help him to become less isolated and to reduce his sense of frustration.

COMMUNICATING WITH THE VISUALLY IMPAIRED PERSON

BACKGROUND REMARKS

There are many degrees of visual loss. In fact, the term "blindness" does not necessarily mean a total loss of sight. The most widely adopted definition of blindness states that "A person shall be considered blind whose central visual acuity does not exceed 20/200 in the better eye with correcting lenses, or whose visual acuity is better than 20/200 but whose field of vision is limited to such a degree that its widest diameter subtends an angle of no greater than 20 degrees." The latter is frequently called "tunnel vision."

Using this definition, a blind person wearing corrective lenses may be able to distinguish size, shape, color and in some instances even read large print. In Minnesota, 76 per cent of all persons served by the State Services to the Blind, however, do not have this great a visual loss. This is not unusual because such services aim to (1) prevent loss of vision, (2) provide non-financial aid and (3) prepare for further loss if that is a possibility. In addition, many persons with diminished vision are eligible for tax deductions and are provided with talking books and braille and large-print materials.

While it is very difficult to assess the extent of visual impairment, it is generally estimated that 1,306,000 Americans are handicapped by visual loss. This number is probably increasing because of a growing number of persons over the age of 65. About 80 per cent of all blind persons lose their sight in adulthood, and 40 per cent of all blindness is caused by cataracts, glaucoma and diabetes. Fortunately, the leading cause, cataracts, can be surgically corrected with a very high degree of success. Glaucoma, on the other hand, is irreversible, but blindness usually can be prevented by medical treatment. Because the early stage of glaucoma does not present noticeable symptoms, it is important that persons over 40 years of age have regular eye examinations that include measurement of intraocular pressure (tonometry).

Nurses must remain alert to changing visual acuity in order to identify new visual problems in their patients, especially those in the older age bracket. Correction to some degree, or prevention of further loss of sight is possible in most individuals. In a study conducted in Minneapolis nursing homes, 577 residents were checked for accurate vision and were given a glaucoma test. A previously undetected visual impairment was found in 46 per cent or 260 patients. Twenty per cent of these required immediate care to prevent further visual loss, and another 20 per cent needed some kind of medical attention. The tragedy of undetected visual problems in elderly persons, even in nursing homes, is that their symptoms are often thought to be oncoming senility. Lack of interest and mind wandering is erroneously attributed to mental deterioration when in reality this behavior may result from auditory loss or visual deprivation or both. When patients do not recognize or do not respond to familiar persons, both hearing and vision should be checked. While all of these conditions may not be correctible, the effects of many can be reduced.

ASSISTING THE VISUALLY IMPAIRED

The nurse's responsibility begins with the application of her knowledge in the recognition of symptoms. She must then refer individuals for medical evaluation and in some cases to an appropriate agency as well. In every state there is at least one agency that provides services to people with visual problems. It may be in the department of welfare in one state and in the department of rehabilitation in another, or there may be a state commission for the blind. There may be volunteer agencies, such as a Society for the Blind. There may also be a rehabilitation center, recreational programs, low-vision aid services and opportunities for sheltered workshop employment. The nurse will need to learn what agencies exist in her own area. Excellent resources are listed in Robert Goodpasture's chapter in the *Handbook of Physical Medicine and Rehabilitation* (see References at the end of this chapter).

A patient's reaction to diminished vision is similar to that in other chronic illnesses—depression, withdrawal, denial, resentment, anger and dependence are all possible reactions. Since eye expression and facial expression are a form of communication, a certain amount of social isolation automatically occurs. The nurse's role is not only to accept the patient's reaction but also to help him seek new goals and learn how to "see" with other senses. Even people who are legally blind may be able to see light and headlines. The nurse can help the patient realize that he has an ability on which to build. People without any vision still have the ability to learn new ways of carrying out daily activities. In addition, vicarious use of another's eyes is often very rewarding. The sighted person can describe art work, cartoons, scenery and so forth. This kind of interdependence is both healthy and rewarding.

When assisting the visually handicapped to walk, it is important to have the patient hold on to your arm just above the elbow. In other words, the nurse does not hold on to the patient. She never pushes or pulls him in one direction or another. She walks normally and naturally, one or two steps ahead so that he follows slightly (see Fig. 7-2). Whenever going up or down stairs, it is important to stop for a moment, state that there are stairs and give the number of stairs. If there are more than three or four steps, simply state that there are several stairs and mention when the last step occurs.

When assisting a person to sit in a chair or get into a car, you can show him

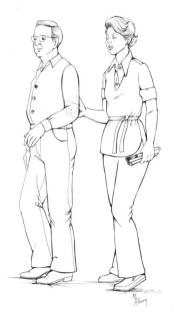

Figure 7–2   Have the visually impaired person hold your arm just above the elbow and walk one or two steps ahead.

the direction to sit by putting his hand on the back of the chair or on the door of the car. Thus, he will know which way the chair is facing or which direction the car door opens. Room doors should always be all the way open or closed to prevent accidents. It is also important that there always be good lighting and that the patient be oriented to a new institution, to his room and its furnishings and to wherever else he might be going. In a hospital, the nurse should state where the slippers, cigarettes, drinking glass and other necessary items are located, and these should not be moved without telling the person of the change.

The nurse may need to read the patient's mail to him. Before doing this, however, it is important to tell him who wrote the letter. If the letter is likely to be of a private nature, he may wish to have someone else read it to him. The nurse may also read books and articles aloud. There are many other helpful measures. She must identify herself as she enters his room. If while walking with a patient you must leave for a minute, make sure that he has something to hang on to, such as a chair or a wall. In this way, he can wait without feeling isolated or lost. When you give a visually impaired person his food tray, describe the place of items in relation to numbers on the face of a clock (see Fig. 7–3). A special dish may be at 11:00. Always be sure to tell him where hot foods are located and pour any liquids for him. Whenever you go through a door, be sure that you state which way the door opens, right or left and in or out.

In some cases the person may use braille. This, of course, requires special training. If the person cannot see the dial on his telephone even with a large number card (see Fig. 7–4) that fits over a dial, he can call the operator and say he is making a braille call. He simply gives the number to the operator who will make the call for him. If the patient cannot identify paper money, it is helpful to have him fold his paper money in different ways. He may fold the one dollar bill lengthwise, the five dollar bill end to end and perhaps not fold the ten dollar bill.

There are many available special services for the blind and the visually handicapped. One recent innovation is called radio-talking books. In many areas this special radio connection can be made to a station; this is often on for 17 or 18 hours a day. There are also templates with cutouts that fit over a check if the

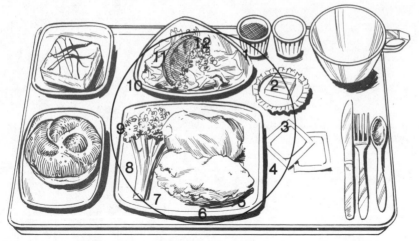

Figure 7–3   Use the concept of a clock face to help the visually impaired person locate tray items.

person has trouble finding where to write the date, the payee and so forth. By writing the American Foundation for the Blind, 15 West 15th Street, New York, New York, 10011, and sending $2.00 along with a canceled check, a template will be specially made. In addition, this organization has a free catalogue of hundreds of items and where they may be purchased. A talking book machine and books are obtained through specially designated local institutions. The Library of Congress will send the name of your state agency. In addition, the *New York Times* and the *Reader's Digest* are printed in large print editions. Another excellent resource is *Reading Aids for the Handicapped,* American Library Association, 50 East Huron Street, Chicago, Illinois 60611. Local resources will be recommended.

In summary, the nurse's responsibility is to recognize symptoms and to see that the individual receives medical care and treatment and that he is referred to other appropriate resources. In addition, she can give emotional support, assist him in walking, provide good lighting, help him to become oriented to his environment and find ways to prevent him from becoming isolated, whether he is in the community or in an institution.

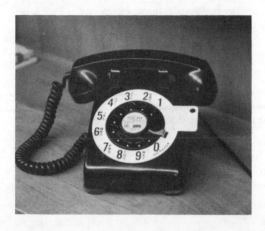

Figure 7–4   Large print card for telephone dial.

LANGUAGE PROBLEMS DUE TO BRAIN DAMAGE

BACKGROUND REMARKS

Goehl defines language as "a system that includes the expressive operations of speaking and writing and the receptive operations of understanding the spoken and written word." When a language disturbance occurs, the in-between mental-linguistic operations are private experiences that have been well described by Patricia Neal, Eric Hodges and others.

Two types of speech disorders may occur in the brain-damaged person — dysarthria and aphasia. *Dysarthria* is a mechanical defect in speech caused by muscle dysfunction due to a loss of sensation or weakness or paralysis. Speech may be slurred or totally unintelligible. Occasionally the vocal cords will be paralyzed also, resulting in "whispering speech." Persons with dysarthria may also have trouble chewing and swallowing, as the same muscles affect these movements, and they must therefore be taught how to swallow.

Aphasia can be generally defined as impaired ability to use or understand symbols of speech and language. This includes not only the ability to speak and to understand speech, but also the ability to read, write, do arithmetic, count, tell time and spell. In addition, a patient may have problems with word recall; that is, he may not be able to say words even though he knows what he wishes to say. He may speak a meaningless group of words and realize that this is not what he means. These problems are not the result of a defect in the peripheral speech mechanism, a defect in peripheral hearing or a defect in general intelligence, nor are they caused by a severe psychological disturbance. They are the result of brain damage.

While this section is mainly concerned with aphasia, two other definitions are in order — agnosia and apraxia. *Agnosia* is a failure of recognition at the conceptual level in a particular sensory modality. For example, a hemiplegic patient may have a visual agnosia (neglect of one side) or a tactile agnosia (failure to identify an object by touch). *Apraxia* is a failure in the ability to direct motor tasks, although the person understands what to do and is physically capable of the task. For instance, a patient may be asked to put out his tongue. While he understands the request, he is unable to reconstruct the necessary motor pattern.

Whenever a hemiplegic person has aphasia, early speech evaluation is recommended, although therapy years later can be helpful. Almost 40 per cent show language problems initially and approximately 80 per cent show eventual improvement. It is widely held that after an acute episode, any improvement during the first six months is due to spontaneous recovery and that recovery after that can be attributed to treatment. According to Goehl, however, "clinical study suggests that the earlier the treatment is begun, the better the chances of recovery." Speech assessment and therapy must take into account the person's previous education, personality, intellectual ability and language status.

It is important to provide an environment that will encourage speech. Reduced speech in the aphasic person is also due to such things as embarrassment, fear of failure, persons who talk for him and those who ignore halting efforts at speech. Families and medical personnel need to encourage speech and to reinforce all efforts at communication. Words are not lost, but they become unavailable to the person afflicted with aphasia. Therefore, hearing short simple sentences concerning immediate events and surroundings can be very helpful. In addition, ambulation, self-care activities and socialization encourage speech.

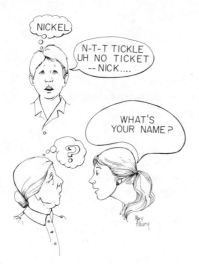

Figure 7–5 Pictorial depiction of aphasia. *Top:* Problem with expression. *Bottom:* Problem of understanding.

Aphasia is manifested in two major ways. The person will have a problem with expression, which includes the ability to speak and write. He will also have difficulty in the reception and understanding of speech and reading (see Fig. 7–5). Most aphasic persons have a problem with both expression and reception, although one may be greater than the other. Sometimes these problems are accompanied by paralysis and a visual field loss, as in the case of stroke. The patient might also have what is known as automatic speech. In this case, the person speaks, but what he says is not under his control.

Before the nurse can find ways of communicating with these patients, she must first of all make some kind of assessment as to what the patient does and does not understand, and what he can and cannot say. Figure 7–6, the Communication Status Chart, is an example of the kind of screening information that can be acquired by a nurse or other professional person who is untrained in speech therapy. The nurse should study items in this assessment tool in order to know the kinds of information that will help her identify problems of her patient. Data from such a tool should be shared by all persons working with a patient and, whenever, possible, should be reviewed by a speech therapist.

COMMUNICATING WITH THOSE WHO HAVE PROBLEMS OF EXPRESSION

The major deficiencies of the person with expressive aphasia will be in the areas of speaking and writing. He may have trouble with grammar, spelling, counting, telling time, using the telephone and naming objects. This, of course, puts the burden of understanding on the nurse, who will need to find ways of searching out the requests that cannot be articulated.

The extreme frustration of having something to say and being unable to express oneself is obviously distressing and causes severe depression in many instances. The nurse needs to make every effort to assist her patients with other ways of expressing himself. She may suggest the use of hand gestures. Simply pointing to what is wanted sometimes can partly alleviate frustration that occurs when the ability to express oneself is impaired. The nurse also encourages speech by saying the word immediately after she knows what it is the patient is

PATIENT'S
NAME: _____ ADDRESS _____ CASE
NO:_____

SEX: M__F__ AGE AT LAST BIRTHDAY:____DATE OF DISABILITY ONSET:____DURATION(FROM ONSET TO DATE):_____

CAUSE OF IMPAIRMENT: CVA___TRAUMA___OTHER_____ AFFECTED SIDE OF BODY: Right___Left___ None_____

HANDEDNESS PRIOR TO INSULT: Right___Left___ Unknown___FORMER VOCATION: _____

FIRST LANGUAGE LEARNED: _____ LANGUAGE SPOKEN IN FAMILY: _____

EDUCATION: Less than 4 years____ 4 to 8 years___9 to 12 years___More than 12 years____Unknown_____

SPECIAL INTERESTS: _____

OBSERVED REACTION TO TESTING: _____

REPORTED REACTION TO ENVIRONMENT: _____

(Write "yes" or "no" after each item) Date	Init'l Screening	Patient Progress			
VISION					
Has Glasses					
Wears Glasses for Distance					
for Reading or Close Work					
If no Glasses, Vision Appears Adequate					
Vision Changed Since Illness-Reported or Observed					
Vision "blurred"					
Vision to Either Side Appears Limited					
Objects Appear Straight Up and Down					
Can Draw Complete Person with Correct Body Image					
HEARING					
Hearing Appears Impaired in R. Ear					
in L. Ear					
Has Hearing Aid (if yes answer one of the following)					
Uses Hearing Aid Always					
Usually					
Occasionally					
Never					
Help to Hearing is Adequate					
Questionable					
Unknown					
TEETH OR DENTURES					
Has Natural Upper Teeth Anterior					
Posterior					
Has Natural Lower teeth Anterior					
Posterior					
Has Upper Denture (partial/complete)					
Has Lower Denture (partial/complete)					
Wears Upper Denture/Partial Usually					
Occasionally					
Never					
Wears Lower Denture/Partial Usually					
Occasionally					
Never					
CHEWING & SWALLOWING					
Can Swallow Liquids					
Can Swallow Solids					
Can Suck					
Drools					
Can Move Tongue Up					
Can Move Tongue Out					
Can Move Tongue to Right Side					
Can Move Tongue to Left Side					
Can Push Cheek Out with Tongue to Right Side					
Can Push Cheek Out with Tongue to Left Side					

GENERAL IMPRESSION: _____

COMMENTS: _____

Figure 7–6 Communications Status Chart. (Courtesy Section of Patient Care Practices, Wisconsin Department of Health and Social Services.)

Illustration continued on following page.

(Write "yes" or "no" after each item) Date	Init'l Screening	Patient Progress			
VERBAL EXPRESSION					
1. Makes vocal sounds.					
2. Articulates speech sounds (including jargon).					
3. Uses isolated words meaningfully.					
4. Uses short phrases meaningfully.					
5. Uses simple sentences meaningfully.					
6. Initiates simple conversation in sentences.					
7. Converses as he did before illness.					
A. Talks or babbles to himself.					
B. Speaks spontaneously but inappropriately.					
C. Mimics speech of others.					
D. Slurs speech.					
GENERAL COMPREHENSION					
1. Matches common objects.					
2. Recognizes common objects without visual clues.					
3. Follows simple commands with visual clues.					
4. Follows simple commands without visual clues.					
5. Listens to simple questions; indicates correct answer.					
6. Listens to a paragraph; indicates correct answer.					
A. Recognizes environmental sounds.					
B. Indicates "Yes" and "No" correctly.					
C. Identifies parts of the body - both sides.					
D. Identifies parts of the body - one side.					
WRITING					
1. Writes or prints own name from copy.					
2. Writes or prints own name.					

3. a. Writes nouns.   )
   b. Writes verbs.   ) Test each
   c. Writes pronouns.)					

4. Writes or prints simple sentences.					
5. Writes or prints a paragraph.					
READING COMPREHENSION					
1. Matches letters of the alphabet.					
2. Recognizes letters of the alphabet without visual clues.					

3. a. Recognizes nouns.   )
   b. Recognizes verbs.   ) Test each
   c. Recognizes pronouns.)					

4. Reads simple questions; indicates correct answer.					
5. Reads a paragraph; indicates correct answer.					
ARITHMETIC					
1. Matches numbers.					
2. Recognizes numbers without visual clues.					
3. Adds simple problem.					
4. Subtracts simple problem.					
5. Multiplies simple problem.					
6. Divides simple problem.					
7. Does simple thought problem, oral or written, depending on ability.					
A. Recognizes time on the clock.					
B. Repeats or writes three or four digit numbers.					
C. Counts money.					
D. Makes change.					

Subsequent diagnosed or suspected episodes since initial screening _____

Figure 7–6 *Continued.*

requesting. For instance, if he is referring to his chair and wants to get into his chair, she can say "chair." However, she should not try to force him to repeat the word. If he is able, he is likely to do so on his own initiative.

The nurse often develops the ability to carry on brief one-way conversations on a topic which she knows is of interest to her patient. She can discuss what she saw his family doing, the pictures he has in his room, the sights out of his window, sports or the tests or various therapies that he is having. Hearing spoken language can be helpful. Periods of rest, however, are equally important, as too much stimulation can be both confusing and tiring.

When speaking to the aphasic patient, it is important to approach from the "good" side, as many have an exaggerated startle response. Understanding will be enhanced if you speak in short, simple sentences, enunciate clearly and use a normal tone of voice. Always be sure that you have the person's attention and that you do not appear to be rushed.

The frustration of communication problems may cause behavior such as crying, swearing or yelling. If one considers how difficult it must be to be totally unable to express oneself, this kind of frustration is understandable. In addition, some of this is not under the patient's control. The nurse should focus her attention not on the behavior resulting from frustration but rather on making every effort to find other ways for the patient to express himself. She can try to have him use a pad and pencil. Although speech and writing impairment go hand in hand, the person may be able to write better than he can speak, so this avenue of communication should be explored. Some institutions have a set of cards that picture the people, the objects and the activities of the hospital. This enables the person to pick out the card that comes closest to expressing his need. Preparing such a set of cards or pictures would be an excellent project for a student or volunteer.

A most unfortunate reaction of personnel to persons who have problems with expression is that they come to the unfounded conclusion that there is also an inability to understand. In many cases, the patient understands very well everything that is going around him. It should be assumed that these persons can understand. Many unfortunate remarks have been made in the presence of a person who has an expressive problem but not a comprehension problem.

The nurse can assist her patients in other ways. She can make every effort to respond to the patient's speech regardless of how minimal. In this way, he will be reassured that his efforts bring forth some kind of response from those around him and will be encouraged to continue to attempt speech. When a patient has expressive difficulty, the nurse can ask questions in such a way that a "yes" or "no" answer is possible. It is important, however, to be cognizant of the fact that some patients say yes when they mean no and no when they mean yes. If you know your patient, this will be evident.

In summary, it is important for the nurse to encourage self-expression through any means available when working with persons who have an expressive difficulty. She needs to accept and respond to any communication that is given, regardless of how minimal or awkward it may be. She must be careful to avoid pressuring the patient into conversation. She can support him by not showing a negative reaction to any emotion that is caused by his extreme frustration. It is helpful to ignore rather than to correct mistakes in word choice. It is important to allow time for the person to search for words when there is a problem of recall and to continue to stimulate conversation. She can assist a patient to review by letting him hear words that have perhaps been forgotten.

COMMUNICATING WITH THOSE WHO HAVE PROBLEMS OF RECEPTION

Persons who have problems in the reception and understanding of written and spoken words may hear meaningless sounds rather than words, or they may simply not be able to put the words together in any meaningful way. Words may even be heard and understood, but they are not retained for a long enough period. Still another patient may understand a word but be unable to connect it to a previously learned meaning. All of these variations are problems of reception and understanding of what goes on around an individual. In receptive aphasia, the nurse must find ways of helping the person to understand.

It is important for the nurse to stand close to her patient so that she can see when she has his attention. If there is a visual field disturbance, often referred to as a field cut, there will be areas which the patient does not see on the paralyzed side. In this instance, the nurse should make a point of standing on the non-paralyzed side of the patient to make sure she is seen. With assistance, some persons can learn to compensate for this problem in certain activities.

If one side of the food tray or place setting is ignored, the patient can learn to look for a brightly colored ruler placed on the edge of the tray or table. If there is a problem reading, a red line can be drawn along the edge of the page and the person can learn to begin reading at the red line or go to the red line, depending on whether the field cut is on the right or the left. It may be hard to compensate for problems in reading when patients also have difficulty with spatial perception, although a ruler placed under each printed line may help the person to keep his place when he reads. Another way to make reading easier is to cut out a window the size of one printed line in the center of a five by eight card. This blocks out the confusion of the surrounding lines.

It may be helpful for the nurse to make generous use of hand gestures. This is much more satisfactory than attempting to prod a patient into verbal expression in response to words he may not have been able to understand. Again, the nurse may ask the patient questions that can be responded to by a yes or no, but again it should be remembered that the patient may say yes when he means no and vice versa.

Assessment of comprehension can be done in a very simple way. The nurse should thoroughly explain to the patient that she is going to try a very simple test and that he should not feel insulted by the simplicity of the questions. In this test, the nurse merely asks the person to point to his eyes, nose, throat, chair, bathroom, door and so forth. If he is able to do this accurately, she can then ascertain if he can follow two directions given at once. In other words, can this patient close his eyes and sit up in the chair? This helps the nurse to identify communication needs for other personnel who will be caring for the patient.

By giving patients extra time, the nurse will encourage greater understanding. Questions and statements should always be simple and concrete, and the fewest possible words should be used. While this is very important, it should never be combined with talking down to a patient. Simplicity does not mean condescension. Understanding may be increased by rephrasing a statement or by simply repeating major words, like the verb and noun of the sentence. Frequently when the patient does not understand, the nurse shouts at him. This is not only inappropriate for persons who have a problem with hearing, but it is also totally ineffective for persons with reception difficulties. When the nurse does speak to a patient, she must be sure to have his attention. She may also need to repeat hand gestures. The physical condition of stroke victims may change from day to day, even hour to hour. While a patient might understand something early in the morning, he might not be able to understand it at noon. She must be careful not to assume he has the knowledge and ability that he does not have. Therefore, all ways of communicating with patients who have varying degrees of understanding must be known by the nurse, since she may need to use them as the immediate situation dictates.

GENERAL ATTITUDES TOWARD PERSONS WITH LANGUAGE PROBLEMS

First of all, the nurse must realize and indicate by her actions and words toward the patient who cannot express himself or understand language that he is not considered deficient intellectually. The fact that he cannot name friends does not mean that he does not know them. Making these distinctions alters the way in which one handles persons with language problems. Too much sympathy can be as damaging as impatience. The major goal of the nurse dealing with a specific patient is to help the patient to express himself, to help him to be understood or to be understood.

To encourage this kind of patient to be as self-sufficient as possible is naturally important. It is important to encourage speech but not to demand it if attempts become too frustrating or too exhausting. This may vary from time to time, and short periods of expectation may certainly be indicated and followed by periods of rest from the strain of attempting to understand or to speak.

Sometimes when the patient is beginning to learn new speech he makes meaningless combinations of words or uses nonsense syllables or swears and speaks in vulgar language. It is vital for the nurse to remind herself that this is not the result of ignorance, mental breakdown, meanness, stubbornness or a basically vulgar personality. She must refrain from responding in a judgmental manner. These are unsuccessful attempts on the part of the person to express himself. The fact that speech comes at all can be considered a success. Praise for efforts as well as successes is important in encouraging the person to try to make further efforts at speech.

Successful ways of communicating with an individual patient should always be incorporated in the nursing care plan, so that everyone does not have to do a special assessment to learn what you already know. Writing these findings on the nursing care plan will spare the patient many hours of frustration as well as save the personnel's time. Entries might include:
- Always try the written word if the spoken word is not successful.
- Always speak in short simple phrases.
- Speak slowly and distinctly.
- Limit the number of adjectives, phrases and complex sentences.

It is not only vital for the nurse to know how to work with these patients, but it is equally vital for families to learn and to practice the suggestions you find helpful. Communication methods on the care plan should be shared with families who in turn may add new insights and ideas to your approach.

It is also important that patients with speech problems not be allowed to sit idly, since this simply allows time for discouragement and depression to increase. Environmental stimulation needs to be provided.

In summary, the nurse has the responsibility, first, to assess the patient for his speech and understanding. Secondly, she has the responsibility to locate ways in which she can communicate with her patient as successfully as possible. Third, she has a responsibility to know where evaluation by a speech therapist can be obtained. If the physician suggests speech therapy and there is not a known therapist in the area, the nurse might send for the Directory of Speech Therapists, published by the American Speech and Hearing Association, 9030 Old Georgetown Road, Washington, D.C. 20014. Finally, she has a responsibility to share her knowledge of the patient both with other personnel and with the patient's family.

REFERENCES

HEARING IMPAIRMENTS

Bender, Ruth E.: Communicating with the deaf. *American Journal of Nursing, 66*:757, 1966.
Chodil, Judith, and Williams, Barbara: The concept of sensory deprivation. *Nursing Clinics of North America, 5*:543, 1970.
Conover, Mary, and Cober, Joyce: Understanding and caring for the hearing-impaired. *Nursing Clinics of North America, 5*:497, 1970.
Corliss, Edith: *Hearing Aids.* National Bureau of Standards Monograph 117, Superintendent of Documents, Washington, D.C., 1970.
Facts About Hearing Aids. Council of Better Business Bureaus, Inc., 1150 17th Street, N.W., Washington, D.C. 20036, 1973.
Gerstman, Hubert L.: Auditory disorders: evaluation and management. *In* Krusen, F. H., et al.: *Handbook of Physical Medicine and Rehabilitation.* Philadelphia, W. B. Saunders Co., 1971.
Humenik, P., Damen, M., and Vines, T.: Rehabilitation of children and adults with hearing impairments. *Canadian Nurse, 62*:38, 1966.
Murphy, Anne J.: A guide for nurses in a hearing conservation Program. *American Association of Industrial Nurses Journal,* October, 1963, p. 21.
Perron, Denise: Deprived of sound. *American Journal of Nursing, 74*:1057, June, 1974.
Rubin, Jack A.: Deafness and its management. *Canadian Nurse, 62*:32, 1966.
Senturia, B., et al.: Otorhinolaryngologic aspects. *In* Steinberg, F. U.: *Cowdry's The Care of the Geriatric Patient.* 5th Ed. St. Louis, C. V. Mosby Co., 1976.
Vernon, McCay: Available training opportunities for deaf people. *Hearing and Speech News, 38*:1, January–February, 1970.
Weiss, Curtis: Why more of the aged don't wear hearing aids. *Journal of the American Geriatric Society,* March, 1973, p. 139.

VISUAL DISABILITY

American Foundation for the Blind: *An Introduction to Working with the Aging Person Who is Visually Handicapped.* New York, 1972.
Barnett, M. Robert: The myth of blindness—the real disability. *Listen,* February, 1966, p. 15.
Bledsoe, C. W.: Rehabilitation of the blind geriatric patient. *Geriatrics, 13*:91, 1958.
Condl, Emma D.: Ophthalmic nursing: the gentle touch. *Nursing Clinics of North America, 5*:497, 1970.
Dyskow, Chris: Training for elderly blind offered. *Heartbeat,* Minnesota Hospital Service Association, September, 1970.
Gallagher, William F.: Rehabilitation of the visually handicapped. *In* Licht, Sidney (Ed.): *Rehabilitation and Medicine.* New Haven, Elizabeth Licht, Publisher, 1968, p. 725.
Goodpasture, Robert C.: Rehabilitation of the blind. *In* Krusen, F. H., et al.: *Handbook of Physical Medicine and Rehabilitation.* 2nd Ed. Philadelphia, W. B. Saunders Co., 1971.
Jackson, George D.: How blind are nurses to the needs of the visually handicapped? *Nursing Outlook, 13*:34, 1965.
MacFarland, D. C.: The blind. *Rehabilitation Record, 7*:2, 1966.
Minneapolis Society for the Blind: *Caring for the Visually Impaired Older Person.* 1936 Lyndale Avenue South, Minneapolis, Minnesota, 1976.
Murphy, Thomas J.: Mobility restoration for the blind. *Journal of Rehabilitation, 32*:20, 1966.
Oerther, Barbara: The blind patient need not be helpless. *American Journal of Nursing, 66*:2436, 1966.

Ohno, Mary I.: The eye-patched patient. *American Journal of Nursing, 71*:271, 1971.
Pigott, R., and Brickett, F.: Visual neglect. *American Journal of Nursing, 66*:101, 1966.
Riffenburgh, Ralph S.: The psychology of blindness. *Geriatrics, 22*:127, 1967.
Smith, Morton E.: Ophthalmic aspects. *In* Steinberg, F. U.: *Cowdry's The Care of the Geriatric Patient.* 5th ed. St. Louis, C. V. Mosby Co., 1976.

LANGUAGE DISORDERS

Belt, Linda: Working with dysphasic patients. *American Journal of Nursing, 74*:1320, July, 1974.
Boone, Daniel R.: *An Adult Has Aphasia.* 3rd Ed. Danville, Illinois, Interstate Printers & Publishers, 1965.
Buck, McKenzie: Dysphasia: the patient, his family, and the nurse. *Cardiovascular Nursing, 6*:51, 1970.
Cohen, Lillian Kay: *Communication Problems After Stroke,* Minneapolis, Sister Kenny Institute, 1971.
Erb, Elizabeth: Improving speech in Parkinson's disease. *American Journal of Nursing, 73*:1910, November, 1973.
Eagleson, Hodge M., et al.: Hand signals for dysphasia. *Archives of Physical Medicine and Rehabilitation, 51*:111, 1970.
Feldman, J. L., and Schultz, M. E.: Rehabilitation after stroke. *Cardiovascular Nursing, 11*:29, March–April, 1975.
Fowler, R. S., and Fordyce, W. E.: Adapting care for the brain-damaged patient. *American Journal of Nursing, 72*:1832, October, 1972, and *72*:2056, November, 1972.
Fox, Madeline J.: Talking with patients who can't answer. *American Journal of Nursing, 71*:1146, 1971.
Fox, Madeline J.: Patients with receptive aphasia: they really don't understand. *American Journal of Nursing, 76*:1596, October, 1976.
Goehl, Henry: Speech and language disorders. *In* Krusen, F. H., et al.: *Handbook of Physical Medicine and Rehabilitation.* Philadelphia, W. B. Saunders Co., 1971.
Hodges, Eric: *Episode: Report on the Accident Inside My Skull.* New York, Atheneum, 1964.
Levenson, Carl: Rehabilitation of the stroke hemiplegia patient. *In* Krusen, F. H., et al.: *Handbook of Physical Medicine and Rehabilitation.* 2nd Ed. Philadelphia, W. B. Saunders Co., 1971.
Moss, C. Scott: *Recovery With Aphasia.* Urbana, University of Illinois Press, 1972.
Skelly, Madge: Aphasic patients talk back. *American Journal of Nursing, 75*:1140, July, 1975.
Taylor, Martha L.: *Understanding Aphasia.* The Institute of Rehabilitation, New York University Medical Center, 1958.

Chapter 8

ASSISTING PATIENTS WITH BOWEL AND BLADDER PROBLEMS

One of the most devastating problems encountered in certain chronic conditions is the loss of bowel and bladder control. Unfortunately, many persons remain incontinent (loss of bowel and/or bladder control) because they have not had the benefit of a training program. The knowledge, the conviction of its importance, the interest and the support of the nurse are essential factors for a successful program.

Many geriatric patients, persons who have suffered a cerebrovascular accident, a brain injury or a spinal cord injury and even those with atonic muscles have had successful bowel and bladder management. Some factors associated with incontinence make management more difficult. They are age over 65 years, a concurrent illness, inability to walk, dependency in the areas of bathing and eating, speech pathology and inability to perform a sequence of three verbal commands (Adams). While patients with these problems may ultimately improve, they are more difficult to train if they have two or more of these problems.

Without some kind of management planning, it is virtually impossible for a person to feel secure in his work or social life. One physician refers to the bladder as a "social" organ. In the case of persons with a spinal cord injury, malfunction of the kidney and bladder was the leading cause of death prior to World War II. A properly managed bladder program, therefore, becomes a lifesaving measure for these patients. The wide-range implications of bowel and bladder care make early consideration of these problems an urgent matter.

Depending on the cause of loss of bowel and bladder control, a patient may either be unaware of the need to void and defecate, or he may have awareness but be unable to control the passing of feces and urine. Loss of control may be caused by a lesion in the spinal cord or distal nerves supplying the bladder and sphincter mechanism, a degenerative disease, brain damage, psychological regression, infection, neoplasm or congenital deformities of the bladder and bowel. Loss of control may be temporary, prolonged or permanent.

The nurse has five major responsibilities in bowel and bladder management, which requires a written plan of care. They are:

1. To determine the person's previous bowel and bladder habits and present status.

2. To initiate measures which assist the patient in his immediate situation.

3. To develop long range goals and a specific plan based upon the person's potential for improvement or deterioration, as the case may be.

4. To provide a continuous evaluation and revision of the plan, so that it meets the patient's current needs.

5. To have the patient participate in setting goals, learning the techniques and keeping his own records whenever feasible.

Once a general program is developed, it is important to have the person dress each day and be as fully occupied and active as possible. Lack of physical and mental stimulation can result in not only loss of control but also indifference to the problem.

BOWEL TRAINING

The goal of bowel training is to achieve control on a regular basis (without laxatives or enemas), usually every one to three days. With a minimum of medication, the nurse can help the patient to establish a regular pattern by stimulating peristalis at a designated time of day.

Before a plan can be started, the nurse needs to know what physical problems may be causing bowel incontinence. In addition, the nurse must obtain certain information and assess it in relation to her patient. Such information would include the following:

1. Does he have any awareness prior to or during a movement?
2. Does the patient have any suggestions regarding his bowel needs?
3. When was the last bowel movement?
4. What is the patient's normal frequency and time of day for a movement?
5. Has the patient been using laxatives, enemas or other means to stimulate bowel movements or to alter stool consistency?
6. What kind of diet and how much fluid does the patient normally take?

The older patient may not have involuntary bowel movements, but is frequently "bowel conscious" and may have the "laxative habit." When this is true, re-eduation of the patient is the first step. This, of course, assumes that the patient is capable of learning. All too often an older person with reduced muscular tone, reduced activity and a reduction in quanitity of food intake expects to have the same bowel pattern as he did when he was 20. It may well be that a bowel movement every two or three days is perfectly normal for such a person. Personnel as well as patients often need re-education concerning the overly rigid emphasis on a daily movement.

Whenever possible, it is important to have the patient participate in the plan. He will determine the time, regulate his diet, and relate it to his daily schedule. Success is more likely if the patient participates. When the patient cannot participate, it may be that the family can give a history of bowel habits in the past. In the case of a spinal cord injury, it is best to wait until the shock of the event has subsided before determining a plan, as timing is crucial to success for these persons. Once the data is gathered, the nurse can begin a plan and then incorporate it into the total nursing care plan.

Stool consistency can affect the success or failure of a bowel program. The ideal consistency of the stool is fairly firm, but soft. A loose stool makes it more difficult to establish control. A medical problem, certain foods, too many laxatives, or even an impaction may cause loose stools. On the other hand, if stools are too firm, irregularity may be the result and ultimately cause impaction. If stools are allowed to be hard over a period of time, the possibility of developing hemorrhoids is increased.

An essential part of the plan, then, is to promote a stool of the proper consistency by regulating diet and encouraging high fluid intake. In some instances medications may be prescribed. Physical activity is also important as it increases muscle tone and stimulates peristalsis.

TOILET EQUIPMENT

Ideally the squat position is most conducive to defecation. Since this is impossible for most persons, any position that approximates this position, such as having the feet elevated, can be of help. Peristaltic activity is apparently greater and gravity assists stool expulsion when the upright rather than the supine position is used at the time of defecation. Whether the patient is able to be in an upright position of course depends on the amount of activity he is allowed, his range of motion, his trunk balance, his tolerance to sitting and the presence of any pressure sores, the severity of spasticity and the general availability of equipment which can provide the proper kind of support.

Regular Toilet. A toilet should be used whenever possible. If maximum support is needed, and the toilet does not have a water tank that can be used as a backrest, a padded backrest can be attached to the back of the toilet (see Fig. 8–1). Additional stability can be attained by securing a safety belt around the patient and the backrest.

A handrail at the side of the toilet can help the patient maintain his balance if he has adequate hand grasp. If a toilet seat is too low for a comfortable transfer (as is often the case for an elderly person), the toilet can be raised. Toilets can be installed at a height of 20 inches from the floor rather than the usual 16 inches, or a raised toilet seat can be purchased and attached to the toilet bowl (see Figs. 8–1 and 8–2).

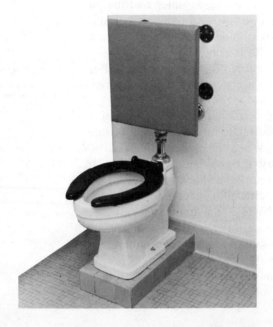

Figure 8–1 Padded backrest for a toilet seat made of ¾ inch thick plywood cut to 19 by 19 inches, padded with foam rubber and covered with sturdy vinyl. (Photo courtesy Sister Kenny Institute, Minneapolis, Minnesota.)

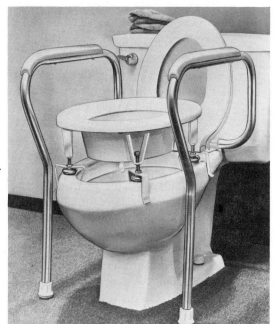

Figure 8–2 Raised toilet seat with armrests. (Courtesy Lumex, Inc., Bayshore, New York.)

Commode. A commode may be substituted for a toilet. This may be used at the patient's bedside, and some types may be rolled directly over the toilet. If the commode has casters, reliable brakes are essential. Adequate arm, foot and back support is essential to provide comfort.

Bedpan. The bedpan is the least desirable piece of toilet equipment. However, when it must be used, certain measures can be taken to minimize its undesirable features. First of all, privacy is essential. If the head of the bed can be elevated, bowel results can be achieved more readily. The bedpan is not only uncomfortable, especially for a thin person, but pressure on bony prominences decreases tissue circulation and can cause pressure sores if a person is allowed to remain on a pan for too long.

Plastic covered foam rubber can be placed between the patient and the bedpan for comfort. If someone must be on the bedpan for as long as a half hour, the maximum amount of time that should be allowed, it may be advisable to use pillows to support the trunk, knees and feet. This can be accomplished by placing pillows under the patient from the head to the bedpan and from the bedpan to the feet. Since pressure on the sacrum cannot be eliminated completely, the skin over this area should be immediately examined for signs of tissue change.

Other Alternatives. The side-lying position with use of incontinence pads or kidney basin are possible alternatives to the bedpan. This might be preferred if the person is unable to sit partially erect, if there is a lack of skin tolerance to pressure, if a decubitus ulcer is present or if there is difficulty in moving the patient onto the bedpan.

Lying on the right side is usually recommended because the descending colon is on the left. The basin or incontinence pads are placed just behind the patient. One or two pads are tucked under the buttocks in order to protect both the patient and the linen from becoming soiled.

THE TIME OF DEFECATION

In most instances the plan is successful if the patient defecates every day or at least every other day. In some persons a two- to three-day schedule is satisfactory. If a schedule is any longer than three days, the prolonged interval encourages the absorption of fluid from the fecal mass and is likely to result in a hard stool, causing a difficult elimination. The setting of the time interval should be based on the patient's previous schedule. It can then be adjusted after an observation period of a week or two.

Regardless of the length of the period between defecations, a specific time of day should be selected. This time can produce more effective results if it takes advantage of the gastrocolic and duodenocolic reflexes, which are most active shortly after eating a meal. This means that the person attempts a bowel movement 20 to 40 minutes after a meal. This should be done daily until it is determined whether the schedule will be daily or every other day. Most persons prefer either morning (after breakfast) or evening (after supper). People who work and prefer to sleep later in the morning are likely to select an evening schedule. Whenever someone changes the time from day to evening, or vice versa, it is likely to take two or three weeks to establish the new time pattern.

Whether a patient uses the toilet, commode or bedpan, he should not be left there longer than 20 to 30 minutes. Prolonged pressure of sitting on a hard surface is not only uncomfortable but can lead to skin breakdown. If there is no bowel response within a 20- to 30-minute period, an unplanned elimination may occur. This is more likely in the early days of the bowel program than later on when a regular schedule has been established.

FOOD AND FLUIDS

In order to maintain a soft formed stool, a high fluid intake (two and a half to three quarts of fluid per day) is recommended. In addition, drinking a glass of hot or warm liquid before a meal, especially breakfast, will facilitate the gastrocolic and duodenocolic reflexes. Some persons drink a glass of warm liquid just prior to defecation. These measures tend to stimulate peristalsis.

Frequency and consistency of stool can be directly affected by the foods we eat. Whenever a dietician is available, she should be consulted. Certain foods tend to increase bowel activity. They include prune juice, lemon juice, oranges and apples, 40 per cent bran cereal (not 100 per cent bran, as this may cause intestinal blockage), figs, stewed prunes and other fresh fruits. Roughage foods such as vegetables, fruits and salads, can be added, increased or decreased according to the consistency of the stool. The more roughage foods, the more likely the stool will be soft. Food preferences must always be considered. Snack foods sometimes assist in maintaining a regular bowel plan. If a snack food is taken in the evening, it is helpful to those who are on a morning schedule. Snack foods eaten in the morning help the person who is on an evening schedule.

Generaly speaking, fluid and dietary adjustments can be very helpful in altering the consistency and frequency of elimination. Such adjustment can often reduce the need for medication.

PHYSICAL ACTIVITY

Activity and exercise generally promote bowel activity. Inactivity not only reduces food needs, but muscular and physiologic responses become somewhat sluggish as well. Both physiologic and psychological functions can be enhanced by seeing to it that the patient has as much independent activity as possible. Many of the therapies during a rehabilitation program may also encourage general bowel function.

MEASURES THAT STIMULATE BOWEL FUNCTION

There are many simple ways of stimulating colonic peristalsis. Drinking hot coffee or tea may be effective. Defecation is sometimes initiated by smoking a cigarette. Suppositories, laxatives, enemas and massage of the anal sphincter are other measures that will encourage bowel response. Some measures may be used temporarily during the establishment of a program. Others may be needed on a permanent basis in order to maintain regularity of the bowel program.

Position. The squat position is the optimal physiologic position for defecation, and the most recent toilet designs take this into account. However, most standard toilet seats and all toilet seats that are raised for ease of transfer make it impossible for the person to squat. It is therefore beneficial to use a foot stool to elevate the person's legs. Those patients who are able can increase abdominal pressure even further by leaning forward.

Suppositories. A suppository is used to initiate reflexes which stimulate peristalsis of the lower colon and rectum, resulting in relaxation of the external anal sphincter. Suppositories act in several ways. They may act through irritation of the rectal wall. Some tend to withdraw fluid from the rectal lining and have a tendency to soften the stool. Others act directly on the mucous membrane to stimulate reflexes which, in turn, result in peristalsis. Still others produce carbon dioxide, which causes pressure in the rectum. Not only do individual suppositories have different physiologic actions, but individuals may respond differently to each kind. If the use of suppositories is required over a long period or on a permanent basis, glycerine suppositories are usually recommended because they are both mild and economical.

Proper insertion of a suppository is essential. Using a finger cot or rubber glove, it should be inserted beyond the internal and external sphincters and rest against the rectal wall. Insertion of the suppository into the stool itself will have no effect whatsoever on defecation. It is recommended that a suppository be inserted approximately 30 minutes before results are desired. The amount of time between insertion of the suppository and elimination will vary according to the individual. In some instances defecation may not occur for as long as two or three hours afterwards. If this occurs, it should be noted and coordinated with the patient's activities.

Medications. Laxative and bulk-forming medications may be ordered by the physician to encourage bowel response. On a permanent basis, though, it is rarely recommended. However, many older people have the "laxative habit." In this instance, vigorous patient education can ultimately result in achieving bowel response without laxatives.

When a laxative is used, it is given in the evening if the patient is on a morning schedule. If the patient is on an evening schedule, the laxative should be given in the morning. Medications are usually used in the beginning of the plan before the kind of diet and amount of fluids are established. Milk of magnesia is probably the most extensively used laxative. Prolonged use of mineral oil is not advised, since it can interefere with absorption of fat-soluble vitamins.

Enemas. Frequent use of enemas should be discouraged as a part of a long-term bowel program. However, enemas may be needed in the early stages of a program, when there has not been a defecation for several days, and in the event of an impaction. Enemas may also be necessary on a more regular basis for patients who have advanced multiple sclerosis.

Instilling only two or three ounces of tap water with a rubber syringe may be all that is needed in many instances. In other cases, the regular, large, tap water or saline enema or a prepared disposable enema may be indicated. When the muscle tone of the anal sphincter is inadequate, a person may be unable to retain the fluid in the rectum long enough to produce results. In this event, a Foley catheter with a large inflatable bulb or #30 rectal catheter with an inflatable rubber bag (the type used for barium x-ray of the lower gastrointestinal tract) may be used to encourage retention of the fluid.

In the event of an impaction (sometimes evidenced by loose stools), digital

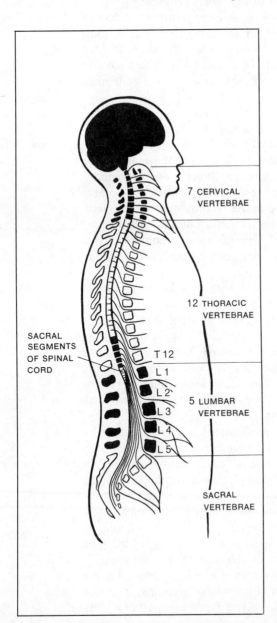

Figure 8–3 Vertebrae *(right)* in relation to the sacral segments *(left)*, which control the reflex arc. Note that an injury at the L1 vertebra level will affect the sacral segments and, consequently, the reflex arc.

removal of the stool may be necessary. It is recommended that first the gloved finger very gently try to break up the stool. After this, a tap water or oil retention enema can be given. If these two measures do not work, digital removal of the stool will be necessary. When this is done, it must be done very gently and with extreme care.

Digital Stimulation. If a spinal cord injury occurs above the sacral nerve roots, the reflex arc is maintained (see Fig. 8–3). In this case massage of the anal sphincter will be effective in initiating defecation. This mild stretching and massage triggers the reflex response involved in evacuation. Anal sphincter massage is contraindicated if the patient does not have reflex arc activity, if spasticity or involuntary contracture of the anal spincter occurs or if there is rectal bleeding.

The procedure for digital stimulation of the anal sphincter is as follows:

1. Put a glove or finger cot on the index finger and lubricate.
2. Insert the index finger in the rectum about 1 to 1½ inches.
3. Use a circular or back and forth motion and stretch the anus slightly.

After some experience, you may notice that touching a certain area in the rectum will trigger a response. This can be determined if you stop moving the finger as the sphincter relaxes. If the sphincter tightens, again move the finger in the same way. It is also helpful to ask the patient to inhale deeply, tighten his abdominal muscles and push down if he has the ability. The procedure may last from one-half minute to five minutes but should not be continued longer than five minutes. Results should occur within 30 minutes after the digital stimulation.

Because some patients react rather quickly to this procedure, it is advisable that the procedure be done on the bedpan, commode or toilet. The patient should of course learn to do the procedure himself whenever possible.

BLADDER TRAINING PROGRAM

The first and most important aspect of a bladder program is a thorough medical evaluation to determine the cause of incontinence or retention. Is it caused by brain damage? By lack of cerebral development? Is it due to a congenital defect? Is it caused by infection? Is it the result of spinal cord injury or neuromuscular disease? Psychological incontinence is not unknown. Neoplasms, stones and other problems of the genitourinary tract are also causes. In addition, it should be noted whether the incontinence is at night, during the day or both. Is there continual dribbling or intermittent voiding?

The ultimate aim of any bladder training or rehabilitative program is to enable the individual to control urination without a catheter if at all possible. This is because prolonged use of a catheter can result in infection and eventual kidney damage. Among World War II and Korean War veterans with a spinal cord injury, not only was renal failure the leading cause of death but 90 per cent of those who died of other causes had pyelonephritis.

Incontinence due to a spinal cord injury or lesion results in a so-called neurogenic or cord bladder. The patient is unaware of the need to void and cannot initiate urination without training. In those whose lesion is above the 2nd, 3rd and 4th sacral segments, the bladder is sometimes able to empty by reflex, and training is aimed at making reflex emptying more efficient. The reflex arc remains intact. These persons have an upper motor neuron lesion and the bladder is often referred to as automatic, spastic or reflex. The reflex bladder will empty suddenly when the stretch receptors reach their threshhold. Sometimes

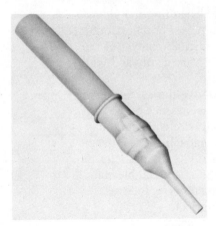

Figure 8–4 One type of external device for a male catheter. (Courtesy Mentor Corporation, Minneapolis, Minnesota.)

the detrusor muscle and the external sphinctor are also spastic, so the bladder does not empty adequately.

In those whose lesion is at the 2nd, 3rd, or 4th sacral segment, there is injury to the reflex arc (review Fig. 8–3). In this case, the bladder is flaccid, and training is aimed at developing methods of emptying the bladder to prevent over-distention and dribbling. These persons have a lower motor neuron lesion and the bladder is often referred to as non-reflex, autonomous or flaccid. The bladder loses its muscle tone and becomes overdistended without any sensations of fullness.

Persons with damage to the cerebral cortex, as in multiple sclerosis, tumor or cerebrovascular disease, have a "mixed" type of bladder in which they have partial sensation and/or partial control. These persons are usually easier to train because of these factors.

Certain patients will probably not be able to become catheter-free. This includes persons with sphincter damage, fistulas, high quadriplegia, advanced multiple sclerosis, multiple myeloma and severe brain damage. In these persons, every means to reduce complications of catheter use must be used. These

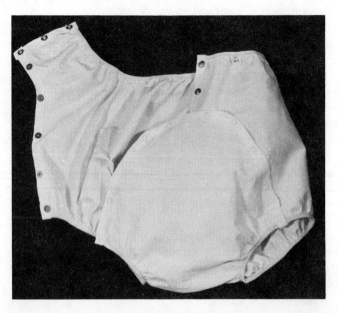

Figure 8–5 A front-opening pair of protective pants which can be worn over any type of absorbent pad.

include a high fluid intake and a scrupulous aseptic technique in catheter care and bladder irrigation. In lieu of a catheter, sometimes an external urinary appliance for men or protective clothing for women can be used satisfactorily (see Figs. 8–4 and 8–5). It is imperative that a male external catheter be applied so that it neither impairs circulation nor causes skin irritation or breakdown. Tapes and straps may cause problems. Application with Rutzen facing cement has been found satisfactory. When a urosheath is used, experimentation with the size and brand may be necessary to locate the right fit.

NURSING MEASURES FOR PATIENTS WITHOUT A CATHETER

The nurse has the responsibility of observing and recording the present voiding pattern. This should be done for two or three days. It may take longer to relate the pattern to activity, fluid intake, a transient illness or emotional stress. Certain observations are essential. What times of day is the patient incontinent? What times is he dry? Does he void in small, moderate or large amounts? Is he aware when there is a need to void? Does he have a sense of urgency when he feels the need to void? Is there dribbling between voidings? Does a problem seem to occur at the initiation of voiding? What is the frequency of voiding? What is the patient's reaction to his lack of control? Is there pain when he voids? Must the patient strain to void?

It is very difficult to estimate the amount of output when a patient is incontinent. However, the following guide may help you to know the amount of output, even though it is not completely precise and depends on whether padding, underpads or other protective linen is used.

DIAMETER OF STAINS*	APPROXIMATE AMOUNT VOIDED
9 inches	50–75 cc.
12 inches	100–125 cc.
18 inches	150–175 cc.
24 inches	200–300 cc.

One of the most helpful nursing measures for patients who do not have a catheter is to provide frequent opportunities to void. Many "accidents" can be prevented by using the toilet, commode or bedpan after meals, after naps, before going to bed and before any activities. Waking the patient in the middle of the night to void often controls night incontinence. The time for awakening is determined by the hour he is found to be incontinent. This also prevents many nighttime falls resulting from patients getting up in a strange and poorly lighted area and having to climb over side rails to use the toilet. This practice is particularly helpful to the elderly, who normally get up at least once and usually twice each night to go to the bathroom.

As assessment and early plans begin, be sure that the patient receives 2500 to 3000 cc. of fluid in order to maintain proper hydration. This can be accomplished by taking one average glassful of fluid every hour from 7 A.M. to 8 P.M. Once the usual time of voiding is established, have the patient void about one-half hour prior to his regular time. First this can be done every hour, then

---

*Bowel and Bladder Training, a filmstrip produced by Trainex Corporation, Garden Grove, California.

every two hours and finally every three or four hours as success occurs. Not all persons will be able to extend their time this long.

It is essential that fluid intake and output be measured when a person is on a bladder training program. This helps to identify the need for fluids as well as the need for voiding and becomes a part of the assessment plan. Once a program starts, it should be evaluated and adjusted every few days until a pattern is established that is in keeping with the patient's physical condition and his ability to maintain it.

Whenever a patient is incontinent, it is important to see that he is clean and dry both for esthetic and physical reasons. It is suggested that the skin be thoroughly cleansed of urine with hexachlorophene soap. Besides cleansing, this soap also provides a protective film over the skin. Only through cleanliness and avoidance of prolonged pressure can skin breakdown be prevented.

For persons who have had mild brain damage, prolonged bedrest or a surgical procedure, a normal voiding pattern after removal of the catheter occurs fairly rapidly. However, if the patient is brain-damaged or is very confused mentally, there is a more difficult nursing problem. In these cases, a rigid toilet schedule must first be set by the nurse mainly to prevent incontinence rather than to control it. Although establishing a bladder training program will be somewhat lengthy and difficult, in many cases it is successful. For the majority of these persons, it is the nurse who becomes trained.

The nurse must observe if the patient's bladder capacity is small. If it is, the patient will need to be taken to the bathroom more frequently. When the patient demonstrates anxiety, it is wise to see if he needs to void. This is especially true of the aphasic person. This might have to be asked every hour or so initially. If the patient's awareness of his need to void is diminished or his ability to wait is lessened, a bedside commonde or the placing of a urinal at the bedside can be helpful. The patient may be unable to initiate use of this equipment on his own, so the nurse will need to assist the patient at regular intervals.

If night incontinence is a problem, withholding fluids after 7 P.M., taking the patient to the bathroom at midnight or leaving a urinal at the bedside can be beneficial. It is also recommended that the patient have adequate daytime activity to increase his cardiac output, which will in turn increase the circulation to the brain, thus helping the patient to be more aware of his needs. Daytime activity can influence the learning of bladder control!

NURSING MEASURES FOR PATIENTS WITH AN INDWELLING CATHETER

When a Foley catheter is used, it is taped to the inner thigh in the case of a female and to the side just below the femoral area to the abdomen in the case of a male (see Fig. 8–6). The latter is recommended when a catheter is used for an

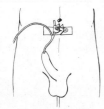

Figure 8–6   Taping of male indwelling catheter to prevent pressure at the peno-scrotal junction.

extended period of time. This minimizes pressure and irritation by increasing the penoscrotal angle. One method is as follows:

1. Using a six-inch length of one-inch wide adhesive tape, press the adhesive surfaces together at the center in order to form a one-inch tab in the center of the tape.

2. Place the tape lengthwise under the umbilicus with the tab upward.

3. Attach another piece of tape (leaving a tab at the end) to the catheter.

4. Pin the two tabs together.

This position should be maintained except when the patient is in the prone position, at which time the catheter is unpinned and the penis is positioned laterally toward the drainage bag. In the case of an orthopedic frame, the penis rests on the canvas strip made for voiding.

The catheter is attached to straight drainage tubing and to a leg bag when the patient is up, or to a bed bag when the patient is in bed. Straight drainage bags should be changed daily, and leg bags should be cleaned with a disinfectant and deodorizer daily. For the male patient, it is important to keep the catheter clean at the exit from the penis to ensure proper drainage of urethral secretions.

When a patient must use a catheter for an extended period of time, it is wise to change it at least once a month. It may be necessary to change it more often; however, with regular bladder irrigation, once a month may be adequate. Change is determined by amount of odor, sediment or obstruction. If a person has a suprapubic catheter—a catheter inserted through a surgical incision above the symphysis pubis (cystostomy)—the frequency of catheter change will be somewhat less.

Catheters may be irrigated by one of two methods. Half-strength normal saline may be injected and aspirated, or a buffered acid solution may be injected into the bladder (usually about 60 cc.) and left there for approximately 15 minutes. Both of these procedures are done once or twice a day according to the physician's directions.

Trail-Off Catheter. Once a patient's physical condition has stabilized and he is able to assume the upright position, the physician will ask that removal of the catheter be tried to see if the patient can learn urinary control with little or no residual urine.

Procedures vary somewhat, but the following is frequently used. Beginning with breakfast, the patient is given 200 cc. of fluid every hour for about three hours. The purpose of this is to build up the amount of body fluid so that the bladder will accumulate approximately 300 cc. within a couple of hours. Next, the catheter is removed and the patient is encouraged to void on a toilet or a commode at regular intervals. The nurse must record the amounts voided and report any incontinence between attempts at voiding.

There are certain aids which will stimulate voiding:

1. There are signs of impending need to void. The patient can learn to recognize these cues in relation to his voiding pattern. Restlessness, headache, chill, flushing, perspiration and a vague feeling of fullness can warn the patient that he needs to void.

2. Methods patients use to stimulate voiding include push-ups, lighting a cigarette, mental concentration, bending forward, stroking inner aspects of thigh or drinking water. Such "tricks" are exceedingly individualized.

3. If the reflex arc is intact, the voiding reflex might be stimulated by tapping the bladder, stroking the inner aspects of the thigh, pulling the pubic hair, anal sphincter massage or manual expression. In the case of a very flaccid bladder, only manual expression will be effective.

4. Manual expression of urine is accomplished by the Credé technique. With the hands flat just below the umbilical area, firmly stroke downward to the bladder six or seven times. This is followed by placing one hand on top of the other above the pubic arch and firmly pressing inward and downward until no more urine can be pressed from the bladder.

If voiding has not occurred within three to four hours, the catheter should be re-inserted. If the patient has voided, there should be a check for residual urine. Use a Foley catheter for this procedure in case the amount of residual urine is not acceptable to the physician. In this case the catheter may be left in. Some authorities recommend that there be no incontinence and that the residual urine be below 100 cc. for a spastic bladder or below 50 cc. for a flaccid bladder. When this is first tried, some physicians order re-insertion of the catheter at night and repeat the same procedure for the next day or two, or until the residual is below 50 cc. If this is not done, it is recommended that the patient stop drinking fluids in the early evening and that he be awakened to void in the middle of the night.

During trial periods, the nurse must be especially cognizant of the possibility of overdistention, which may be exhibited by restlessness, perspiration, chills, flushing or paling, marked elevation of blood pressure, cold extremities, distended bladder or severe headache. These are the symptoms of *autonomic hyperreflexia,* which occurs in persons with a spinal cord lesion below the level of injury and can be triggered by a distended bladder, a fecal impaction, skin stimulation and other autonomic responses. When autonomic hyperreflexia occurs, it must be treated as a medical emergency. A physician must be called. The cause must be removed, but care must be taken not to cause more stimulation. For instance, in the case of a distended bladder, a new catheter is inserted and urine is released very slowly and in small amounts. The patient's head should be elevated and blood pressure should be monitored every five minutes.

Hourly intake of fluid and attempts to void every two or three hours continue throughout the day. This information must be accurately recorded in relation to time, fluids, meals and activities, until a patient is well established. Residuals are checked daily in the initial phase of this program, then twice a week and ultimately every other week.

Whether the patient with a spinal cord injury can remain catheter-free will depend on three possibilities: (1) whether his bladder will empty by automatic reflex activity after filling to a certain capacity, (2) whether the bladder will empty by stimulation of the intact reflex by external stimuli or (3) whether the bladder can be manually expressed by the Credé technique.

If the first attempt at trial off-catheter is not successful, it does not indicate that future attempts will be unsuccessful. It merely means that the program should be abandoned for a brief period and restarted within a week or so. During these periods patients need a great deal of encouragement and psychological support.

INTERMITTENT CATHETERIZATION

Intermittent catheterization is a physiologic method of facilitating the return of bladder function. The goal is to establish bladder continence for persons with a neurogenic bladder without the use of an indwelling catheter.

In some instances, the person's ability to void varies from time to time, requiring intermittent catherization. If the person does not have a urinary tract infection, intermittent catheterization is frequently preferred. Persons try to void first and are then catheterized. When strict asepsis is used, persons may be catheterized q.i.d. for months. In fact, the lowest incidence of infection occurs among those using intermittent catheterization, according to several studies.

While procedures vary, they usually have these features in common: (1) urine culture done two or three days prior to intitiating the trial period to make sure there is no infection; (2) normal daily fluid intake of about 2000 cc. taken from about 7 A.M. to 7 P.M.; (3) after the catheter is removed, the patient is asked to void every four hours and is catheterized for residual after each voiding; and (4) as the residual decreases, the intervals between catherization are increased. One physician reduces the number of times of catheterization to once a day when the residual is 100 cc. or less, then weekly for a month and ultimately stops if the residual remains less than 100 cc.

Food and Fluids.   In addition, it is usually suggested that the urine be kept acid in order to reduce the likelihood of urinary tract stones, and to prevent the growth of bacteria in the urine. Some foods, such as cranberry juice, can help accomplish this. Because the patient often must drink large quantities of fluids (women may only be able to take 2500 cc., while men usually can tolerate 3000 cc.), it is important to vary the kinds of fluids and find those that are particularly liked. Carbonated fluids sometimes seem to irritate the bladder, so non-carbonated fluids are recommended. Any form of alcohol is contraindicated. Some milk is necessary, but only in very small quantities because of its high calcium content, which fosters formation of stones. Some physicians do not allow patients with a spinal cord injury to have dairy products for up to five years. An excess of fruit juices will alkalize the urine and may cause a problem in bowel consistency. It is best to vary the kinds of fluids in order to maintain a balance of the effects of each.

CONTROL OF INCONTINENCE BY ELECTRONIC STIMULATION

Continence of the bladder has been achieved in selected cases of cerebral palsy, hemiplegia, multiple sclerosis, demyelinating disease, upper and lower motor neuron injuries and meningomyelocele by the use of a bladder stimulator. A bladder pacemaker is implanted in the bladder. When it is time to void, this is activated by the patient, who controls an external transmitter (about the size of a transistor radio). In upper motor neuron injuries, this has been successful in less than 50 per cent of the cases. The successful cases have also had a sacral block. The latter procedure actually transforms the bladder to a lower motor neuron bladder. See Chapter 9 regarding sexuality in the patient with a lower motor neuron injury.

As neuromodulation devices and surgical techniques become more refined, it is anticipated that a greater number of persons will become "continent" by these means.

SUMMARY

Bowel and bladder training programs are essential to the success of each person's ultimate rehabilitation goals. These programs must be incorporated into the total nursing care plan, so that all shifts of nursing personnel are assisting the patient in a consistent and meaningful way. Whether the patient ultimately achieves bowel and bladder control will of course be determined by the cause of his loss of control, the extent of brain damage and any infections or other complications which exist. Nursing intervention in this area needs to be individualized, ingenious and rigorous.

REFERENCES

Abramson, Arthur S.: Advances in the management of the neurogenic bladder. *Archives of Physical Medicine and Rehabilitation, 52*:143, 1971.

Adams, M., Baron, M., and Caston, M. A.: Urinary incontinence in the acute phase of cerebral vascular accident. *Nursing Research, 15*:100, 1966.

Altshuler, A., et al.: Even children can learn to do clean self-catheterization. *American Journal of Nursing, 77*:97, January, 1977.

Clark, C. L.: Catheter care in the home. *American Journal of Nursing, 72*:922, May, 1972.

Comarr, Estin, A.: Practical urological management of the patient with spinal cord injury. *British Journal of Urology, 31*:1, 1959.

Delehanty, Lorraine, and Stravino, Vincent: Achieving bladder control. *American Journal of Nursing, 70*:312, 1970.

Donahue, P., and Van Deusen, A.: Intermittent catheterization in neurogenic bladder rehabilitation. *ARN Journal, 1*:8, March–April, 1976.

Feustel, Delycia: Autonomic hyperreflexia. *American Journal of Nursing, 76*:228, February, 1976.

Glen, E. S.: Effective and safe control of incontinence by the intra-anal plug electrode. *British Journal of Surgery, 58*:249, April, 1971.

Grosicki, Jeanette P.: Effects of operant conditioning on modification of incontinency in neuropsychiatric geriatric patients. *Nursing Research, 17*:304, 1968.

Guyton, Arthur C.: *Textbook of Medical Physiology.* 4th ed. Philadelphia, W. B. Saunders Co., 1971, pp. 442–445 and 751–752.

Habeeb, Marjorie, and Kallstrom, Mina: Bowel program for institutionalized adults. *American Journal of Nursing, 76*:606, April, 1976.

Halverstadt, D. B., and Parry, W. L.: Electronic stimulation of the human bladder: 9 years later. *Journal of Urology, 113*:341, March, 1975.

Kira, Alexander: *The Bathroom.* New York, Viking Press, 1976.

Kuhn, Hannah, et al: Intermittent catheterization as a rehabilitative nursing service. *Archives of Physical Medicine and Rehabilitation, 55*:439, October, 1974.

McGuckin, Maryanne: Urine cultures — key to diagnosing urinary tract infections. *Nursing '75, 5*:10, December, 1975.

Merrill, D. C., and Conway, C. J.: Clinical experience with the mentor bladder stimulator. I. Patients with upper motor lesions. *The Journal of Urology, 113*:335, March, 1975.

Merrill, D. C.: Clinical experience with the mentor bladder stimulator. III. Patients with urinary vesical hypotonia. *The Journal of Urology, 113*:335, March, 1975.

Merrill, D. C.: Urinary incontinence treatment with electrical stimulation of the pelvic floor. *Urology, 5*:67, January, 1975.

Sister Kenny Institute Staff: *Introduction to Bowel and Bladder Care.* Minneapolis, Sister Kenny Institute, 1975.

Smith, Donald, R.: *General Urology.* 8th Ed. Los Altos, California, Lange Medical Publications, 1975.

Stafford, Noval: Bowel hygiene of aged patients. *American Journal of Nursing, 63*:102, 1963.

Swezey, Robert L., and Hallin, Roger: Technics for chronic drainage of bladder. *Archives of Physical Medicine, 48*:201, 1967.

Talbot, Herbert, S.: Management of neurogenic dysfunction of the bladder and bowel. *In* Krusen, F. H., et al.: *Hankbook of Physical Medicine and Rehabilitation.* 2nd Ed. Philadelphia, W. B. Saunders Co., 1971.

Tillery, Betty, and Bates, Barbara: Enemas. *American Journal of Nursing, 66*:534, 1966.

Tudor, Lea L.: Bladder and bowel retraining. *American Journal of Nursing, 70*:2391, 1970.

Whelan, John: *Urological Nursing Procedures.* Rehabilitation Monograph 43, New York Institute of Rehabilitation Medicine, New York University Medical Center, 1970.

Winter, C.: *Nursing Care of Patients with Urologic Diseases.* 3rd Ed. St. Louis, C. V. Mosby Co., 1975.

Winter, C., et al.: Urinary calculi. *American Journal of Nursing, 63*:72, 1963.

Woodrow, Mary, et al.: Suprapubic catheters: a direct line to better drainage. *Nursing '76.* Part I, *6*:40, October, 1976; Part II, *6*:40, November, 1976.

Chapter 9

MAINTAINING SEXUALITY

How do age, disease and disability affect a person's sexuality? Until very recently, patients all too often received information that originated from commonly accepted myths mixed with whatever beliefs and attitudes were held by the nurse or the doctor on the case. More frequently, however, the subject was either ignored or evaded because of lack of factual information and/or embarrassment on the part of patients, physicians and other involved persons. It is, of course, unknown how much suffering, unnecessary stress and sexual dysfunction this has caused.

A few examples will illustrate the widespread nature of the professional evasion of the subject. In a patient booklet on Multiple Sclerosis, under the heading "Sex," it reads, "Do the best you can." That is all; it then goes on to the next heading. The 3 million people who have coronary atherosclerotic heart disease have received no better suggestions until recently. When Hellerstein and Friedman reviewed 33 cardiology texts, they found only 1000 words on the subject. That is approximately two printed pages! A final example of neglect in the area of sex is the nursing home patient. Personnel continue to report the use of drugs, isolation and discipline when they are confronted with a resident who shows interest in sexual expression.

Nurses are usually ill-prepared to deal with this subject and frequently resort to saying "Ask your doctor" when questioned about it by patients. Unfortunately, this answer may either deter the patient from bringing up the subject to anyone again, or the physician may turn out to be no better prepared to give helpful answers than the nurse. Recently schools of medicine have attended to the subject of sexuality better than schools of nursing. According to Lief, only three medical schools had formal training in human sexuality in 1960, but 106 of 114 medical schools included courses on sexuality in 1974. In contrast in 1973, SIECUS (the Sex Information and Education Council of the United States) surveyed 176 baccalaureate schools of nursing and found only one respondent offering a course in human sexuality, and even in this school, the course was an elective. Since nursing personnel are with patients a greater amount of time than other members of the health care team, it becomes essential that the nurse do everything to help the person to receive accurate information and to work through any problems that exist. This does not mean that the nurse must become a sex counselor, unless she has had more specialized training, but it does mean that she is able to discuss the subject knowledgeably and without embarrassment.

Basically, this means that the nurse must at least:

1. Know the biological, psychological, social and cultural aspects of sexuality.

2. Know how sexuality is affected by aging, disability, and certain diseases.

3. Work through her own background, feelings, values and convictions in relation to sexual behavior and alternative sexual practices.

4. Listen to the patient to identify his or her feelings, values and areas of concern.

With the knowledge, attitudes and skills resulting from the above, nurses will be able to assist persons without imposing their own values or behaviors by (1) using the person's values as a beginning, and (2) sharing appropriate information to meet the person's needs. When courses in human sexuality are not available, the reader is directed to the references at the end of this chapter.

SEXUALITY AFTER SPINAL CORD INJURY

A frequently held myth is that disabled persons, especially the paralyzed and disfigured, have no need for sexual expression. This belief is perpetuated from various quarters. First of all, society at large tends to regard the disabled as nonsexual beings. Secondly, parents of children with congenital or acquired problems often believe that the sexuality of their children should not be developed, and they therefore attempt to provide an asexual social environment. In addition, patients themselves are deeply afraid of being inadequate sexually. Finally, when physicians and nurses have inadequate sex education themselves, they are also affected by these powerful influences. Fortunately, some outstanding physicians and health professionals are providing impetus to improved education of both professionals and patients. The paraplegic and quadriplegic have received particular attention.

PHYSIOLOGICAL EFFECTS OF A CORD INJURY

Male. Bors and Comarr have studied spinal cord–injured persons extensively. Among males, they found the following relationships between types of injury and sexual capability:

INJURY	PERCENTAGE OF MALES HAVING CAPABILITY OF:		
	(A) ERECTION	(B) COITUS	(C) EJACULATION
Upper motor neuron injury — complete	93%	70%	4%
Upper motor neuron injury — incomplete	99%	80%	31%
Lower motor neuron injury — complete	25%	20%	18%
Lower motor neuron injury — incomplete	90%	90%	50–90%

The male erection may originate in two ways, by reflexogenic or psychogenic stimulus. A reflexogenic erection may occur spontaneously or it may be the result of local external stimulation. A psychogenic erection occurs in response to psychic stimulation such as odor, imagination or a visual encounter. The small number (25 per cent) of men having a complete lower motor neuron injury who are capable of having an erection have psychogenic erections only. Those with a complete upper motor neuron injury capable of having an erection (93 per cent) have reflexogenic erections only. Between 90 and 99 per cent of those with incomplete lesions (upper and lower motor neuron) can experience both reflexogenic and psychogenic erections.

Of the 529 males surveyed, only 3 per cent sired children. Even cord-injured males who can ejaculate seldom have sperm that have morphology and motility within the normal limits required for procreation.

Female.   The sexual effects of spinal cord injury to a woman are fewer. A woman, while she may lack sensation, does not lose function. Regardless of the level of injury, she continues or regains her menstrual cycle and has the potential to become pregnant. Women with adequate pelvic measurements can usually deliver vaginally whether they become pregnant before or after their injury. While a woman usually loses the ability to have an orgasm, she is still capable of sexual satisfaction. Many cord-injured women report that substitution of pleasurable sensations in other parts of the body along with satisfying their partner's needs is both fulfilling and gratifying.

SEXUAL EXPRESSION AND MARITAL ADJUSTMENT

Some patients are able to broach this subject to the team member with whom they feel most comfortable during their rehabilitative program. Others are not. In order to place sexuality in perspective as one aspect of the total care program, it is wise to indicate to the patient early in the rehabilitation program that sexual counseling is available. This acknowledges that it is not a taboo subject and that the staff is ready to talk about this aspect of their lives, and it leaves the timing for such discussions up to the patient.

During counseling sessions, less emphasis is placed on orgasm, erection and ejaculation, and the more crucial elements of the relationship and communication between partners are stressed. These are, of course, the same issues in marital counseling, whether the couple is able-bodied or not.

Depending on the level of injury, whether the lesion is complete or incomplete and the individual characteristics of the patient, alternative sexual practices that satisfy both partners can usually be found. Manual stimulation or the use of a vibrator may help to produce a more effective erection in males. Manual clitoral stimulation or a prosthetic device may be used for women. Oral-genital sex may be satisfying. Catheter-dependent persons may or may not remove their catheters during coitus. If the catheter is not removed from the male, it may be folded back over the penis.

Generally speaking, when a relationship is strong, a couple will be able to experiment with various sexual activities until they find ways that are gratifying and esthetically pleasing to both partners as well as being physiologically possible. The divorce rate among disabled persons reflects the soundness of the relationship just as it does among non-disabled persons. If one partner in a troubled marriage becomes disabled, the possibility of a divorce is fairly great, as such a stress added to an already stressful situation may well become intolerable. When a relationship is strong, the difficulties and adjustments created by a disabling accident can usually be overcome without divorce. For those who marry after their injury, the divorce rate is low. In these cases, the adaptations to the injury are known and made prior to the marriage.

When consideration of the other partner is uppermost in each partner's mind, it seems that even an event as traumatic as a spinal cord injury cannot cause separation. If separation does occur, it is usually for reasons other than the spinal cord injury itself.

EFFECTS OF HEART ATTACK AND OTHER DISEASES ON SEXUALITY

The aim of this section is merely to suggest through example the large numbers of patients whose sexuality is affected or threatened by a disease or its treatment. The nurse encounters these persons daily, in the obstetrics department, the intensive care unit, the surgery unit, the rehabilitation unit, the nursing home, the ambulatory clinic and in the home.

It is fairly well known that the heart beats faster, respirations increase, and blood pressure rises during sexual activity. If this is true, is sexual expression after myocardial infarction safe? This question is asked by thousands almost daily, but many persons do not ask the question out loud or to the right person. With little or no information and out of fear of having another attack, unknown numbers of patients refrain from sexual activity after heart attack. Others refrain because they experience some physical symptoms such as chest pain during coitus. When patients cannot or do not discuss these problems with their physicians, it may be due to reticence on the part of the physician. When the physician does not initiate the subject, the patient is likely to sense the physician's discomfort and be unwilling to explore the subject. Thus, sexual dysfunction may be perpetuated when it may be totally unnecessary or at least correctable.

Hellerstein's studies show that the cardiovascular cost of many daily activities, such as driving a car, walking to work, or arguing at dinner, is comparable to that of sexual activity with a spouse. Other studies show that those who participate in an active conditioning program can maintain an active sexual life. Certainly the biologic and psychologic variables of each patient must be assessed before recommendations are made. However, it seems that most patients can maintain their sexuality if they maintain their general physical condition. Some modification in behavior may be recommended, such as avoiding coitus sooner than three hours after eating or drinking an alcoholic beverage, having coitus in the morning when the body is more rested or using a medication before coitus.

Many other conditions that permanently affect a person's health or function will influence sexual expression, physically and/or psychologically. Much of what was described under spinal cord injury can be applied and adapted to other neurological diseases. In addition, persons who have diabetes and those who have had a colostomy (or other ostomy), a mastectomy, a hysterectomy or a prostatectomy may have perceived changes as well as real changes in their bodies affecting sexuality. If we are to implement the concept of holistic care, sexual counseling must become an integral part of health care. The reader is referred to Nancy Fugate Wood's excellent book, *Human Sexuality in Health and Illness,* for more detail in the physical and psychological aspects of many conditions, as well as counseling suggestions.

SEXUALITY AND THE AGING PROCESS

MYTHS

Regardless of facts to the contrary, some older persons, families of the aged and health care professionals still believe that at middle age or soon after, both sexual desire and sexual capability disappear. This causes guilt and embarrassment for those who maintain their sexuality and unhappiness to the many older persons who accept society's myth and make it a self-fulfilling prophecy. In addition, it separates the sexuality of a person from the rest of the physical and psychosocial being. This is particularly obvious in health care settings, such as the nursing home.

Why are these false beliefs held? It is not entirely clear, but many reasons can be identified. While a person may reject one false belief, he may tenaciously cling to another. For instance, some people equate sex with procreation, and as a result have had a fairly inactive sexual life. To these persons, when procreation capability ceases, sexual activity also ceases. Secondly, we live in a youth-oriented society that emphasizes physical attractiveness, which is equated with sex. Those who think in these terms may ridicule the sexuality of older persons on the basis of wrinkles and reduced musculature. One psychiatric theory traces the attitudes of society to repressed oedipal and incest taboos, a remnant of a child's disbelief that his own parents make sexual love. There are even beliefs that exertion from coitus can damage health. Couples who have had a poor relationship for years may find age an acceptable excuse to discontinue sexual relationships. Finally, in the case of widowed persons seeking a new spouse, children may fear a reduced inheritance and use society's myths to demean and dissuade such an alliance.

All of these factors place the older person in conflict with society. Whether they reject or adopt society's expectation of being asexual, they experience anxiety and stress from the conflict between the sexual role carved out by society and their own individual needs. This is an obvious example of "Ageism," the prejudice against the elderly so well described by Robert Butler.

FACTS

While Kinsey and other more recent researchers have provided us with insights from much data, the studies done by Eric Pfeiffer, of the Center for the Study of Aging and Human Development at Duke University, and by Masters and Johnson may be considered landmarks in this area. They confirm that both the ability and the desire for sexual expression can continue into the eighth decade when general health is good and if there is an available partner. While knowlege of factual information alone cannot change people's attitudes, it is a first step toward accepting the sexuality of older persons and providing suitable environments for the expression of that sexuality. Ultimately, it may even help us to enjoy a less distorted old age of our own.

Masters and Johnson point out that the aging male may talk himself out of effective sexual functioning because of certain physiologic changes that will somewhat alter his sexual responses. Their studies show that, while the male may notice a delayed erective time, decreased ejaculatory pressure and other changes, "he does not lose his facility for erection at any time." They go on to say that some of the physiologic changes are advantageous and may actually improve a sexual relationship. Because the older male has greater control of the ejaculatory process, he may be increasingly able to satisfy his partner.

The female also experiences physiologic changes. The vagina becomes less elastic and less moist. Occasionally some women experience uterine pain during intercourse, but fortunately, this problem can be treated. Hormone therapy and vaginal lubricants are used with success. The woman can continue to experience orgasm into her old age also. Many women report greater sexual satisfaction after the menopause than before. The demands of raising a family, worry about pregnancy, and changes that sometimes result from the Pill no longer exist, and release a woman from tensions that once interfered with sexual enjoyment.

The Duke University studies bear out the latter point. Fifteen per cent of their study sample showed a steady increase in sexual activity and interest with age. Since these studies are longitudinal, such findings cannot be attributed to wishful thinking or poor memory. They report that 40 to 65 per cent of those 60 to 71 years of age engage in fairly frequent intercourse; only 10 to 20 per cent of those over 78 years were still active sexually. In most instances, both the male and the female agreed that when there was a cessation of intercourse, it was due to the male.

Dr. Joseph Freeman states that "Rapid changes in sexual pattern of the elderly suggest psychiatric disorders, particularly depressions which are susceptible to proper treatment." It is well to keep such a possibility in mind, as we are probably all guilty of attributing a superficial or stereotype reason for behavior changes in the elderly.

Other findings show that 2 out of 3 males and only 1 out of 5 females over 65 years of age are active sexually. This difference is caused by the reduced number of available men at this age, greater reluctance on the part of women to engage in sex outside of marriage and belief in some of the myths noted earlier.

In summary, research into both physiologic functioning and sexual practice indicates that sexual interest and ability continues throughout the life span when partners are available and in generally good health. Religious, social and family influences unfortunately may not encourage expression of this aspect of the human personality when a person grows old.

SEXUALITY IN INSTITUTIONAL CARE

The availability of privacy for the expression of sexuality in a home for the aged or a nursing home does not always exist. When one marriage partner is a resident and the other is not, when the spouses are in different sections of an institution, and when unmarried persons occasionally develop a relationship, three major problems arise for the persons involved. First of all, rarely is the setting suitable for either physical comfort or privacy. Secondly, institutions are often concerned that families may object to residents' engaging in sexual activity. Indeed, some may, but many do not. Lastly, personnel may take it upon themselves to supervise, report, chastise or separate any couples who may desire closeness.

It is important that staff become knowledgeable on this subject. It is also important that institutional philosophy and policies be made known to all personnel. The Patient's Bill of Rights as it stands today, while not specific in this area, seems to give residents the "right" to privacy, but few actually have it. Some states are making such privacy mandatory by legislative action. For many persons, the subject is difficult to discuss, as it causes so much discomfort. Therefore, personnel must be helped to deal with the sexuality of residents. If both personnel and residents share similar attitudes, regardless of what those attitudes are, very few problems will arise. It is therefore wise for potential employees or potential residents to know how the institution handles this aspect of a resident's life prior to admission or employment. Nonetheless, in the future it will be essential for administrators and staff to explore this area, to examine their own attitudes and to consider how to provide an environment in which residents can maintain their sexuality.

One other problem, very different in nature, arises in nursing homes with some degree of regularity; namely, a patient will behave in ways that embarrass others. They may expose themselves or make overtures to personnel or other residents who are uninterested in their advances. Such behavior may be caused by a variety of factors, such as mental or physical deterioration, fear, frustration or anger.

In such cases of irregular behavior, it is first of all important to assess the patient for any physical problem. For instance, the person may be merely scratching an undetected dermatitis of the genitalia, or he may be experiencing a serious personality change due to a brain tumor. If the behavior does not seem to have a correctable physical cause, personnel need to know how to minimize the patient's unacceptable actions. Negative ways of doing this include diverting, lecturing, cajoling or using medication or restraint. In many instances, however, such measures are likely to enhance the behavior and will invariably demean the patient as well as reduce his self-esteem. Nurses who have succeeded in either reversing or minimizing improper behavior recommend the following:

1. Look for a cause.
2. Reveal no sign of shock or value judgment.
3. Control the behavior with firmness but without causing shame or embarrassment.
4. Search for ways of altering the environment that might reduce patient frustrations.
5. Determine a desirable behavior and then decide how to reinforce it, in order to help to diminish the undesirable behavior.
6. Discuss the matter and any ameliorative plans with the patient.

These nursing measures will help to maintain an openness to finding both alternative causes for the innappropriate behavior and alternative approaches for reshaping it along more desirable lines.

SUMMARY

This chapter has dealt with a most neglected aspect of rehabilitative and continuing care: human sexuality. In order to deal with this more adequately, health care professionals need to have greater knowledge about this aspect of personality and to develop a self-awareness that allows them to deal with patients therapeutically.

REFERENCES

Anderson, Catherine J.: Sexuality in the aged. *Journal of Gerontological Nursing*, *1*:6, November–December, 1975.

Anderson, Thomas, and Cole, Theodore: Sexual counseling of the physically disabled. *Postgraduate Medicine*, *58*:117, July, 1975.

Bors, E., and Comarr, A. E.: Neurological disturbances of sexual function with special references to 529 patients with spinal cord injury. *Urologic Survey*, *10*:191, December, 1960.

Boyarsky, Rose E.: Sexuality. *In* Steinberg, F. U.: *Cowdry's The Care of the Geriatric Patient.* 5th Ed., St. Louis, C. V. Mosby Co., 1976.

Bregman, Sue: *Sexuality and the Spinal Cord Injured Woman.* Minneapolis, Sister Kenny Institute, 1975.

Butler, Robert N.: *Sex After 60: a Guide for Men and Women for Their Later Years.* New York, Harper and Row, 1976.

Comarr, A. E., and Gunderson, B. B.: Sexual function in traumatic paraplegia and quadriplegia. *American Journal of Nursing, 75*:250, February, 1975.

Eisenberg, M. G., and Rustad, L. C.: *Sex and the Spinal Cord Injured: Some Questions and Answers.* 2nd Ed. Veterans Administration Hospital, 10701 East Boulevard, Cleveland, Ohio, 1974. Superintendent of Documents, Washington, D.C. 20402.

Evans, R. L. et al.: Multidisciplinary approach to sex education of spinal cord injured patients. *Physical Therapy.* 56:541, May, 1976.

Felstein, Ivor: *Sex in Later Life.* New York, Pelican Books, 1970.

Gregory, Martha F.: *Sexual Adjustment: A Guide for the Spinal Cord Injured.* Accent Special Publications, Accent on Living, Inc., P.O. Box 726, Bloomington, Illinois 61701.

Hanlon, Kathryn: Maintaining sexuality after spinal cord injury. *Nursing '75, 5*:58, May, 1975.

Hellerstein, H., and Friedman, E.: Sexual activity and the post-coronary patient. *Medical Aspects of Human Sexuality, 3*:70, March, 1969.

Jaeger, Dorothea, and Simmons, Leo: Improprieties in patients. *Nursing '72, 2*:30, February, 1972.

Kreger, S. M.: Sexuality and disability. *ARN Journal, 2*:8. January-February, 1977.

Kroah, Janet: How to deal with patients who act out sexually. *Nursing '73, 3*:39, December, 1973.

Lief, Harold, and Payne, Tyana: Sexuality — knowledge and attitudes. *American Journal of Nursing, 75*:2026, November, 1975.

Lobsenz, N. M.: *Sex After Sixty-five.* Public Affairs Pamphlet No. 519, 1975. Public Affairs Pamphlets, 381 Park Avenue South, New York, New York 10016.

Masters, M. H., and Johnson, V. E.: *Human Sexual Inadequacy.* Boston, Little, Brown and Co., 1970.

Mooney, T. O., Cole, T. M., and Chilgren, R. A.: *Sexual Options for Paraplegics and Quadriplegics.* Boston, Little, Brown and Co., 1975.

Pfeiffer, E. and Davis, G.: Determinants of sexual behavior in middle and old age. *Journal of American Geriatrics Society, 20*:151, April, 1972.

SIECUS Guides. A series of pamphlets on sex published by the Sex Information and Education Council in the United States, 1855 Broadway, New York, New York, 10023.

Woods, Nancy Fugate: *Human Sexuality in Health and Illness.* St. Louis, C. V. Mosby Co., 1975.

Chapter 10

PATIENT AND FAMILY LEARNING—THE TEST OF TEACHING

Robert F. Mager in his book *Developing Attitude Toward Learning* poses three questions every teacher must ask before a teaching plan is started. They are, "Where am I going? How shall I get there? How will I know I've arrived?" These three questions are basic to any meaningful teaching plan, whether it is directed to students or to patients and families, whether it is related to immediate needs or whether it is future-oriented to the home.

The subject of patient and family teaching has something in common with nursing care plans: Everybody talks about it but very few nurses do much about it. In order to identify reasons for this lack, several studies have been conducted with the cooperation of staff nurses. The most common problems were found to be (a) lack of knowledge of what content was required by a patient; (b) lack of teaching skill; (c) lack of clarity between doctor and nurse roles; (d) insufficient time; and (e) failure to assume the responsibility of teaching.

From personal experience at various institutions which cannot claim an outstanding record of patient teaching and from the various studies done on this subject throughout the country, it becomes eminently clear that before anything can be done about improved patient teaching, the nurse must first of all accept teaching as a nursing responsibility. This chapter is written with the assumption that patient and family teaching is a part of the nursing role. This chapter is also written with the assumption that nurses need more information about the relationship between teaching and learning before they can be expected to fulfill this role.

It is vital that teaching not be left to chance. Thus, it must be assigned to a specific person. While it is important that everyone share the teaching role, it is vital that one person be designated to be ultimately responsible for the outcome. In order to have a meaningful patient education program, it is important that a teaching plan become a part of the total nursing care plan. The rate of learning and the patient's level of knowledge can be recorded. The teaching plan will be revised and evaluated as time goes on.

Before we consider patient education, let us first consider various characteristics that distinguish teaching from learning along with a few factors that influence both.

LEARNING

DEFINITION

For our purposes, learning will be defined as a change in behavior. This can mean a change in a concept, an attitude or a skill. When learning is viewed in this light, it becomes possible to measure learning by observing changes in the learner. Thus, the nurse can ultimately test the effectiveness of her teaching. For our purposes, it is helpful to think of evaluating teaching by evaluating learning. When learning does not take place, the nurse will reassess needs with her patient and re-evaluate her approach.

Rehabilitation is a learning process—a change in concepts, attitudes and skills. Some patients are so aware of this that they prefer to be called students or clients once they are no longer acutely ill. Readers will note that much of the content of this book can be used by both the nurse and the student patient.

CHARACTERISTICS OF LEARNING

Several characteristics of learning must be considered by every teacher. First of all, learning does not take place unless there is some activity (mental or physical or both) on the part of the learner. The learner is not simply a sponge that absorbs new knowledge, attitudes or abilities. He must be active rather than passive. In this sense learning is creative, because the learner actually must integrate what is taught into a new behavior.

This integration and the speed with which it occurs will be dependent upon several factors. Learning will be influenced by the individual's intellectual ability. It is well to remember that many persons learn more than their intellectual ability might indicate. The reverse of this is also true. Learning will also be influenced by previous experiences which may have had a negative or positive influence. It will be influenced by background knowledge which may include both accurate and inaccurate information. Skill learning will be affected by motor ability. The person's attitude toward the content as well as his reaction to the teacher can inhibit or encourage learning as the case may be. Finally, it is important that the learner can see some useful purpose in the material being presented if both learning and retention are to take place.

BLOCKS TO LEARNING

Adults have special learning problems that frequently go unheeded in health education of patients and families. The idea of school is very disagreeable to many adults. The idea of learning may produce a sense of inadequacy and anxiety because an adult often equates knowing with being adult. In order to learn, one must first acknowledge that there is a lack of knowledge in a particular area.

Adults may have other emotional reactions toward learning. Previous school experiences may have been unpleasant and call up a sense of insecurity. Adults may have negative feelings toward authority. This can be exhibited by general resentment. The nurse should be extremely sensitive to this possibility and guard against any authoritarian overtones. Adults also have individual emotional responses to words, situations, institutions and people. These reactions may be due to their own past experiences or to those of family members or friends, or they may be due to inaccurate knowledge. Since the learner may look at a situation as he perceives it, not necessarily as it actually is, the nurse must be aware of this possibility. She can attempt to assess and discuss it in order to prevent it from interfering with learning. ,

Adults will naturally resent being placed in any situation in which they are treated like children. They have had the ability to run their own lives, and they want to maintain this in every way possible. The nurse teacher can build on this when she teaches independent activities.

Besides general adult qualities that may influence learning, there are problems that affect learning when the person is also a patient. For instance, impaired vision may be a very important problem if the patient is diabetic and must learn to read an insulin syringe. Impaired hearing is an obvious impediment to learning in any situation. In the latter event, greater visual learning would be appropriate. Illness might cause a shorter attention span, and any teaching should be adjusted accordingly in order to achieve maximum learning. Brain injury, inadequate kidney dialysis, medications, a febrile state and other conditions can cause mental cloudiness, perceptual inaccuracies, or both, which will impede comprehension.

In addition to the patient's physical problems, there will be emotional reactions to the illness and to an altered personal role. These reactions will influence the quality and speed with which learning will take place. Anxiety is probably one of the most obvious and most common emotional reactions which will affect learning. The patient may be anxious about his future, he may be anxious about the outcome of his disease, he may be anxious about the amount of pain and discomfort that he is likely to have, he may be anxious that he will be unable to do the things he is taught. If he does not learn readily, he will feel stupid and fear possible ridicule. Anxiety may be manifested in many ways and vary in degree but it can cause confusion, reduced learning and general ineffectiveness of a patient education program. Frustration from inability or difficulty in learning new things may in turn impair the person's desire to pursue learning, resulting in depression, anger or denial. In these instances, an ex-patient who has experienced and overcome these same problems may be the best teacher, as the discouragement is confronted by the very existence of such a person.

The patient must want to learn. The desire and motivation to learn is not always as strong as we would wish it to be. Since motivation is not something that can be readily changed by another person, we must not feel overly discouraged when we have problems in this area. What motivates one person may not motivate another. Those who had to support a family during the depression are more readily motivated by money because it decreases their anxiety about hunger, loss of self-esteem and lack of employment. Fewer persons who were reared in the last decade or two are likely to have this kind of response to money as a motivator.

Basic research into understanding the person who is highly motivated is still lacking. The late Dr. Abraham Maslow was actively engaged in the study of "those who come out of their self and make the world a part of themselves." These highly motivated people may or may not have a physical disability. Many healthy people are disinterested in taking adequate care of themselves. This helps us to remember that the problem of motivation has much more to do with what goes on inside the patient than on the outside. Since this particular aspect of human beings is not a simple one, the nurse must engage in her work on the premise that "individual experiences are never identical." Not only are no two patients alike, but she must also be aware that the patient is not reacting and responding in the same way that she is to a given experience. It is her job, however, to try to discover what does move the patient to action and what does seem to increase his desire to learn. She can then capitalize on these desires and use them as ways to help him to learn.

Even when motivation is present, another factor, readiness—both physical and mental—must be considered. Once the patient's physical condition has stabilized, the nurse will discuss some of the necessary skills to be learned. She may ask direct questions about his feeling toward what is to be learned. In rehabilitation, one can be particularly sure that the patient is ready for teaching when he seems ready to relinquish the patient role and expresses both a desire and a need to know how to care for himself.

Poor memory may also block or delay learning. For some, repetitive teaching may be helpful. Severe brain damage may of course make it impossible for some persons to understand or to retain what they have learned. Constructional apraxia, a condition that sometimes follows stroke, may seem like a memory problem but is actually a perceptual motor disorder. In this instance, the person can tell you what he should do but is unable to actually do it. It is vital that the patient have a speech and psychological assessment whenever there is brain damage, so that the nurse's teaching can be appropriate to that person's capabilities. Review Chapter 7 for greater detail in dealing with these conditions. The articles by Fowler and Fordyce listed at the end of this chapter will also be of inestimable assistance in this area.

TEACHING

DETERMINING NEEDS

If we think of teaching and learning as a process, it becomes readily apparent that that process is an interaction between teacher and learner. It is based on the learner's needs. In determinging these needs, the nurse will observe the kinds of problems a patient has and try to project how this will be altered in the home environment. The patient knows himself and his home and will be able to see other needs. What the nurse sees as a need and what the patient sees as a need then become the goals of teaching.

When the nurse is attempting to determine the patient's needs, she has really three basic ways of locating them. First of all, she can observe the patient's physical functional ability. She will also note his mental capabilities. As the patient attempts to perform various tasks, especially in self-care, she will be able to determine where he needs help. Therefore, observation of the patient's present performance as well as knowledge of his functional and mental abilities are articulated first. Second, the nurse can look into the future and try to ascertain some of the problems that will arise outside of an institutional situation (home, work, transportation and public facilities). These are then added. Third, the patient must participate actively throughtout the entire process. He may see different priorities than those perceived by the nurse, and he will most certainly see additional problems. In almost every instance, the patient's priorities in terms of choice of topic, sequence of material and amount to be learned each time should be adopted and accepted. In rehabilitation settings, the nurse and patient often make verbal contracts regarding these matters.

SETTING OBJECTIVES

Once the needs have been determined, objectives can be stated. In setting objectives for patient teaching, it is imperative that they clearly express what the patient needs to learn and what the patient needs to know rather than what the nurse is going to teach. For example, an objective stated in terms of teacher activity might be "to teach the patient to feed himself." This is the kind of objective that makes evaluation of learning almost impossible. The nurse's teaching might be very fine, but one would not know what the patient learned. Therefore, the objective should be stated in terms of the patient—"to be able to feed himself." This can be measured. One can ultimately see if the patient is able to feed himself.

Thus, the key to stating objectives is to state them in terms of what the patient is to learn. This is done through the use of action verbs such as feed, walk, desire and so forth. Verbs such as think, feel and consider cannot truly be measured because they are a matter of value judgment on the part of the teacher rather than a patient behavior. Remember, when writing an objective, express what the patient should be doing, not what you as a nurse instructor are doing.

CONTENT

Content will obviously be geared to the physical and mental condition of the patient and cannot be discussed in any detail except as it relates to a specific patient. In helping a patient learn to care for himself if he has right hemiplegia, there are certain obvious content items which must be included. If he is to learn to take care of himself, he must learn to be able to do his own personal hygiene, feed himself, care for himself at the toilet and dress himself.

It is important that the patient have the functional potential to do what is to be taught. In addition, the nurse must make sure that a patient is able to do certain preliminary steps before he is taught a skill. For instance, if a patient must learn a transfer procedure, he obviously must have trunk balance, be able to turn, be able to follow directions and be able to come to a sitting position.

Regardless of what the subject is, it is well to remember that the patient must first have a general overview of what you are going to teach. His feelings and needs can be explored at this time. Second, it is important to begin with simple concepts and later move on to the more complex ideas. Third, it is important to teach skills in a logical sequence of steps. In some instances, it might be best to teach just one or two steps at a time. For instance, if a patient is learning to come to a sitting position, at first it may be best for him to learn to turn over by grasping the side rail or the side of the mattress and to use the unaffected leg to help the affected leg. Once he has mastered turning over, he can then learn to move from the side lying to the sitting position. Selection of the size and number of teaching steps is naturally determined by the fatigue factor and by the intellectual ability of the patient.

ESTABLISHING A CLIMATE CONDUCIVE TO LEARNING

Whether the patient is merely taught or whether he actually learns is greatly related to the climate established by the teacher. First of all, much teaching is, can be and should be done informally and spontaneously as patient questions arise. However, teaching cannot be left entirely or even partially to chance. Content and objectives must be determined and adjusted according to whether the actual teaching takes place in an informal or formal manner, with one patient or with a group. This is far less important than the climate in which the patient learns. The latter will definitely affect learning.

Learners feel more comfortable when they have been consulted and have had some part in selecting the priorities and sequence of the material to be covered. Certain qualities can make the teaching situation humane and provide the patient with the kind of understanding and emotional support that help him to learn. The following attitudes and actions on the part of the instructor will be helpful in providing a desirable atmosphere.

• Begin by reviewing the mutually agreed upon objectives so that there is no misunderstanding of the purpose.

• Always reward patients for their responses and do this immediately. If they have done something correctly, praise them for the correctness and express warmth and genuine delight. If they have done something incorrectly, praise them for their efforts. All attempts to learn should be encouraged in every possible way.

• When a patient does something incorrectly, do not say, "That's wrong" or "You'll have to try it again." Sensitive persons are easily discouraged. Say such things as, "If you do it this way, it will be easier for you" or "You'll find the next time it will be less awkward if you do it the other way."

• Provide instruction in sequence and quantity that will allow for as many successes as possible. If too much is given at any one time, the patient is almost assuredly going to have a lot more failures. The aim is to minimize the number of failures.

• Give the student an opportunity to have some control over the length of the instructional session. You might say to him at the beginning, "Tell me when you get tired and feel that you have learned enough for today."

• Skills should be practiced in private rather than in public whenever feasible. This saves embarrassment when someone wonders if other people think he is stupid, slow or awkward. Such discomfort discourages efforts.

• Attempt to relate new information to his future life whether it be work, the role of a father or mother, preventing future hospitalizations and so forth.

Remember, research is telling us that learning takes place where people feel comfortable, where they are not frightened, where they do not have a lot of negative reactions. Few of us were taught this way, and unfortunately we do not have a large number of positive experiences upon which we can draw. However, learning is favorably influenced by the teacher who has a humane message in her attitude as well as helpful content in her words.

METHODS OF TEACHING

There are many methods of teaching—some are formal and some are informal. Generally speaking, there is the standard lecture method which is merely a presentation of facts and materials to one or more persons. Second, the discussion method provides for a verbal exchange between one or more persons. Greater interaction between instructor and learner can enhance more pertinent learnings. A very important method of teaching in health care is the demonstration and return demonstration. This, of course, is particularly appropriate to skills and is one that is used continually in the field of rehabilitation.

In reality, the nurse probably combines and adapts these three methods of teaching. In most subjects it is imperative to present some facts in order to provide some basic understanding and general knowledge. In addition, the nurse must provide for interaction with the patient, so that time must always be allowed for discussion. Another method that can be incorporated with other methods of teaching is the problem-solving technique. By having the patient identify a problem and some of the principles within a given learning situation, his future ability to work out problems at home can be developed.

In many instances, group teaching is more effective than individual teaching. It also has the virtue of saving teaching time. When group teaching is used, it is always helpful to follow-up individual patients to find out what differences in learning occurred so that individual help can be given in areas of less understanding.

Regardless of the method of teaching and regardless of whether the teaching is to an individual or a group, the nurse must be aware of the following problems, as they can interfere with the patient's learning and understanding.

• Speak loud enough and distinctly enough for the patient to hear.

• Use simple terms when speaking to patients because technical terms can interfere with learning. If you have a highly educated patient who wishes to speak in more technical terms, this is different. However, for the usual patient, remember to use lay terms. If you must use technical terms, be sure to define them.

• Plan content so that it proceeds from simple to complex ideas.

• Encourage questions at frequent intervals, and allow time for discussion of the answers.

• Permit a certain amount of ventilation of feelings.

• Do not ramble from the subject and try to remain with your objectives unless the patient finds it necessary to clarify other material before you can return to the particular objective of the day.

• Be sure there is good lighting and that the patient can see. Stand away from your work whenever you are demonstrating a procedure. All too frequently the nurse forgets that the patient cannot see what she is doing.

• Make sure that there is no noise interference from radios, Muzak, television, visitors and other patients, since these not only distract but also interfere with hearing.

• Vary your teaching as much as possible by the use of motion, color, personal reference or reference to other patients who have succeeded and found certain information helpful.

• Provide reading materials for the patient, either from textbooks, patient manuals or patient monographs on the subject. This is a particularly important feature of learning. It reinforces what was taught while you were in the presence of the patient by allowing him an opportunity to review the material and to think about it in greater detail.

• In teaching someone with a memory problem, use excessive drill to produce overlearning, and provide environmental cues such as colors and signs.

The use of visual aids and written materials can improve understanding in most instances. The nurse who has audiovisual materials at her disposal is indeed fortunate.

Whether it be slides, 8 mm. or 16 mm. films, filmstrips or transparencies, it is always worth locating good audiovisual materials. Naturally, few general staff nurses will have time to locate such materials for her teaching. She might, however, ask her supervisor or inservice director for materials that will enhance her teaching. For instance, there is a series of nine single concept films for paraplegia education (for patients) available from the National Medical Audiovisual Center in Georgia. This is only one example of films that are prepared for patients. This is a growing field, and as time goes on, more and more films will become available. When professional films are reviewed, patients should be considered because some films are appropriate for several audience levels.

In general, selection of methods of teaching is based on the needs of the patient, the manner in which the content can best be presented, the ability and condition of the patient and the resources of the institution.

EVALUATION OF TEACHING

Basically, evaluation of teaching should be called evaluation of learning and rightfully belongs under learning rather than teaching. It is a teacher responsibility, however, and for this reason is included under teaching. In order to evaluate, one must return to the original objectives and observe the patient to see if he has learned the skills, attitudes or knowledge that were originally established.

It is possible to prepare written examinations for some learning. This of course cannot be the responsibility of the general staff nurse. Preparing a good examination is both difficult and time consuming. In the case of intensive home training, such as patients who learn to do their own kidney dialysis, a written examination is an extremely effective method of evaluation. These are prepared by experts well in advance of the teaching.

In lieu of a written test, the nurse might ask questions. She should avoid questions which can be answered by yes or no because they give such limited information. Questions can be asked in such a way that the patient must give more complete answers. For example, "How do you plan to arrange your bedroom for most effective transfer?" or "What activities will prevent contractures?" Another way of evaluating learning is by asking and seeking expressions of feelings about what has been taught and general reactions to the subjects at hand.

Still another method of determining the amount of learning and assessing the need for further teaching is the home visit. The visiting nurse will observe if the patient is actually incorporating what is learned into his daily life. They will discuss any necessary adaptations and plan for future assistance as necessary. The next chapter will deal in greater depth with planning for home care. If one views chronic disability and illness as a family affair, both the patient and his family will be included in the teaching and the evaluation of learning. Home visits, therefore, will include assessment of broad aspects of the patient's life.

Even when a person has learned to care for himself, he or she may return home and switch methods or do only some of what was taught. Anselm Strauss has identified several reasons for this. Patients may feel that the procedures they learned in the hospital take too much time, require too much energy, make them too visible to others, cause too much isolation, cause too much pain, or are too costly financially. While the nurse can try to be aware of such factors, she may have virtually no control over them. She may try to identify the factors that are preventing the patient from following through on what he has learned, assess the potential harm and then work with him in terms of his motivations and perceptions.

PREPARING TEACHING PLANS

The following teaching plans are not meant to be all inclusive for each patient. They are, however, meant to exemplify the various facets of teaching which will occur during various stages of illness. One of the plans is related to a patient's stay in an acute hospital; one is related to patient follow-up in the home. The third teaching plan is related to care in an extended care facility. They are presented to indicate the variety of patients who will need teaching, and they also serve to demonstrate that teaching is a necessary part of all stages of a patient's illness as well as of his follow-up care. Each teaching plan could be adapted to patients with other conditions.

TEACHING PLAN 1

Setting: Patient's Home

Patient: 70-year-old woman who had right radical mastectomy two weeks ago. Lives alone

Objective: To gain maximum function of right arm

CONTENT	TEACHER ACTIVITY	PATIENT ACTIVITY
Physiology of disuse and exercise	Visit 1 on Monday: Discuss objective with patient	
Arm exercises	Describe problems of disuse and the result of exercise	
	Demonstrate exercises	Return demonstrate the exercises
		Identify daily activities which utilize these arm movements
	Leave pamphlets *After Mastectomy* and *Help Yourself to Recovery*°	Perform exercises t.i.d.
	Visit 2 on Thursday: Identify problems with pain and edema, gradually increasing range of motion and frequency of exercises	Describe problems and successes with daily activities
	Determine need for further visits	

°Available from American Cancer Society, 219 E. 42nd Street, New York, New York   10017.

TEACHING PLAN 2

Setting: Extended Care Facility

Patient: 40-year-old man with multiple sclerosis

Objective: To maintain maximum function of hands and arms

CONTENT	TEACHER ACTIVITY	PATIENT & FAMILY ACTIVITY
Range of Motion exercises of shoulder, elbow, wrist and fingers	Day 1: Explain purpose of exercises	
	Demonstrate exercises	Have patient return the demonstration on one side
	Discussion during return demonstration	Have wife return the demonstration on the other side
	*Leave monograph, *Range of Motion Exercises, Key to Joint Mobility.* Read pp. 9–12 and 17–36	
	Days 2–6, discuss and observe performance at intervals	Days 2–4: During the next few days, repeat return demonstrations until both patient and wife can perform the exercises.
		Days 4–6: Patient does exercises t.i.d. without reminding

---

*Available from Sister Kenny Institute, Chicago Avenue at 27th Street, Minneapolis, Minnesota 55404.

TEACHING PLAN 3

Setting: Hospital for Acute Disease

Patient: 57-year-old woman with emphysema just recovering from pneumonia

Objective: To perform postural drainage exercises

CONTENT	TEACHER ACTIVITY	PATIENT ACTIVITY
Anatomy and physiology of respiratory tract	Day 1: Discuss teaching objectives	Discuss
Pathology of emphysema	Give patient the booklet *Living with Asthma, Chronic Bronchitis, and Emphysema.** Read pp. 1–12	
Postural drainage exercises		
Factors affecting respiratory disease		Read pp. 1–12
	Day 2: Before lunch, question patient about reading	Describe anatomy, physiology and pathology of condition
	Using books, review various positions for postural drainage	Demonstrate postural drainage positions
	Before supper, supervise postural drainage with discussion	Postural drainage
	Day 3 and 4: Assist patient t.i.d. a.c. as needed, until performed as instructed without reminding.	Postural drainage t.i.d. a.c. independently

*Available from Riker Laboratories, Inc., Northridge, California.

SUMMARY

Patient learning is a key element in the patient's ultimate success and ease in adaptation to both major and minor changes in living. The nurse's role in accomplishing this goal is vital. Where there is a lack of understanding between the teaching role of the doctor and the nurse, it must be discussed and clarified so that the patient does not suffer merely because responsibilities are not clear. Teaching plans are essential in terms of what is being taught as well as who is responsible for the ultimate learning. Finally, the success of any teaching program depends on what the patient has learned and the application of that learning in his daily living.

The focus of the nurse must not be on herself; it must be on what the patient is learning. She must be able to answer the questions that were asked in the first paragraph of this chapter. Where am I going? Answer: Toward the patient's needs which are stated in my objectives. How am I going to get there? Answer: By creating a climate that has a positive effect emotionally and by using teaching methods that are appropriate to the subject. How will I know I've arrived? Answer: When the patient can demonstrate he has learned.

REFERENCES

Audiovisual Aids Utilized in Teaching Rehabilitation Nursing. Published by *American Journal of Nursing,* Educational Services Division, February 24, 1970.

Batterman, Betty, et al.: Hypertension. Part II. Treatment and nursing responsibilities. *Cardiovascular Nursing, 11*:41, September–October, 1975.

Coulter, Pearl P.: The role of the nurse in the prevention of illness and in health teaching. *In* Christopherson, V. A., et al.: *Rehabilitation Nursing: Perspectives and Applications.* New York, McGraw-Hill Book Co., 1974.

Cullin, Irene C.: Techniques for teaching patients with sensory defects. *Nursing Clinics of North America, 5*:527, 1970.

Fowler, R., and Fordyce, W.: Adapting care for the brain-damaged patient. *American Journal of Nursing, 72*:1832, October, 1972, and *72*:2056, November, 1972.

Hall, Edward: *The Silent Language.* Greenwich, Connecticut, Fawcett World Library, 1966.

Hayakawa, S. I.: *Language in Thought and Action.* New York, Harcourt Brace Jovanovich, 1964.

Hurd, Georgina G.: Teaching the hemiplegic self-care. *American Journal of Nursing, 62*:64, 1962.

Huston, Janet: Overcoming the learning disabilities of stroke. *Nursing '75, 5*:66, September, 1975.

If you ask me: What encourages general duty nurses to teach patients? *American Journal of Nursing, 60*:1236, 1966.

Larsen, George: After-stroke optokinetic nystagmus. *American Journal of Nursing, 73*:1897, November, 1973.

Mager, Robert F.: *Preparing Instructional Objectives.* Palo Alto, California, Fearon Publishers, 1962.

Mager, Robert F.: *Developing Attitude Toward Learning.* Palo Alto, California, Fearon Publishers, 1968.

Overs, R. P., and Belknap, E. L.: Educating stroke patients' families. *Journal of Chronic Disease, 20*:45, 1967.

Pfaudler, Marjorie: After-stroke motor skill rehabilitation for hemiplegic patients. *American Journal of Nursing, 73*:1892, November, 1973.

Pohl, Margaret: *The Teaching Function of the Nursing Practitioner.* Dubuque, Iowa, Wm. C. Brown Co., 1973.

Redman, Barbara, and Daly, Susan: Patient teaching for home hemodialysis. *In* Bergersen, Betty S., et al.: *Current Concepts of Clinical Nursing.* St. Louis, C. V. Mosby Co., 1969.

Redman, Barbara: *The Process of Patient Teaching in Nursing.* St. Louis, C. V. Mosby Co., 1972.

Schwartz, Doris: *The Elderly Ambulatory Adult.* New York, Macmillan, 1964.

Storlie, Frances: *Patient Teaching in Critical Care.* New York, Appleton-Century-Crofts, 1975.

Strauss, Anselm: *Chronic Illness and the Quality of Life.* St. Louis, C. V. Mosby Co., 1975.

Stryker, Ruth Perin: *Back to Nursing.* 2nd Ed. Philadelphia, W. B. Saunders Co., 1971, Chapter 7.

A Treasury of Techniques for Teaching Adults. National Association for Public School Adult Education, 1201 16th Street, NW, Washington, D. C. 20036.

Chapter 11

PLANNING FOR DISCHARGE

Nursing is an integral part of all stages of patient care, regardless of the setting. Although the same nurse will not accompany a patient from hospital to rehabilitation center to home, the need for nursing care nonetheless continues in each place. If adequate information accompanies the patient from place to place or agency to agency, care can be continued just as if the same nurse had come along. The aim, therefore, is for nursing to extend itself beyond the institution and to provide for uninterrupted care, usually referred to as continuity of care. It is anticipated and generally conceded that the patient will reach his or her highest potential after discharge, not during hospitalization.

At a recent conference, a paraplegic lecturer startled his audiences of rehabilitation nurses by stating, "My rehabilitation just began in the hospital. Ninety per cent of my rehabilitation occurred after discharge." He continued to humble his audience. "The nursing goals at discharge were not relevant six months later. I can do things none of my doctors, therapists or nurses thought I could do." Let this be a warning to all care givers—sometimes our discharge goals are not high enough. Lack of imagination and the fear of being unrealistic often lead to low expectations on the part of health professionals. The discharged person with drive and motivation may continue to adapt and rehabilitate himself over a period of years, reaching goals that only he thought himself capable of.

On the other hand, the person who has a progressive degenerative process may have only increasing dependence and decreasing activity to look forward to. In fact, some individuals may need to have goals that center on helping them to cope with stresses resulting from their condition. More important than goals, therefore, is an accurate description of what the person can do, what he cannot do and where assistance is required.

Modern health care practice assigns the responsibility for uninterrupted care to the institution or agency. Continued supervision after discharge must be considered a part of the care given at the institution. It is considered a "moral, medical and economic" necessity for optimum care. Patients who do not have follow-up care often suffer additional and unnecessary problems, and re-admissions are all too frequent. Re-admissions are costly in terms of dollars, in terms of physical drain and regression of the patient, and in terms of the negative emotional impact on and discouragement of both the patient and the family.

In the latter part of 1974, it was made mandatory for long-term care facilities to have a discharge plan for all Medicare and Medicaid patients. Basically, such a plan includes (1) assessment of medical, nursing, social and emotional needs, (2) evaluation of a rehabilitation potential, and (3) a review of available care alternatives. This regulation also requires documentation of procedures and persons responsible for discharge planning. While one could argue that discharge is not a realistic goal for many older persons, some rehabilitation goals are almost always possible to achieve. This regulation can influence the lives of nursing home patients by changing the focus of goals of care. No matter how successful a rehabilitation program has been, it may be of little ultimate value if the patient is not prepared to function outside the protective environment of an institution. If patients encounter problems with which they are unable to cope, they will not only become discouraged but they will also lose some of the function already learned. Many studies indicate that a large number of "rehabilitated" patients regress when follow-up care is absent. Such regression is usually prevented when a public health nurse works with the patient while he is adapting to home and to the many overwhelming physical and psychological experiences that occur when life with a disability begins.

Successful continuity of care may mean a referral to a public health nursing agency. Many nurses have not had public health experience and cannot anticipate the needs and problems that require the specific services of a public health nurse. In the case of the disabled, this can be particularly damaging because of the long-term effects on the patient.

The role of the public health nurse is basically that of case finding, referral and follow-up. The public health nurse teaches patients, counsels them, helps them to adjust to using equipment, helps them to adapt to home problems (many of which cannot be anticipated) and seeks additional consultation when indicated. One of the major contributions is to work with the family as well as the patient. In the case of follow-up care of a person with a disability, a major role is to assist both the patient and family to cope with the reality and the consequences of that disability.

Because the lack of accountability is viewed as causing lack of or poor continuity of care, the Steering Committee of the NLN Division of Nursing Services recommends the following:

1. Appoint one person, preferably on a full-time basis, to work with staff members in developing plans for the next stage of nursing care, even as the present stage is being provided.

2. Develop well-defined, clearly written procedures for patient referral, and interpret them to the entire staff.

3. Confer on the appointed person the administrative authority to carry out the continuity program.

4. Delegate to the appointed person responsibility for effective planning and ongoing communication with appropriate service agencies.

In addition to the above, continuity of care requires the coordination of services, which may be few or many. The person may need only a physician and a nurse, or the services of a social worker, vocational counselor, physical therapist and speech pathologist may also be required.

DISCHARGE TO WHERE?

During hospitalization, information about the patient's home, his family members and the general family relationships is obtained. The social worker will be deeply involved in this aspect of care. Ultimately, the patient, the family, the doctor and the social worker come to a joint decision as to whether the person will go home or elsewhere. If the decision is to live at home or in special housing, evaluation of the success of their decision will be a responsibility of the public health nurse. In some instances, temporary arrangements may be made for purposes of evaluation.

Generally speaking, most authorities feel that a disabled person benefits most by living at home with his family. In some instances, however, the family situation may make this impossible. Family members may be unable to take care of the disabled person because of their age, lack of mental ability, lack of physical capacity and other responsibilities. If the patient does not get along with his family, living at home could be detrimental. If living at home is detrimental either to the patient or to the family, other arrangements must be made. In most instances, however, the home is tried first before other arrangements are made.

If a person is not discharged to his home, he can consider several other alternatives, especially in metropolitan areas. Besides state institutions, there are non-institutional or non-custodial living centers. Some nursing homes offer an environment that may be appropriate. There are special residential centers in some cities where disabled persons can live relatively independently. Foster homes are frequently available. Low-rent housing units for the semi-independent are often an answer. Living in small groups may be preferred by disabled persons. Sometimes a young person will choose to live at home for a while but will then want to try a residential center with others his own age, just as any young adult may wish to leave home. All of these possibilities must be evaluated according to the individual's place in the family, preferences, financial resources, condition and family relationships.

THE BEGINNING

Just before writing this chapter, I talked to a young paraplegic man who had left the Sister Kenny Institute about two months previously. I asked him what he wished he had known when he was first injured. He answered immediately, "Tell them to tell us that we can do all of the things we did before." He added, "For months I didn't realize that I would be able to have a home, a job, friends or family, or even that I would be able to go fishing. Knowing this would have helped me to accept the permanence of my disability."

For this and other reasons, planning for care at home must begin as close to the time of admission as is possible. Naturally, it must be postponed during any acute illness in which the matter of life or death is a question. Throughout the hospitalization and during a rehabilitation program, thought must be given to how the patient will care for himself at home. Plans will be re-assessed according to new information as it is gathered. For example, it may initially seem wise for the patient to go home. As the social worker, the nurse or the psychologist learns to know the family situation, however, it may become evident that family relationships could be harmful rather than helpful to the patient. In this event, discharge planning would obviously be altered. On the other hand, a family that initially seems non-supportive may appear this way because of lack of confidence and fear about how to manage home care. In this event, the family will learn and probably be able to cope with the situation.

In the beginning, estimates of future functional potential are usually possible. While this will also be re-evaluated, overall future needs are usually clearly indicated. More detailed needs will emerge as time goes by. In addition, the fi-

REQUEST FOR HOME EVALUATION

To: _____
   [name of agency]

From: Rehabilitation Institute
   Re: _____
       [name, address and telephone number of patient]

Date: _____

The above patient is presently at our center. In order to plan his future program, we would greatly appreciate your assessment of the home.

Hospital Data

Diagnosis & disability: _____

_____

Date of admission: _____

Person or relative to contact: _____

_____

Insurance: _____

1. What are the family's concerns about the patient, his disability and his return home?

2. Who is likely to assume the responsibility for care of the patient and what seems to be the attitude of this person about this responsibility?

3. Who is in the family and what is the health status of other family members?

4. Does the emotional and physical environment seem conducive to the patient's progress and adjustment after discharge?

5. When is it most convenient for family members to be available for teaching?

6. Additional comments:

_____
                                    [signature of interviewer]

Return To: [name of nurse or social worker,
              address of institute]

Figure 11-1   Request for Home Evaluation form.

nancial impact on the family will be explored, usually by the social worker, and resources will be recommended.

THE FAMILY

During any hospitalization, whether short-term or long-term, it is important to include the family. During the hospitalization of a person who will be disabled, the inclusion of the family becomes even more essential. When the family lives in town, it is not difficult to arrange for interviews with the person who has primary responsibility for planning home care. Depending upon the institution, this will be done by a nurse, a social worker or a psychologist. If the family lives out of town, this person must gather information either by questionnaire or by telephone between visits.

It is this author's feeling that sending a questionnaire to a family is impersonal and may give partial and sometimes misleading information. For example, some family questionnaires ask such questions as, "Do you expect to take care of the patient after discharge?" If the family checks "yes," they do not even have an opportunity to learn what this will entail.

When the patient lives out of town, there are two major ways of exchanging information with the family. The first is a direct phone call to obtain an initial impression about their attitude toward the patient, the disability and the possibility of a return home. At this time, the family has an opportunity to ask questions which can be answered directly. It is then possible to find out when the family can come to the institution for an interview as well as for necessary instructions. This provides an opportunity to find out about the health status of other family members and the kinds of problems they have, and to discuss ways of alleviating some of these problems.

A second way of contacting the family is through the local public health nurse. For instance, a Request for Home Evaluation (Fig. 11–1) may be sent to the local public health nursing agency. The public health nurse will obtain the information requested and add other impressions determined as a result of her personal contact. While such information is admittedly second hand, it does provide a dimension that neither a phone call nor a questionnaire can.

EVALUATION OF THE PHYSICAL ENVIRONMENT

If the patient is going to use a wheelchair, crutches or braces, the home must be evaluated in terms of obstacles and safety for use of such equipment. The three most common architectural problems encountered by the patient at home concern the entrance to the home, the bathroom and the bedroom. Many barriers to a normal life are not due to the disability but to the width of doorways, the thickness of carpeting, the number of stairs and so forth.

When the family begins to think about their home in terms of a person with a disability, they will be asked to evaluate their house. This is done by asking the family to draw a written floor plan of their house and to fill in information similar to that requested in the Home Questionnaire (Fig. 11–2). This information should be brought or mailed to a specific person at the rehabilitation institute, hospital or nursing home. If any major alterations are necessary, the family will need time to make them.

HOME QUESTIONNAIRE

FOR

_____

[*name of person*]

I. Number of floors of home _____ Split-level? _____ Apartment? _____
basement? _____ ground floor? _____ second floor? _____

If house has more than one story or is split-level:
No. steps to upper level: _____
Width of steps: _____
Depth of steps: _____
Height of steps: _____
Are the steps covered? _____ If yes, what is the covering? _____
Is there a railing? _____ If yes, on which side? _____

II. Entrances:

Front	*Back*
No. steps: _____	No. steps: _____
Width of steps: _____	Width of steps: _____
Depth of steps: _____	Depth of steps: _____
Height of steps: _____	Height of steps: _____
Railing? _____	Railing? _____
Which side? _____	Which side? _____

III. Bathroom:

Please sketch arrangement of bathroom, location of window and the direction
in which the door swings open.

Floor on which the bathroom is located: _____
Dimensions of room: _____
Width of door: _____
Is there a tub? _____ Is there a shower? _____
Are the wall studs located where sturdy installation of a hand rail is
possible? _____

IV. Bedroom:

Floor on which bedroom is located: _____
Dimensions of room: _____ Width of door: _____
Is there a threshold? _____

V. Other comments or questions:

If you are not coming for a visit during the next week, kindly mail this to:
[*name of appropriate person at institute,*
name of institute,
address of institute]

Figure 11–2   Home Questionnaire form.

HOMEMAKING INFORMATION

Name_____

1. Do you plan to perform homemaking activities?

2. Number and ages of family members at home:

3. Will you have to help with the housework when you return home?

4. Kitchen:

   a. Dimensions and arrangement (diagram on separate sheet).

   b. Amount and height of counter space:

   c. Type of stove (gas, electric), and location of dials:

   d. Cupboard arrangement:

   e. What appliances do you own?

5. Laundry:

   State the kind and location of laundry, drying and ironing equipment. If you have a washer and dryer, do they load from the top or front? Is the ironing board adjustable?

6. Cleaning:

   Number of rooms:_____

   Type of cleaning equipment:_____

   Kinds of rugs and floors:_____

Figure 11-3   Homemaking Information form.

The use of such a questionnaire is obviously a formalized way of obtaining information and is necessary for persons who have a severe disability or who are dependent on a wheelchair. Patients with very little disability, however, may have an equally difficult time in leading an independent life even when a problem is temporary. For example, a 72-year-old diabetic man who had had severe vascular problems of the legs was discharged from a general hospital. He was told that because of his legs and his cardiac condition he was not to go up or down stairs for about four weeks. He lived alone in a fourth floor walkup. No one had inquired whether he could carry out the medical orders, and he had not mentioned it. Perhaps he did not think about it in his desire to leave the hospital to save money. How was he to obtain groceries? How was he to visit the doctor? How was he to get his prescribed exercise? He was discharged without any discharge planning and without a public health nursing referral. When he was readmitted because of his inability to carry out his treatment program, his problem came to light.

In the case of a person with a colostomy or ileostomy, the room of concern is, of course, the bathroom. The nurse taking care of such a postoperative patient needs to be informed of the facilities and conveniences that should be available for independence and care. It would be fruitless to cite further examples. Suffice it to say that when a patient leaves an institution, management of care (self-care or care by an attendant) must not be left to chance.

If the patient is a homemaker, further information is required. The form Homemaking Information, shown in Figure 11–3, is an example of the types of questions asked by the occupational therapist. The nurse may have some responsibility for providing resources in this area if occupational therapy services are unavailable. (See the bibliography for resources at the end of Chapter 17.)

TRANSPORTATION

If the patient is told to return to a clinic, whether it be for speech therapy, physical therapy, vocational evaluation or general medical follow-up care, how the patient will get there must be considered. Will the patient's family be able to take him? Will he require a special conveyance? Will he have to employ an ambulance or special medical bus, or will he have learned how to drive his own car with adaptive equipment? (The latter will be discussed in greater detail in Chapter 18.)

JOBS AND SCHOOL

While the person is still in the hospital, consideration must be given to his future. Will he or she be able to work or go to school? What financial assistance will be needed? Special education during hospitalization for those in grade school and high school is usually available through the public school system. Prevocational evaluation along with psychometric testing can also be completed when an interdisciplinary team is available.

After discharge, vocational plans will be pursued in greater detail. Referral to the State Division of Vocational Rehabilitation would of course be the first step. The public health nurse can be of immense assistance if these problems have not been explored prior to discharge, and will assist in various ways if the referral has been made. (See Chapter 18 for additional information.)

METHODS OF ESTABLISHING UNINTERRUPTED CARE

As the health team has become more aware of its responsibility toward the patient after discharge, various methods of accomplishing it have emerged. A special worker is sometimes assigned the responsibility. Some hospitals have instituted a position called the liaison nurse. Other job titles such as the nurse coordinator, the referral nurse or the extended care nurse are also used. Regardless of the title, the nurse with this position has the responsibility of working with the patient, his family and the health team, and of coordinating referral to community resources. Almost every state and large community has a list of agencies available. The liaison person will naturally have this information at her finger tips and will explore every resource that seems appropriate for a particular situation.

In some instances, the liaison nurse visits the home prior to a patient's discharge and once or twice after discharge. This does not preclude referral to a public health nurse unless the problem is only temporary and can be handled in these few visits. In fact, it is usually this nurse who communicates with the public health nurse.

Another way of providing continuity of care is for a liaison nurse to be on the staff of a public health nursing agency. In this instance, the public health nurse visits patients in the hospital prior to discharge. The head nurse helps to identify patients with referral needs. The public health nurse then talks to doctors and to various members of the health team and prepares the patient for home. This system has an advantage because it also allows the public health nurse to attend interdisciplinary conferences and nursing care conferences prior to discharge. In this case, she makes the actual referral to the nursing agency as well as to other appropriate agencies.

Regardless of the system used, whether the nurse in the institution goes to the home, whether the public health nurse comes to the hospital or whether communication takes place by telephone or written form, there are basic essentials to all continuity of care. The first is that someone in the hospital be assigned the responsibility of providing the patient with the best possible transition from institution to home, from institution to institution or from station to station within the institution. If this responsibility is not specifically assigned to someone, it seldom gets done. It may be the responsibility of the head nurse or it may be the responsibility of the nurse clinician, a clinical specialist or a liaison nurse. That it is assigned to someone as a regular part of their work is more important than who does it.

The second essential in any working plan for continuity of care is that the name of a specific person must be available. It is very difficult for a public health nurse to find out about a patient if she knows only that he was discharged from a particular hospital. If the hospital was large, it is especially difficult. By the time she finds out which station to call and locates the nurse who took care of the patient (and it is probably her day off), the entire process of referral becomes frustrating and cumbersome. This can be avoided if the person sending a referral signs her name. This ensures exact identification of the person having information about the patient.

The third way of providing continuity of care is through a written referral form. These are sometimes called discharge reports, transfer forms or information transmittal forms. These forms may have the same pitfalls discussed in relation to nursing care plans. The kind of form is far less important than what is put on it. They may be small and inadequate for the rehabilitation patient, they may require detailed information or they may merely consist of a Xeroxed copy of the nursing care plan. If the care plan was adequate, it clearly identifies the data gathered, specific problems and successful approaches. At institutions where there is copious book work and no one seems to have time to make out a lengthy referral form, a note can be added to the Xeroxed nursing care plan. This may be quite adequate and is most certainly better than no information, which is all too often what the public health nurse receives. Figure 11–4 is an example of a Patient Assessment Record. This can be used in a variety of ways—as a record to be used by the community nurse, as a referral to or from a public health agency or as a referral to or from an institution.

PATIENT ASSESSMENT

PATIENT'S NAME:	FACILITY/AGENCY	PATIENT'S RECORD NUMBER

HOME ADDRESS:	REFERRED FROM:	DATES FROM TO

PATIENT'S SOCIAL SECURITY OR MEDICARE NUMBER:	DIAGNOSES:

PATIENT'S MEDICAID NUMBER:	

OTHER HEALTH CARE COVERAGE: SPECIFY	

PREVIOUS LONG TERM CARE FACILITIES-NAME(S):	DATES FROM TO	

SUMMARY OF ADMISSIONS AND DISCHARGES THIS FACILITY/AGENCY

DATES OF ADMISSION			DATES OF DISCHARGE			PLACE: 0. HOME, NO REFERRAL 1. HOME, REFERRAL TO AGENCY: SPECIFY 2. OTHER HEALTH CARE FACILITY: SPECIFY 3. FUNERAL HOME: SPECIFY	DATES OF ASSESSMENT			LEVELS OF CARE
MONTH	DAY	YEAR	MONTH	DAY	YEAR		MONTH	DAY	YEAR	

INSTRUCTIONS: CHECK ALL BOXES WHICH APPLY. FILL IN ALL SPACES AS INDICATED

BIRTH DATE:
MONTH   DAY   YEAR

BIRTH PLACE: SPECIFY STATE OR COUNTRY
☐ USA
☐ Other

SEX:
☐ Male
☐ Female

RACE:
☐ White ☐ Other: Specify
☐ Negro

RELIGIOUS PREFERENCE: ☐ None
☐ Catholic   ☐ Protestant
☐ Jewish   ☐ Other: Specify _____

MARITAL STATUS:
☐ Single   ☐ Divorced
☐ Married   ☐ Separated
☐ Widowed   Duration of Status _____

FAMILY INCOME: ☐ Unknown
☐ $15,000 or more   ☐ $5,000 - $6,999
☐ $10,000 - $14,999 ☐ $3,000 - $4,999
☐ $7,000 - $9,999   ☐ Less than $3,000

EDUCATION: ☐ No Schooling
☐ Graduate College ☐ High School Diploma
☐ Undergraduate Col. ☐ Elementary/High School
  Degree or Yrs.____   Grades Completed _____
☐ Trade, Tech. or   ☐ Special Education
  Vocational   Yrs. _____

USUAL OCCUPATION: ☐ Housewife
Specify   ☐ Never Employed
_____

EMPLOYMENT STATUS: ☐ Never Employed
☐ Currently Employed ☐ Retired
☐ Sick Leave   ☐ Pension
☐ Currently Unemployed ☐ No Pension

DISCHARGE PLANNING:
☐ Discharge Anticipated: ☐ Discharge Not
  To Where?   Anticipated: Reason

NUMBER OF LIVING CHILDREN: _____
Son(s) _____   Daughter(s) _____

USUAL LIVING ARRANGEMENTS:
☐ Home - Apartment   ☐ Alone
☐ Rented Room(s),   ☐ With Spouse
  Commercial   ☐ With Others: Specify
☐ Domiciliary/Personal
  Care Facility   _____
☐ Health Care Facility _____
  Type _____   _____

ATTENDING PHYSICIAN: NAME	TEL. NO.	PERSON TO BE NOTIFIED: NAME	TEL. NO.
ADDRESS		ADDRESS	RELATIONSHIP
ALTERNATE PHYSICIAN: NAME	TEL. NO.	OTHER PERSON TO BE NOTIFIED: NAME	TEL. NO.
ADDRESS		ADDRESS	RELATIONSHIP
ATTENDING DENTIST: NAME	TEL. NO.	PHARMACY: NAME	TEL. NO.
ADDRESS		ADDRESS	
ATTENDING PODIATRIST: NAME	TEL. NO.	FUNERAL DIRECTOR: NAME	TEL. NO.
ADDRESS		ADDRESS	

HARVARD CENTER FOR COMMUNITY HEALTH AND MEDICAL CARE   JULY, 1975

Figure 11–4 Four-part Patient Assessment and Referral form. (Courtesy Harvard Center for Community Health and Medical Care. Developed under DHEW grant #HS-01162.)

Page 2

INSTRUCTIONS: CHECK ALL BOXES WHICH APPLY. FILL IN ALL DIAGONALS AS INDICATED. "DESCRIBE HELP" IS TO INCLUDE NUMBER OF HUMAN ASSISTANTS AND/OR TYPE OF MECHANICAL AID.

Patient's Name _____

Patient's Number _____

Name of Facility _____

FUNCTIONING STATUS ITEMS

MOBILITY LEVEL — DATE
- Goes Outside Facility/Home
- Moves About Inside Facility/Home
- Confined to Bed and Chair
- Confined to Bed

DESCRIBE HELP

WHEELING — DATE
- Does Not Wheel-Walks
- Wheels Self
- Is Wheeled by Others
- Does Not Wheel (Confined to Bed or Bed and Chair)

DESCRIBE HELP

WALKING
- Walks
- Does Not Walk — (Bed and Chair)
- Confined to Bed

DESCRIBE HELP

TRANSFERRING
- Transfers Self
- Is Lifted
- Does Not Transfer (Confined to Bed)

DESCRIBE HELP

BATHING
- Bathes Self
- Is Bathed

DESCRIBE HELP

STAIRCLIMBING
- Climbs Stairs
- Does Not Climb Stairs

DESCRIBE HELP

DRESSING
- Dresses Self
- Is Dressed
- Is Not Dressed

DESCRIBE HELP

EATING/FEEDING
- Feeds Self
- Is Spoon Fed
- Fed via Syringe, Tube, I.V., Clysis

DESCRIBE HELP

TOILETING
- Uses Toilet Room, Day and Night
- Uses Toilet Room & Bedpan, Urinal and/or Commode
- Does Not Use Toilet Room

DESCRIBE HELP

BEHAVIOR PATTERN
- Appropriate
- Inappropriate - Once a Week or Less Often
- Inappropriate - More Often Than Once a Week

DESCRIBE INAPPROPRIATE BEHAVIOR

BOWEL FUNCTION
- Continent
- Incontinent less than once a week
- Incontinent more than once a week
- "Ostomy" or other problem

TYPE OF OSTOMY CARE OR OTHER PROBLEM

COMMUNICATION OF NEEDS
- Communicates Verbally — English
- Communicates Verbally — Other Language
- Communicates Non Verbally
- Does Not Communicate

DESCRIBE LANGUAGE BARRIER OR NON-VERBAL COMMUNICATION

BLADDER FUNCTION
- Continent
- Incontinent - less than once a week
- Incontinent more than once a week
- Indwelling Catheter
- "Ostomy" or other problem

TYPE OF OSTOMY CARE OR OTHER PROBLEM

ORIENTATION: Time, Place and Person
- Oriented
- Disoriented—Some Spheres Some Time
- Disoriented—Some Spheres All Time
- Disoriented—All Spheres Some Time
- Disoriented—All Spheres All Time

INDICATE SPHERES AFFECTED

HARVARD CENTER FOR COMMUNITY HEALTH AND MEDICAL CARE   JULY, 1975

Figure 11–4 *Continued.* (2)

Page 3

INSTRUCTIONS: CHECK ALL BOXES WHICH APPLY
FILL IN ALL SPACES AS INDICATED.

Patient's Name _____
Patient's Number _____
Name of Facility _____

IMPAIRMENT ITEMS

	NO IMPAIR-MENT	IMPAIR-MENT	COMPLETE LOSS	COMPENSATION, TYPE OF IMPAIRMENT	DATE				
SIGHT					**THERAPIES:** SPECIFY FREQUENCY				
HEARING					PHYSICAL				
SPEECH					OCCUPATIONAL				
	NO TEETH MISSING	SOME OPPOSING TEETH	NO TEETH OR NO OPP. TEETH	TYPE OF DENTURES: NONE, UPPER, LOWER, BOTH	SPEECH				
DENTITION					INHALATION				

PARALYSIS/PARESIS   ☐ None
Type   Date of Onset   Location (If applicable)

SOCIAL SERVICE				
OTHER: SPECIFY				

EXTREMITY	MISSING LIMBS Date of amputation, Type: (BE, AE, BK, AK), Prosthesis: (P)	FRACTURED HIP(S) Date, Repair (R) or Prosthesis (P)	OTHER FRACTURES/ DISLOCATIONS Date, Specific Bone or Joint	EXTREMITY	JOINT MOTION Specify (—) or Within Normal Limits (WNL) or Indicate joint and disorder: Limited Motion (LM) Contracture (C), Instability (I), or Pain & Swelling (P&S)			
UPPER R		////////		UPPER R				
L		////////			L			
LOWER R				LOWER R				
L					L			

MEDICALLY DEFINED CONDITIONS

Present (✓)	CONDITION	Onset Month	Year
	Alcoholism		
	Anemia — Type:		
	Angina/M.I.		
	Arthritis — Type:		
	Cardiac Arrhythmia —Type:		
	Congestive Heart Failure		
	Diabetes Mellitus		
	Drug Abuse — Type:		
	Hypertension — Type:		
	Malignancy — Location:		
	Mental Illness — Type:		
	Neurological Disorders— Type:		
	Respiratory Disease (Chronic) — Type:		

RISK FACTOR MEASUREMENTS

FACTOR	INDICATE DATE AND READING			
Height (Record once)				
Weight				
Blood Pressure				
Blood Cholesterol				
BUN				
Albuminuria				
Blood Sugar (Specify Test)				
Dig. Level (Specify Test)				
Hemoglobin or Hematocrit				
Prothrombin Time				
Serum Potassium				
Other: Specify				

Cigarette Smoking (✓)   # PER DAY
Never Smoked _____ Currently Smokes _____
Ex-Smoker __ Does Not Smoke, History Unknown _____

COMMENTS/ADDITIONAL INFORMATION:

HARVARD CENTER FOR COMMUNITY HEALTH AND MEDICAL CARE   JULY, 1975

Figure 11–4 *Continued.* (3)

Page 4

INSTRUCTIONS: FILL IN ALL SPACES AS INDICATED					Patient's Name _____

Patient's Name _____
Patient's Number _____
Name of Facility _____

DATE					DATE				
MEDICATIONS: WRITE EACH MEDICATION IN ITS THERAPEUTIC CATEGORY. INDICATE DOSE. FREQUENCY AND ROUTE OF ADMINISTRATION.					**SPECIAL NURSING PROCEDURES**: SPECIFY FREQUENCY, SITES AND/OR TREATMENT IF APPLICABLE				
Analgesics/Narcotics					Decubitus Care: Site(s)				
Antacids									
Antibiotics/ Anti-Infective									
Anticoagulants					Dressing(s): Sites:				
Anticonvulsives									
Antihypertensives					Eye Care: Specify				
					Oxygen R_x: Type				
Bowel Regulators					Restorative Nursing: Bowel and/or Bladder Training: Specify				
					ROM Exercises: Sites				
Cardiac Regulators					Other: Specify				
Diuretics/ Electrolytes					Restraints: Sites of Application				
					Teaching: Ostomy Care: Type				
Insulin/ Hypoglycemics					Self Injection: Specify				
Sedatives/ Barbiturates					Other: Specify				
Tranquilizers/ Antidepressants					Other Special Nursing: Specify				
Vasodilators					**PROFESSIONAL VISITS**: INDICATE NUMBER OF TIMES PATIENT HAS BEEN VISITED SINCE LAST ASSESSMENT				
Vitamins/Iron					Attending M.D./D.O.				
Others: Specify					Other M.D./D.O.				
					Dentist				
					Podiatrist				
					Other: Specify				
NUTRITION					**PSYCHOSOCIAL ITEMS**: SPECIFY FREQUENCY				
Diet: Specify					Visitors				
Food/Fluid Intake: No Problem (√) Problem Specify					Recreation/Activities Program				
					Reality/Remotivation Program				
Supplemental Nourishments: Specify					Religious Services				
Dining Location: Specify					Other: Specify				

HARVARD CENTER FOR COMMUNITY HEALTH AND MEDICAL CARE   JULY, 1975

Figure 11–4 *Continued.* (4)

NURSING CARE REFERRAL ATTACHMENT

June 5, 1977

This 22-year-old man was struck broadside by a car while riding his motorcycle on April 24, 1975 and was immediately quadriplegic with a C6 fracture. He was on our PM & R service from August 25, 1975, to January 30, 1976, when he had intensive rehabilitation. During this time he had a suprapubic cystostomy.

The patient has permanent paralysis of his lower extremities. He is dependent in bladder and bowel function and, in addition, has partial paralysis of his upper extremities. He will need part-time nursing care. He has had decubitus ulcers on his knees, tibial crest and sacrum. These areas remain sensitive and will have to be watched closely, as will the ischial areas. He must wear socks at night to protect his feet, and the socks must be on straight. He can be positioned on abdomen at h.s. with pillows under chest, thighs and legs. Catheter must be checked to be sure it's free when on abdomen. He can be up in a wheelchair from four to eight hours now, but ischial areas should be checked q.d. for redness.

He has a suprapubic catheter, which should be changed q. 4 weeks. It should be irrigated b.i.d. with saline, followed by instillation of 30 cc. renacidin q.d. He must continue to force fluids to 3000 cc. daily.

Bowel program consists of Dulcolax tab, 1 at h.s. on Sunday, Tuesday, and Thursday, and Dulcolax suppository and commode on Monday, Wednesday, and Friday a.m. He sometimes requires milk of magnesia p.r.n. the night before bowel movement.

He will need range of motion once daily, since he gets no exercise in the electric wheelchair. He is completely dependent in self-care when in bed, requiring total care for washing, dressing and transferring. He gets up in the wheelchair with use of Hoyer Lift. He has special adaptive wrist devices that allow him to shave, brush his teeth and practice writing. He can feed himself with help of plate guard, adaptive wrist device and special fork, and must be allowed to do this. Food must be cut. He needs a long drinking tube.

During former hospitalization he had periods of deep depression and withdrawal almost to the point of muteness, and he threatened several times to commit suicide. He is now struggling to find reasons for living and answers to such questions as, "Why did this have to happen to me?" His relationship with his family has not been a smooth one, but we have noticed some positive signs in this area. His mother is Italian and talks about taking him to Italy to have a miracle performed to restore him. In our contact with her, we found her to be very cooperative and very appreciative of anything done for her son. His father appears to be very accepting of having his son at home.

The consultant in psychiatric nursing has been working with him and will send you a more detailed report.

The patient is planning to assist his father in a snowmobile business—already in operation—from his parents' home. A telephone is available, and other adaptive measures to allow him to do bookkeeping are being planned.

He plans to go home from June 12 to June 16 on a trial leave. A home visit by you on the 15th of June would be most beneficial.

Equipment already at his home:
- 2 canvas corsets
- Bye-bye decubiti cushion
- Electric wheelchair
- Right- and left-hand splints
- 2 Dermatec pads
- Special plate guard, special fork and long drinking tube
- CO_2 operated hand splint
- Flotation pad and mattress
- Hi-Lo Bed

Figure 11–5 Dictated Nursing Care Referral Attachment.

A frequently overlooked tool is the dictating machine. This allows the nurse to give the information in less time than if she wrote it. Figure 11–5 is the attachment dictated about one patient at a rehabilitation hospital. As one can see, the information would be welcomed by any public health nurse following the patient after discharge.

The other side of the coin is the Public Health Nursing Report. Figure 11–6 is an example of the report of public health nursing visits to the home. This was sent back to the referring hospital. Instead, a Xeroxed copy of her own records could be mailed back to the appropriate person.

In reality, almost every chapter of this book deals with some area that must be considered in discharge planning. Repetition therefore is inadvisable. Nonetheless, there are specific questions that require the attention of the nurse who is responsible for discharge planning. While they originate from the basic nursing care plan, they stretch beyond it—the key to continuity of care! The following are major areas of concern:

1. Will the family and patient have an adequate opportunity to receive help while they are working out their initial problems of adjustment?

2. Will the family be able to adapt the physical environment to provide maximum independence for the patient?

3. What are the financial abilities of the family, and where can they obtain financial assistance? A social worker is essential in this area.

4. What equipment will be necessary for the patient?

5. What must he know in order to take care of himself?

6. What family teaching is essential to his care?

7. What additional resources must be sought—for example, an attendant? a

---

PUBLIC HEALTH NURSING REPORT

Patient's Name _____

6/8/76—On my first visit the family indicates they are eager to have their son home.
6/15/76—The patient was up in the wheelchair when I visited. They have been doing very well this weekend. I checked his equipment and they said they are a little clumsy in giving him care, but they will learn. He is irrigating his bladder twice a day and doing the instillation. He is taking his meds but he said his Inversine had been changed to twice a day and he has been perspiring profusely. He has been drinking large amounts of water. We discussed pressure areas and his care. They are very eager to have him discharged now. The sister will also learn how to give him his care.

A young paraplegic who I thought would be a very good friend lives nearby. Maybe an association like this will help keep up his interests at home. He wanted to know whether I would be able to change his catheter. I told him this must be done by the doctor at the clinic. I told him that I would be available and help them in any teaching in his care.

Signature of Nurse _____

Figure 11–6   Public Health Nursing Report. (Follow-up of patient described in Fig. 11–5.)

housekeeper? a home health aide? school referrals? outpatient treatment? medical follow-up? vocational training? social organizations? recreational groups?

8. What members of the health team will be needed after discharge?

9. Where can the patient go to obtain further information?

The overwhelming number of adjustments and changes will take place at a pace that is sometimes too rapid. Is it any wonder that persons with a disability need assistance after discharge? Follow-up may be more intense during the first few months after hospitalization, but regular visits from the nurse, often on an annual basis, are desirable for continued care in the future.

SUMMARY

Continuity of care is essential if the goals of the original rehabilitation program are to be fulfilled. It goes beyond the immediate discharge needs and acts as an available resource for changing needs. A heavy burden of responsibility lies with the nurse to assume responsibility for providing referrals for follow-up care. This must be an assignment within an institution, and it must be done prior to discharge, not on the last day as an afterthought while the patient is packing his clothes to leave. Evidence continues to mount that patients regress physically, emotionally and socially when follow-up care is not available. This not only has economic implications for our community but also indicates a lack of quality in our overall health program. While this chapter has emphasized the severely disabled person, the concept of discharge planning and continuity of care is no less important for the many patients who enter and leave our general hospitals and for those geriatric patients who go to nursing homes or other congregate care facilities. The nursing responsibility is the same.

REFERENCES

American Hospital Association: *Discharge Planning for Hospitals*. 840 North Lake Shore Drive, Chicago, Illinois 60611, 1974.

Anderson, E. M., and Irving, J.: Uninterrupted care for long-term patients. *Public Health Reports, 80*:271, 1965.

Barnard, M. E.: Here's how to plan for discharge of patients. *Modern Nursing Home, 28*:44, June, 1972.

Chien, Ching Piao, and Sharaf, Myron R.: Factors in the discharge of chronic patients. *Hospital and Community Psychiatry, 22*:24, August, 1971.

Collier, A. C., et al.: Rehabilitation center visiting nurses join forces in home care program. *Hospitals, 43*:92, 1969.

Commission on Professional and Hospital Activities: *Quality Assurance in Long-Term Care Facilities*. Ann Arbor, Michigan, 1975.

Community Service Society of New York: *Continuity in Care for Impaired Older Persons*. Department of Public Affairs, New York, 1965.

Conti, Mary Louise: Continuity of care for elderly discharge hospitalized patients. *In* Burnside, Irene: *Psychosocial Nursing Care of the Aged*. New York, McGraw-Hill Book Co., 1973.

Coombs, R. P.: Active-care hospital nurse expands her role. *Canadian Nurse, 66*:23, 1970.

David, Janis, Hanser, Johanne, and Madden, Barbara: *Guidelines for Discharge Planning*. Attending Staff Association of Rancho Los Amigos Hospital, Inc., Downey, California, 1968.

Gaspard, Nancy J.: The family of the patient with long-term illness. *Nursing Clinics of North America, 5*:70, 1970.

Holmes, Thelma M.: The changing role of the public health nursing services in the rehabilitation of patients. *In* Stewart, Dorothy, and Vincent, Pauline: *Public Health Nursing*. Dubuque, Iowa, Wm. C. Brown Co., 1968.

Jarrahizadeh, Ali, and High, Carol: Returning long-term patients to the community. *Hospital and Community Psychiatry, 22*:2, February, 1971.

Juntti, M. J.: Problem solving in arranging for comprehensive home care. *Nursing Forum, 8*:103, 1969.

Katz, Sidney, et al.: *Effects of Continued Care: A Study of Chronic Illness in the Home.* DHEW Publication No. (HSM) 73–3010. Superintendent of Documents, Washington, D. C., December, 1972.

LaRocco, A.: *Planning for Hospital Discharge: A Bibliography With Abstracts and Research Reviews* (HSRD-70-17). Rockville, Maryland, National Center for Health Services Research and Development, 1970.

Lowman, Edward, and Klinger, Judith: *Aids to Independent Living.* New York, Mcgraw-Hill Book Co., 1969.

Metropolitan Health Planning Corporation: *Conference on Discharge Planning.* 908 Standard Building, Cleveland, Ohio 44113, October, 1970.

Mitch, Anna D., and Kaczala, Sophie: The public health nurse coordinator in a general hospital. *Nursing Outlook, 16*:34, 1968.

National League for Nursing: *Continuity of Nursing Care from Hospital to Home.* New York, 1966.

Peabody, S. R.: Assessment and planning for continuity of care from hospital to home. *Nursing Clinics of North America, 4*:303, June, 1969.

Phoenixville Community Nursing Service: *A Study of the Feasibility of Home Rehabilitation of the Chronically Ill and Aged by a Visiting Nurse Association in a Small Community.* Phoenixville, Pennsylvania, 1966.

Robinson, Geraldine: From the hospital, where? *Nursing Outlook, 15*:47, 1967.

Saunders, Ethel, and Swinyard, Chester: The public health nurse's role in rehabilitation. *Nursing Outlook, 9*:426, 1961.

Sherman, John B.: Transfer of nursing home patients. *Michigan Medicine, 69*:579, 1970.

Tobis, Jerome S., and Zohman, Leonore: Follow-up study of cardiac patients on a rehabilitation service. *Archives of Physical Medicine and Rehabilitation, 51*:286, 1970.

Turner, Charlotte, and Mahoney, Robert: After hospitalization. *In* Stewart, Dorothy, and Vincent, Pauline: *Public Health Nursing.* Dubuque, Iowa, Wm. C. Brown Co., 1968.

Wensley, Edith: *Nursing Service Without Walls.* New York, National League for Nursing, 1963.

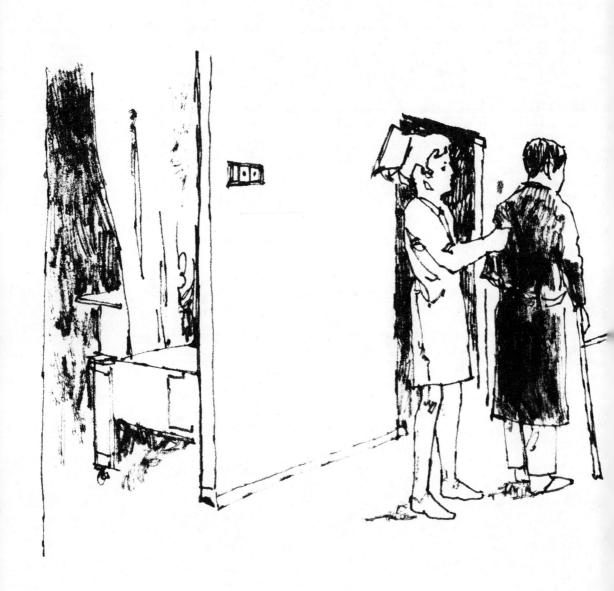

Unit III
NURSING SKILLS

Chapter 12

BODY MECHANICS—BASIC KNOWLEDGE FOR ALL NURSING PERSONNEL*

A knowledge of body mechanics and proper use of the body can be applied to activities performed every day. How we vacuum the carpet, how we pick up a dropped pencil, how we walk, sit, stoop and stand, how we get into a car and how we perform other everyday movements can affect us in many ways. Through better use of our body and better knowledge of a few basic principles of movement, all of us can reduce the amount of effort expended each day. We can reduce fatigue and strain as well as minimize the danger of injury to ourselves and to our patients. Practical application of such principles will enable both the patient and health personnel to conserve energy, to preserve muscle tone and joint mobility and to develop habit patterns of moving and lifting that will not cause trauma to muscles, ligaments and joints.

For the nurse such activities as bed making, moving a patient from chair to bed, moving a patient on and off a stretcher, bathing a patient and giving back care can be accomplished smoothly, efficiently and without fatigue. Many of us, however, go off duty with a backache. The effects of moving and lifting improperly can be more serious than just the backache. In one year in the United States, 12.5 persons in every thousand—over two million people—sustained back injuries and in some cases permanent disabilities as the result of improper lifting.

A sizable number of these injuries were incurred by nursing personnel who move and lift patients every day. These persons either did not know how to move and lift properly or were careless in their techniques. It is more likely that the knowledge had not been practiced often enough to become an automatic skill such as driving a car. Those who have sustained back injuries know that conscious effort and practice of proper body movement can prevent years of discomfort, disability and expense. This can become a test of our commitment to the rehabilitation principle of prevention. At any rate, health workers need to learn *and to perform regularly* methods of moving and lifting patients based on principles of body mechanics. This means, very simply, using the whole body—trunk, head and extremities—in a way that provides maximum efficiency and minimal strain. The same principles apply to patients and personnel alike.

---

*The author is indebted to the Sister Kenny Institute for permission to reprint parts of the section on equipment from their monograph *Moving and Lifting Patients: Principles and Techniques,* by Judith Andre Yates (1970).

It is obvious that the need for this information becomes even more crucial when working in an operating room, an orthopedic unit, a nursing home or a rehabilitation center. Not just a few but most patients will be dependent physically. As a result, the nurse will be moving and lifting not occasionally, but constantly. In addition, this area of knowledge relates to transfers, ambulation and sitting activities and so must be taught to patients, families and attendants. It is therefore essential that the nurse have a thorough grasp of the principles of body balance and the techniques in proper use of the body.

PRINCIPLES UNDERLYING USE OF THE BODY

BODY MECHANICS

Biomechanics, to use the broader and more accurate term, is the science dealing with the effects of energies and forces (both internal and external) on a body in motion or at rest. Very simply stated, it relates the forces in muscles, bones and joints with externally applied loads (the pull of gravity or some applied resistance). The motion and position of the body affect its ability to work against applied forces. From this rudimentary definition, it becomes clear that our concerns over movement, position and load are related to the complex sciences of mechanics, anatomy, musculoskeletal physiology and kinesiology (the science of body movement).

CENTER OF GRAVITY

The force of gravity is the mutual attraction that an object and the earth have for one another in a vertical direction. This force influences all human movements and can make motion easier whenever one can work with it rather than oppose it.

The magnitude of gravity depends upon the mass of the object. The point at which the mass is centered is called the center of gravity. The force of gravity is theoretically applied at this point because a suspended object will remain in balance if it is suspended at its center of gravity.

When an object is symmetrical, the center of gravity is at its geometrical center. The human body is, of course, not symmetrical. In the standing position, the center of gravity of the human being is located at about 55 per cent of the body's total height, in the pelvic cavity slightly anterior to the upper part of the sacrum. In moving and lifting, knowing the location of the center of gravity is important, since the lower the center of gravity the greater is an object's stability. Applied, this means that greater stability can be attained when the center of gravity is lowered by bending at the hips and knees.

The line of gravity is an imaginary vertical line passing through the center of an object perpendicular to its base of support. In the human being, a perpendicular line intersecting the body through the center of gravity and passing through the body's base of support is the human line of gravity (see Fig. 12–1). In moving and lifting, muscular effort must be increased to prevent falling whenever the line of gravity and the center of the base of support shift away from each other. Applied, this means that balance is most easily achieved when the body is erect and the base of support is widened.

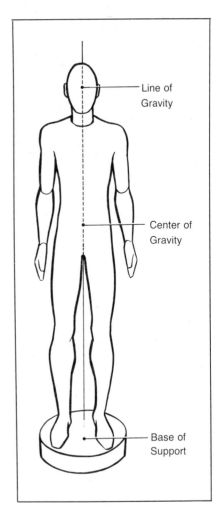

Figure 12–1 Locations of the line of gravity, the center of gravity and base of support.

Whenever you can, always push or pull an object instead of lifting it. If an object rests on the floor (such as a piece of furniture) it is mechanically easier to move it by pushing it. This is because you use your leg muscles and the weight of your body to make the effort. In addition, the forward movement of the body makes the change in your center of gravity almost automatic.

If an object is on an elevated surface (such as a patient on a bed or a box on a table), it is mechanically easier to move it by pulling it toward you. This is because one uses the flexor muscles of the arm to make the effort. In addition, the working surface of the bed or table blocks the movement of your body from going any way but backward, so any forward movement is limited by the extent of your reach. In this case, you alter your center of gravity by moving an object closer to you and/or bending at the hips and knees. In other words, *if you cannot push efficiently with your body, you must pull with your arms.*

If two or more persons are needed, and one of them must push, it is the person pushing who should direct the move, because he will have the greater amount of muscular strain. The number of assistants will vary according to (1) your capabilities and (2) the difficulty with which the patient moves. Never attempt to move an object or a patient alone if there is any doubt about your ability to do it without excess muscular strain.

FRICTION

Friction is a force opposing the movement of an object over a surface. When moving a patient or an object, the speed can be increased and the muscular force can be reduced if this resistance is decreased or eliminated. Applied, this means that when you move a patient in bed, you can lessen the resistance by reducing as much as possible the area of the patient's body that contacts the bed surface. The use of a sheet for lifting is helpful because the sheet can be raised slightly to decrease the amount of friction, and thus the patient can be moved more easily.

SUMMARY

Basically, there are three concepts that must be kept in mind whenever you move and lift. First, consider the location of your center of gravity; second, imagine the location of your line of gravity; and third, determine the necessary base of support. Understanding the relationship between these factors is essential whether you are moving and lifting at home or at work. This will enable you to use groups of muscles in concert with one another.

Applying the following principles will help prevent muscle strain, injury and fatigue. Remember that when these principles are *not* adhered to, some muscles are underused while others are overworked because they must compensate for faulty motions.

1. The relationship between the size of the base of support (your feet) and the location of the center of gravity (your pelvic area) determines stability.

2. Stability can be increased by lowering the center of gravity, by widening the base of support or by doing both (see Fig. 12–2). In other words, lower your pelvis or put more distance between your feet (front to back and sideways), or do both.

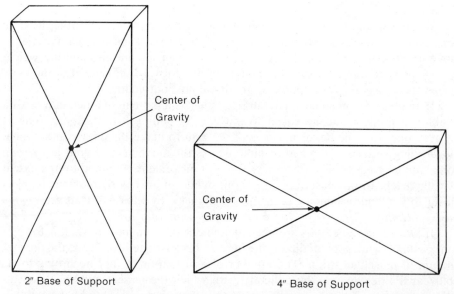

2″ Base of Support   4″ Base of Support

Figure 12–2   The stability of a 2 by 4 inch block is increased by lowering the center of gravity and widening the base of support.

3. When weight is added, the center of gravity shifts in the direction of the added weight. To compensate for this, carry or hold an object close to your center of gravity.

4. Reduce the amount of friction between surfaces.

POSTURE AND GUIDELINES FOR PREVENTING INJURY

STANDING POSTURE

Basically, good body mechanics means good preventive maintenance of your body. The effects of daily improper use of muscles or even an acute strain are seldom immediate. Most injuries and problems are cumulative and result from constant abuse.

While good posture helps a person to look and feel better, it also helps to make the body work more efficiently and operate with minimum strain. Correct posture means keeping the segments of the body in good alignment at all times—that is, during sitting, standing and walking. Sleeping posture is especially important for people with back strain and paralysis, and is essential for patients who must remain in bed for any length of time. The latter will be discussed in greater detail in Chapter 13.

In good standing posture, the feet are slightly apart, the toes face forward, the knees are slightly flexed and the stomach and buttocks are tucked in. The shoulders are held back and the chin is parallel to the floor.

If your job entails standing for long periods of time—in the operating room, for example—it will help if you shift your weight from one foot to the other and move your feet frequently in order to contract the muscles of the legs which in turn promotes circulation. If you have an opportunity to sit when on duty, it is important to do so whenever possible. There are many opportunities to sit down such as when stopping to visit patients. This also helps the patient! On the other hand, if you have a desk job, take every opportunity to stand and walk.

When you must stoop, be sure that you bend at the hips and the knees or alter the height of your work so that it is at a level that is as comfortable as possible. When you bend to reach your work, always remember to use your leg muscles, not your back muscles. *The muscles in your legs are meant to do the body's work. The back muscles are not.* Always try to avoid reaching. Use a stable step stool whenever you must reach for anything that is above your head. Keep your work close to you so that you do not have to stretch toward it. When you move or lift something from the standing position, remember to broaden your base of support. Put your feet apart with one slightly in front of the other, so that you *broaden the base of support from front to back as well as from side to side.* This also allows you freedom to move in all directions.

SITTING POSTURE

Sitting posture is extremely important and even more so for the inactive person who must use a wheelchair. A seat should provide both thigh and back support. It should be possible for the person to have the feet flat on the floor (or footrest); the head should be erect and the knees, ankles and hips should all be at right angles. In addition there should be space behind the knees so that circulation is not cut off by pressure from the edge of the chair seat.

There are four points which must be taken into account in order to attain proper sitting posture (see Fig. 12–3). First of all the seat height should be considered. Alterations must be made if there is undue pressure behind the knee or if the patient is unable to rest his feet flat on the floor. A small foot stool can be used under the feet to relieve pressure behind the knees when the seat is too high. A cushion may be placed on top of the seat to raise the patient if the seat is too low.

Secondly, the size of the seat is important. If it is too deep, a cushion can be placed at the patient's back. If it is too wide, a pillow can be placed between the patient and the armrests on each side to enable him to sit up properly. If the width and depth of the seat is too small, one would need a different size chair.

Arm height is also important to good sitting posture. If the patient tends to lean over in order to lower his arms to the armrest, chair arms can be raised by placing a pillow on each.

Fourth, the height of the back of the chair is important. In order to provide back support, the height should come to at least the lower part of the scapula at the level of the armpit.

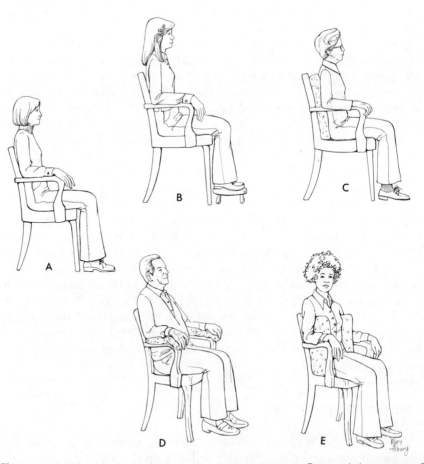

Figure 12–3   Adjustments to obtain correct sitting posture. *A*, Correct sitting posture. *B*, A foot stool to prevent pressure behind the knees. *C*, A pillow or cushion at the back to compensate for a seat that is too deep. *D*, Pillows or cushions under the arms to compensate for low armrests. *E*, Pillows or cushions at the sides to compensate for too wide a seat.

Can You Identify Errors in Body Mechanics?

(Mark C for correct and I for incorrect and give the reason—answers are at end of chapter.)

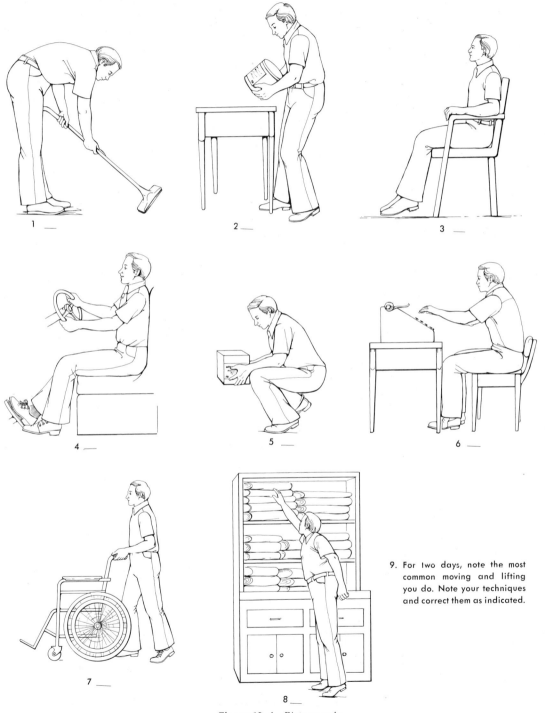

9. For two days, note the most common moving and lifting you do. Note your techniques and correct them as indicated.

Figure 12-4 Picture quiz.

When a person rises from a sitting position, the principles of gravity can be used to advantage. It becomes a great deal easier for anyone to rise without strain if he leans forward and places one foot slightly in front of the other one, which is placed well under the sitting surface. In this way, he has widened his base of support and shifted his center of gravity by leaning forward. This is useful to practice in our daily lives, very helpful to any weak patient who gets in and out of a chair and essential to learning standing transfer techniques. If the person holds onto a bed, chair or table for additional support, it must be sturdy and secure so that it will not move out from under the person.

These simple tricks of the trade will help any patient. We often forget to tell patients who have had major or minor surgery, those with heart conditions, the elderly and countless others how to move. This can immensely help their mobility and the ease with which they get in and out of bed and in and out of chairs. In addition, teaching patients in this manner not only helps them to move more comfortably and be more independent, but it also saves unnecessary strain on the nurse and family because the patient needs less assistance.

Before going onto the next section, check yourself by answering the eight-point picture quiz in Figure 12–4. Afterwards, compare your answers with those given at the end of the chapter.

MOVING A PATIENT UP AND DOWN IN BED

One of the most common daily activities of the nurse is to move a patient up in bed. This can be difficult for the nurse, and it can be hard on the patient. Certain things can be done to make this a smooth and easy process.

Whenever the patient can assist, he should be asked to do so. One way is to have him bend one or both legs and push down with his feet and arms to bring himself up in bed. If one arm is paralyzed, it should rest across his abdomen so that it doesn't drag and make the motion more difficult. A patient might find it easier to grasp a short side rail, which is available on almost all beds today, while pushing himself up in bed with his feet.

It is common for the nurse to help the patient to move whenever the patient has a certain amount of generalized weakness. He can usually assist in the move even though the effort is too great for him to do it alone. In this case, the nurse should put both arms under the buttocks of the patient, bend slightly at the knees, brace her knees on the side of the bed and ask the patient to bend his knees and move simultaneously with her count.

If the patient is very weak, two assistants are usually needed. If the patient is very heavy, or if he is unconscious, a third person may be needed to move the patient's legs. Be sure the bed is flat before starting the procedure, which is as follows:

1. Cross the patient's arms over his abdomen.
2. Two assistants stand on the same side of the bed. One assistant places her hands and forearms all the way under the upper part of the patient's trunk so that one hand is under the shoulder and one hand is placed just above the elbow. The other assistant places one hand and forearm under the buttocks just below the pelvic crest and the other at approximately the location of the greater trochanter. This person should keep her arms close together so that the patient's buttocks will not sag (see Fig. 12–5). A third assistant may be needed to support the head or the lower extremities.

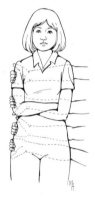

Figure 12-5   Position of hands for moving a patient.

3. Just prior to moving the patient up or down in bed, he should be moved to the side of the bed closest to the assistants in order to minimize the reaching (see Fig. 12-6). The "1–2–3–lift" signal enables the assistants to act simultaneously and permits the patient to remain in proper body alignment.
4. Always tell the patient what you are going to do and the direction in which he is to be moved. Also, explain to him that he will be moved at the count of three so that he can assist in the movement.
5. Ask the patient to raise his head (if possible) during the move. This reduces weight and resistance.
6. The person who lifts the heavier part of the patient's body calls the signals: "1–2–3–move."
7. During the move
   a. Turn your body slightly so that you face the direction opposite to that in which the patient is being moved, with your weight on the outside foot which is also forward (see Fig. 12-7). Both persons should be in the same position and have the same foot forward.
   b. Bend at the hips before the count is given.
   c. Stabilize your pelvis by contracting the abdominal and gluteal muscles.

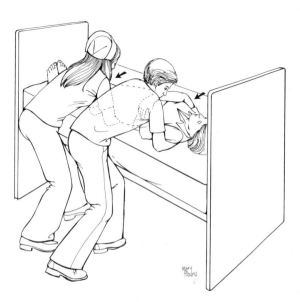

Figure 12-6   Move patient close to your side of the bed to prevent unnecessary strain from reaching.

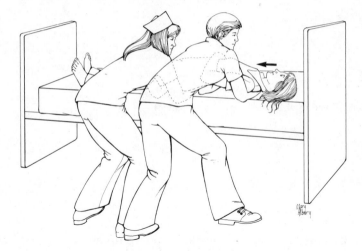

Figure 12–7 Turn body slightly toward the opposite direction of the move, placing your weight on the outside leg, which is forward.

d. When the count is given, shift your weight to your back foot as you move the patient. Avoid any rotation of the trunk to protect the spine.

In this particular method, you will be facing away from the direction in which you are moving the patient and must, therefore, take care not to bump his head on the headboard of the bed. This method is easier than facing in the direction that the patient is moving, because you are pulling (using your arm flexors) rather than pushing (using your arm extensors). In addition, there seems to be better balance and somewhat less strain on the back. Although some persons prefer to face the other way, it is recommended that you try this procedure.

Whenever a patient is unable to help himself to turn and move, it is helpful to use a folded sheet placed under the patient from his shoulders to below his knees. When this is used, the assistants stand facing each other on opposite sides of the bed. The edges of the sheet are rolled inward close to the patient's body. The move is, as already described, on the count of three.

During any move it is vital that you do not twist or turn your spine. If you must turn, be sure that you turn by shifting the position of your feet rather than by twisting your trunk and spine.

SUMMARY OF BASIC RULES OF BODY MECHANICS

1. Give yourself a broad base of support by keeping your feet apart, one slightly ahead of the other.

2. Make maximum use of your center of gravity by moving close to your work or by holding any objects close to you.

3. Protect your back by (a) never twisting and (b) using your leg muscles to move and lift.

4. Contract your abdominal and gluteal muscles to stabilize the pelvis prior to moving an object. This also protects the ligaments and joints from strain and injury.

5. Minimize friction between the moving object and the surface over which it is being moved. This will require less energy from all.

6. Get someone to help or use a mechanical device if there is any question that your load is too heavy or difficult.

SELECTED EQUIPMENT USED FOR LIFTING PATIENTS

BATH CHAIR LIFT (SEE FIG. 12–8)

The bath chair lift aids in lifting a person into a tub. It is used in the nursing home quite commonly.

Procedure for Bath Chair Lift

The lift is positioned so that the ring seat height is at the same level as the transfer chair height. After transfer, the lift is raised to a height where the feet clear the edge of the tub. The chair then rotates around and over the tub and lowers into the bath water until the frame rests on the tub bottom. The backrest raises up to allow comfortable use of the entire tub.

The lift is available from:

> Invacare Corporation
> 1200 Taylor Street
> Elyria, Ohio 44035

HYDRAULIC LIFT (SEE FIG. 12–9)

The free-standing manual or electric hydraulic lift makes it possible for one person to lift and move the completely dependent patient safely and with little

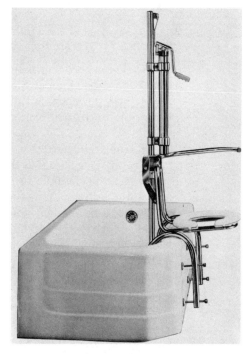

Figure 12–8 Bath chair lift can be used in the home. (Courtesy Invacare Corporation, Elyria, Ohio.)

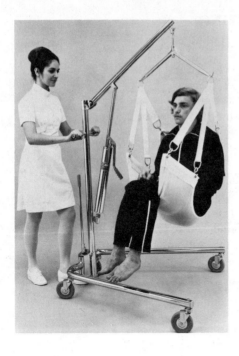

Figure 12-9 Portable hydraulic lift for bed transfers. Simple accessories make it adjustable for both bath and car transfers. (Courtesy Invacare Corporation, Elyria, Ohio.)

physical effort. Most lifts have a one-piece sling seat with web straps that hook to a wide-angle swivel bar. (An additional headpiece is usually available to support the patient unable to lift his head.)

Before introducing the patient to the hydraulic lift, be thoroughly familiar with its use. Have someone lift you so that you know how the patient feels. Demonstrate the lift to the patient before using it with him. If the patient wears glasses, remove them if the swivel bar rides close to the patient's face.

Procedure for Moving from Bed to Wheelchair

• The wheelchair is first braked and positioned parallel to the bed and the sling is positioned under the patient extending from his shoulders to his knees.

• Push the open end of the lift's horseshoe base under the side of the bed. Lower the horizontal bar so that the straps reach the sling. Lock the hydraulic valve.

• Hook the shortest web strap into either of the two holes in the top part of the sling, making sure that the hooks are turned away from the patient. Hook the center strap in the hole in the middle of the sling and the last strap in the last hole at the bottom. Adjust straps to fit the patient.

• Have the patient hold on to the straps or place his arms across his abdomen. Make sure that his arms are clear of the hooks. Pump the hydraulic handle with long, slow, even strokes until the patient's buttocks are clear of the mattress. Grasp the steering handle and roll the lift out from the bed, guiding the patient's legs as necessary.

• Turn the lift toward the wheelchair and roll its base around the chair. Release the check valve by turning it slowly. Push against the patient's knees to tip the wheelchair slightly, and slide the patient gently down the back of the chair so that his buttocks rest far back in the chair when finally seated.

• Close the check valve as soon as the patient has come to rest and the straps are loose enough to be detached. Position the patient comfortably and detach the web straps. The sling may be left in position for readiness in moving the patient back into bed.

The hydraulic lift is available from:

Ted Hoyer and Company Inc.
2222 Minnesota Street
Oshkosh, Wisconsin 54902

and

Invacare Corporation
1200 Taylor Street
Elyria, Ohio 44035

PATIENT ROLLER (SEE FIG. 12–10)

The use of a patient roller makes it possible for two persons to move the patient from bed to litter with minimal effort. It is not recommended for persons with a paralysis or spinal cord injury. The device consists of aluminum rollers attached to a frame covered with fiber glass or similar material. While moving over the roller, the trunk and lower extremities are kept in a straight line, so that little flexion, extension or lateral motion of the head or trunk occurs.

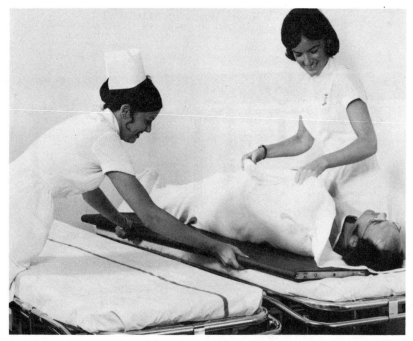

Figure 12–10 Davis Patient Roller is used to transfer persons from litter to bed, x-ray table or surgical table. (Courtesy Chick Orthopedic, Oakland, California.)

Procedure for Using the Patient Roller

The roller is placed on an ordinary litter which is positioned lengthwise against the side of the bed. One assistant stands next to the bed; the other next to the litter. One assistant uses a turning sheet to roll the patient toward her. The other assistant slides the transfer device under the patient so that it supports his head, trunk and lower extremities. The patient can then be moved over the roller and onto the liter.

Davis Patient Roller is available from:

> G. H. Chick Company
> 821–75 Avenue
> Oakland, California 94621

STRETCHER LIFT (SEE FIG. 12–11)

A hydraulic stretcher lift is available that acts as an ordinary litter and also enables only one person to lift a helpless person. It consists of a litter frame that is adjustable for height and a special sheet with webbed straps.

The special sheet is placed under the patient and then buckled to the frame. The patient can then be transported as on a litter. This piece of equipment is not recommended for the patient who needs firm support for back stability. It is, however, recommended for treatment rooms, operating rooms and x-ray departments where orderlies and personnel are unavailable for lifting.

The stretcher lift (Surgilift) is available from:

> Hamilton Industries
> P. O. Box 137
> Two Rivers, Wisconsin 54241

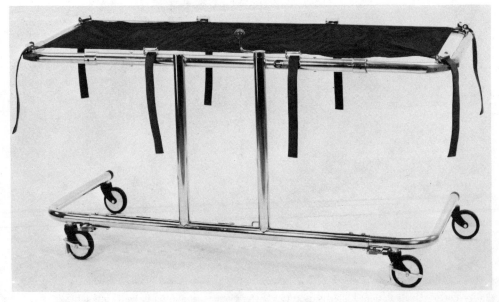

Figure 12–11   Surgilift. (Courtesy Hamilton Industries, Two Rivers, Wisconsin.)

Answers to Quiz: Can you Identify Errors in Body Mechanics?

1. I Back muscles instead of leg muscles are being used to bend. Feet are together instead of apart.
2. C Load is held close to the center of gravity.
3. I Chair seat is too high, and there is consequent pressure on circulation behind the knees.
4. C There is good back support.
5. C Stooping to lift—leg muscles, not back muscles, are used.
6. I Chair seat is too small and work is too far away from worker.
7. C Good posture.
8. I Stretching for load. Step stool is needed.

REFERENCES

Bilger, A. J., and Greene, E. H.: *Winter's Protective Body Mechanics.* New York, Springer Publishing Co., 1973.
Body Mechanics Applied to Nursing, Study Unit 4. New York, Blakiston Division, McGraw-Hill Book Co., 1969.
Brunnstrom, S.: *Clinical Kinesiology.* 3rd Ed. Philadelphia, F. A. Davis Co., 1972.
Flitter, H. H.: *An Introduction to Physics in Nursing.* 6th Ed. St. Louis, C. V. Mosby Co., 1972.
Ford, Jack R., and Duckworth, Bridget: Moving a dependent patient safely, comfortably: Part 1—Positioning. *Nursing '76, 6:*27, January, 1976.
Ford, Jack R., and Duckworth, Bridget: Moving a dependent patient safely, comfortably: Part 2—Transferring. *Nursing '76, 6:*58, February, 1976.
Foss, Georgia: Use your head and save your back . . . body mechanics. *Nursing '73, 3:*25, May, 1973.
Wirta, R. W., and Taylor, D. R.: Engineering principles in rehabilitation medicine. *In* Krusen, F. H., et al.: *Handbook of Physical Medicine and Rehabilitation.* 2nd Ed. Philadelphia, W. B. Saunders, 1971.
Work, R. F.: Hints on lifting and pulling. *American Journal of Nursing, 72:*260, February, 1972.
Yates, Judith A.: *Moving and Lifting Patients: Principles and Techniques.* Minneapolis, Sister Kenny Institute, 1970.

Chapter 13

POSITIONING METHODS AND SKIN CARE*

All too often a patient develops complications independent of his illness. This tragedy causes pain, expense and delays, or limits the total rehabilitation program. A pressure sore, for example, can develop after several hours of constant pressure to a skin surface. It may then take thousands of dollars and many weeks or months to restore skin and underlying tissue health from this one error. A joint contracture can result from remaining in one position for a relatively short period, but it will take months to correct, or it may even cause permanent deformity. To rehabilitate a patient because of chronic disease or disability is one thing, but to have to rehabilitate him for problems that could have been prevented by nursing measures is a tragic waste.

Whether the patient is acutely or chronically ill, whether he is in a hospital, nursing home, rehabilitation center or his own home, proper preventive positioning will be necessary. In order to maintain correct posture, to prevent contractures and to prevent pressure sores, proper standing, sitting and bed positions are essential to the prevention of musculoskeletal problems. The fact that a decubitus ulcer can develop in less than 24 hours tells us that we cannot wait for someone else to set up a turning schedule. Contractures and foot drop occur within a few days when muscles, tendons and joints become less flexible due to lack of use, lack of alternative positions and incorrect posture. Even "correct" positions become incorrect if they are maintained over too long a period of time. Knowing the unfortunate results of only a few hours of neglect should rouse us to preventive measures and constant vigilance.

POSITIONING—A METHOD OF MAINTAINING POSTURE

Posture is usually discussed in relation to standing and sitting positions, as in the previous chapter. We less frequently speak of bed posture—good posture when lying in bed. Since posture refers to the alignment of body parts in relation to one another, it is a relevant consideration for any position. Good posture is

---

*The author is greatly indebted to Doris Bergstrom, Catherine Coles and Ann Lundberg, who originally prepared the material on bed positioning in a manual called *Basic Positioning Procedures,* published by the Sister Kenny Institute, Minneapolis, 1971.

extremely important in the lying position because it not only helps preserve the patient's well-being but also prepares him for the time when he will be on his feet again.

PRINCIPLES OF GOOD POSTURE

To understand good horizontal (lying) posture, let us first review what is good vertical (standing) posture. The feet must be together with toes and knees facing forward, the arms are relaxed and at the side; the trunk is straight; and the head is held high. Now envision the body in the same alignment but on a horizontal plane, lying supine on a firm bed. This is good lying posture. The surface of the bed is firm in order to support the body parts; thus, postural requirements for standing can be simulated. If the patient's feet are placed against a footboard, it keeps them at a right angle to the legs with the toes pointing toward the ceiling. A small pillow under the patient's head gives support without pushing the head forward.

In order to achieve correct sitting posture, the feet should rest flat on the floor, or there should be proper foot support. The hips and knees should be positioned so that they are approximately at right angles, with the body weight distributed evenly over the thighs and buttocks. The lower back should rest against the back of the chair so that the segments of the spine are directly above the ischia. Forearms should be supported at the elbow level without causing elevation or drooping of the shoulders. Head support is not needed for the patient with normal neck musculature. (See Chapter 12.)

In the semi-reclining position, head support is needed in order to promote comfort and good posture. This position is often used when the patient cannot achieve full trunk elevation or has limited hip range of motion, vascular insufficiency, trunk musculature weakness or generalized weakness. The nurse needs to know the degree of elevation tolerated.

RESULTS OF INCORRECT POSITIONING

When the patient is lying on an ordinary spring and mattress, his hips sag from two to five inches, forming an angle of about 120 degrees at the hip joints. This can result in hip contractures. The semi-Fowler's position forms an angle of about 110 degrees. Continued use of this position can cause the same problem. With correct positioning on a firm mattress, the hip joint angle is 150 degrees, and this lessens the possibility of hip contracture.

The force of gravity pulls a paralyzed foot into a foot drop position, and the calf muscles and heel cords shorten, complicating future attempts at walking. Use of pillows under the patient's knees or continued elevation of the knee gatch can, in a few days, produce knee contractures and increase the extent of hip contracture. Heel cord tightness and flexion contractures of the knee and hip produced by improper bed positioning result in a variety of gait and posture problems.

Multiple pillows under the patient's head and shoulders round the back and push the head forward. These facts have critical implications for the proper use of pillows and bed gatching. Generally, when a patient gets out of bed after a period of time, he will have the same position he was allowed to have in bed

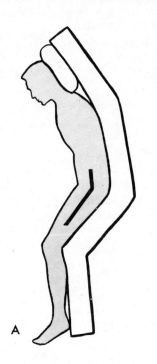
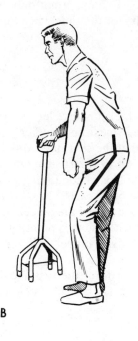

Figure 13–1 Bed posture (A) and standing posture (B) may become the same!

(see Fig. 13–1). Stiff and contracted joints will not improve upon standing. There-fore, let bed posture imitate good standing posture!

Incorrect posture and position can also cause skin problems. Measures which contribute to maintaining range of motion such as positioning also result in better skin care. A flexed position of the joints can cause the skin of one part to be in contact with the skin of another part, as for example, in the claw-like hand position of the hemiplegic. The dead tissue and debris that collect in the hand create a need for more rigorous skin care.

In certain other conditions, such as diabetes, arteriosclerosis, peripheral vascular disease and rheumatoid arthritis, circulation is reduced. Since the skin and tissues are not receiving adequate nutrition, they are more susceptible to damage than is normal skin tissue. Such tissue also heals more slowly. It is not recommended that such persons sit or lie with their knees or ankles crossed or sit so that the edge of a chair presses on the back of their legs. Neither should such individuals sit or stand for prolonged periods of time. In addition, pressure from the weight of the body, clothing, casts or appliances must be avoided or at least reduced.

A POSITIONING PLAN

Whether the patient is at home or in an institution, a plan for positioning is essential. It is incorporated into the plans for other elements of the patient's care. Basically, it requires (1) assessment of the patient, (2) selection of positions and equipment appropriate to the individual, (3) selection of a time schedule and (4) adjustment of the plan.

ASSESSMENT OF THE PATIENT

The nurse must be first concerned with the overall condition of her patient. She must ask such questions as, will a specific medical or surgical condition affect his positioning plan? Is the patient unconscious? Does he have pain? Does he lack sensation? If so, in which areas and to what degree? Does he lack muscle function? Is there any paralysis? Is there spasticity? Does he have edema? Is there any rash, redness, irritation or infection of the skin? What is his body type? That is, does he have enough muscle tissue to protect bony prominences? Is he continent or incontinent of the bowel and bladder? To what extent is he capable, mentally and physically, of assisting in his own positioning? Are there contractures? Does he already have a pressure sore?

Some of these questions have very special implications for the nurse. The question of contractures is one in particular. It is the nurse's responsibility to know that certain joints are susceptible to the development of contractures, how to tell if the patient has lost full range of motion and what to do to help prevent contractures. This subject is discussed in greater detail in Chapter 14.

A contracture is a shortening and tightening of soft tissue, resulting in limited motion of a particular joint. Contractures occur in any part of the body whenever that part is not regularly carried through its full range of motion. They may occur in limbs or structures where there is no pathological condition. The two most common sites for contractures are the flexor aspects of joints and the adductors of the shoulders and hips.

Contractures develop when a joint remains in one position for as short a period of time as three or four days. Certain factors contribute to immobility and subsequent contracture. They include lack of consciousness; paralysis or weakness of a limb; spasticity (uncontrolled movement), which tends to keep an extremity in one position unless forcibly moved; pain, which makes a person avoid movement; the force of gravity (for example, when a patient lies supine and his feet tend to drop downward and the legs tend to rotate externally); and immobilizing devices such as casts and braces.

SELECTION OF POSITIONS AND EQUIPMENT

The nurse considers the patient's overall condition, his specific diagnosis and her assessment in selecting the positions and equipment to be used. First, she rules out any contraindicated positions. She then selects positions which she considers important for preventing complications and promoting the comfort of her patient. If she is in doubt, she should check with the physician to ascertain if any positions she has selected are contraindicated. The positions selected will then determine what kind of equipment will be needed. Equipment will be discussed later in the chapter.

DEVELOPING A POSITIONING TIME SCHEDULE

While a positioning schedule is important for most patients, we are particularly concerned here with the patient who is physically ill or unconscious, one who cannot respond, one who has pain on being moved (such as the newly postoperative patient) or one who has severe loss of muscle function or loss of sensation. These patients need special positioning care because they either cannot change positions by themselves or they do not feel discomfort from being in one position for too long a period of time. In these cases, a written schedule for change of position is necessary. The nurse should not need a physician's order. This is a preventive nursing measure.

Observation is the key to setting up the time schedule. This is the only way to determine the tolerance of the patient's skin and underlying tissue. It is best to begin with a two-hour period for each position that has been selected. By the end of this period, the area on which the patient has been lying or sitting should be examined. Skin redness will develop, especially over bony prominences. Usually this will disappear within half an hour. The nurse should also feel gently for any lumps, which would indicate changes in tissue below the surface. It is generally safe to have the patient resume lying in the same position if redness is no longer present and no congestion or lumps are palpated.

If the patient has dark skin, be sure to examine him in good light, as color changes are less obvious. In the case of edema, the skin becomes lighter in color, and to test for erythema, you should feel the skin for warmth. Gentle palpation of the tissue may help to locate impending decubiti.

If skin redness persists for several hours, it indicates that a pressure sore is very likely developing. If further pressure to such an area is not avoided, a lesion may develop within a few hours. The patient should, therefore, stay off any area if there is persistent redness. If this is impossible, measures should be taken which will keep the area free from pressure. The nurse should massage *around* the reddened area to increase circulation.

After a position change, massage is used to stimulate circulation in the area where there has been pressure, giving special attention to areas over bony prominences (see Fig. 13–2). A cream or lotion can facilitate the massage.

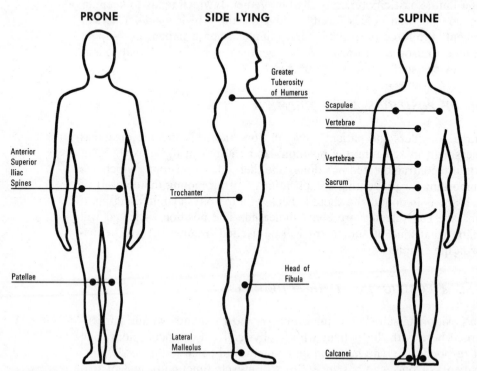

Figure 13–2 Bony prominences most susceptible to skin breakdown according to position. (Courtesy Sister Kenny Institute, Minneapolis, Minnesota.)

POSITIONING SCHEDULE

HOUR	POSITION	COMMENTS
6:00 A.M.— 8:00 A.M.	left side lying	breakfast—feeds self
8:00 A.M.—10:00 A.M.	supine	bed bath, including range of motion; bowel program every other day
10:00 A.M.—11:00 A.M.	prone	back care; work up tolerance; now tolerates 40 minutes (turn to right side)
11:00 A.M.— 1:00 P.M.	right side lying	dinner—feeds self
1:00 P.M.— 3:00 P.M.	left side lying	visiting
3:00 P.M.— 4:00 P.M.	prone	range of motion; tolerates 40 minutes; try to increase (turn to supine)
6:00 P.M.— 8:00 P.M.	right side lying	visiting
8:00 P.M.—11:00 P.M.	left side lying	evening care
11:00 P.M.— 3:00 A.M.	supine	sleeping
3:00 A.M.— 6:00 A.M.	right side lying	sleeping

Figure 13-3   Positioning schedule. (Courtesy Sister Kenny Institute, Minneapolis, Minnesota.)

In general, the nurse should start massaging around a bony prominence, work closer to the prominence and finally massage over the prominence (if the skin is normal). Massage is best done by using the pads of the first two or three fingers and working with firm but not hard pressure. Movements should be circular and done about four or five times over the area.

If there is persistent redness, a sign that a pressure sore is in the process of development, or if the skin is already broken, massage is done only around and not directly over the area. Massage should be gentle, so that any injured tissue is not further irritated.

Friction massage is useful to prevent the tightness of scar tissue which occurs in areas where pressure sore healing has taken place. Again, care must be taken not to injure the healed tissue. Since scar tissue will break down more readily than normal tissue, timing schedules must generally be shorter if such areas exist.

If there are no signs of impending skin breakdown, the periods spent in each position can gradually be increased at the rate of about a half an hour at a time. The nurse should allow at least two or three days after each increase to determine the tolerance to the increased period of time. In general, remaining in one position for three to four hours is considered to be a maximum safe period for persons who require a positioning schedule.

A positioning schedule should be written in order to guide the entire nursing staff. It must be planned around positions appropriate to the patient's activities—eating, bowel program, visiting hours, medical treatments, and so forth (see Fig. 13-3). Family members should also be instructed as to methods and frequency of position changes.

The patient who lacks sensation but who is able to change his own position must be impressed with his responsibility in preventing prolonged pressure. He should be taught to observe the condition of his skin daily or more often, as necessary. A long-handled mirror can be used to check the back, buttocks and groin area. The patient can set an alarm clock to waken himself for changes of position during the night. For periodic relief of pressure on the ischial tuberosities during sitting, the patient with sufficient upper extremity function should be taught to do a pushup at intervals throughout the day. If possible, periodic standing is preferable because it reduces other effects of immobility.

It is important that the patient be made as comfortable as possible within the limits set by each position. A tolerance must be developed for positions which permit good body alignment and prevent tightness or reduce existing tightness. Sometimes the length of time spent in one position needs to be limited purely from a standpoint of comfort. As the patient becomes accustomed to a position, the time can then be increased.

Boredom can be a problem. During the time the patient is positioned, he must remain relatively inactive. Sometimes he becomes excluded from the environment. Mirrors can be arranged so that the patient can view activity outside his room or he can watch television. Visitors can also be encouraged. For the long-term patient, positioning on a litter or prone cart should be included in the plan in order to provide an opportunity for greater socialization and recreation.

Prone lying is often objectionable to the patient because of the limited view of the environment. It is a position, however, that needs to be included unless it is contraindicated medically. Many persons become accustomed to sleeping in a prone position at night or during a daytime nap.

It is important to interject at this point that positioning is equally important when a person must sit all day. Change of position in this instance means relief of pressure. At 20 to 30 minute intervals, persons in wheelchairs must shift position and do several sitting push-ups, using the arms of the wheelchair for support. This not only prevents decubitus ulcers but it strenghtens arm muscles as well.

ADJUSTMENT OF THE POSITIONING PLAN

The first positioning plan will usually require adjustment. Evaluative observation should be made on a day to day basis until a plan is formed that is satisfactory to the patient and appropriate for prevention of pressure sores and contractures. Once this is established, a weekly evaluation is usually adequate. The nurse should determine from the patient how well a position is tolerated and for what period of time. She also should observe the effectiveness of each position. For example, she will check to see whether joint range is being reduced, maintained or increased. It is important to check the patient's range of motion in each joint.

Revisions of the plan are often indicated as the general condition of the patient changes. For example, a patient who regains consciousness or who has improved muscle function will begin to change his own position. Changes in the placement of positioning equipment may be indicated as range of motion or skin condition improves. As the patient's mental and physical condition improves, he may be able to assume new positions, increase the time spent in each position or discontinue whole parts of the plan.

For the chronically ill and disabled, however, a positioning schedule along with preventive pushups may be necessary for the rest of the person's life to prevent pressure sores and contractures.

THE THREE BASIC BED POSITIONS

In considering the position of a patient, be it in bed or in a chair, one must consider the head, the trunk, the upper extremities and the lower extremities. The three basic bed positions can be adapted in many ways. For example, a side lying position can be a partial side lying position, so that the patient is neither supine nor actually on his side. Such adaptations are individualized according to the comfort and the condition of the patient and are aimed at preventing any stress or strain of the body by providing adequate support.

THE SUPINE POSITION (SEE FIG. 13–4)

A correct supine position is achieved as follows:

1. *Head*—A small pillow which does not force the head forward and the chin downward can be used for comfort.
2. *Trunk*—Align the body so that the spine is straight.
3. *Upper extremities*
   a. The affected arm may be placed in a variety of positions.
   b. The wrist should be extended and a hand roll used. The roll should be placed at a slant so that the thumb and fingers go around the roll, with the thumb opposite the index finger.

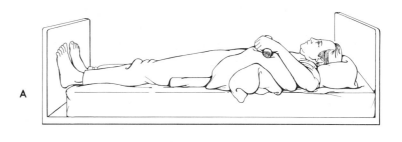

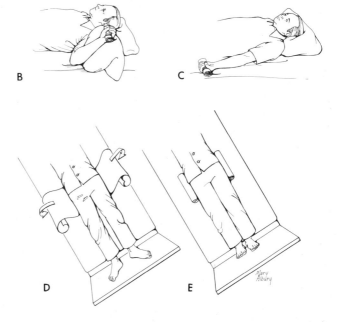

Figure 13–4 Supine positioning. *A,* Basic supine position with hand roll, arm support, hip trochanter roll, heel space and foot support. *B* and *C,* Alternate arm positions. *D,* Direction of trochanter roll. *E,* Trochanter roll in place so that hips are not externally rotated.

4. *Lower extremities* — For the supine position, always position the feet first.
   a. Support the feet at a right angle. Splints may be used to accomplish this position. If a footboard is used, be sure that there is space between the edge of the mattress and the footboard so that there is not undue pressure on the heels.
   b. Support the lower extremities by preventing the hips from rolling to an outward position by using trochanter rolls. The direction of the roll of a trochanter roll should always be underneath, as the arrow indicates in Figure 13–4.

SIDE LYING POSITION (SEE FIG. 13–5)

To achieve the correct side lying position, positioning should be in the following manner:

1. *Head* — Use a full size pillow under the head to promote comfort and proper alignment.
2. *Trunk* — If the patient is paralyzed or has severe involvement of one side, such as hemiplegia or a fractured hip, he should not be placed on that side. If it is desirable to keep pressure off the ankle, knee, hip and shoulder, use additional pillows.
3. *Upper Extremities*
   a. There are alternate positions of the top upper extremity. The top arm can be placed in front of the patient on a pillow at his side. The bottom arm is

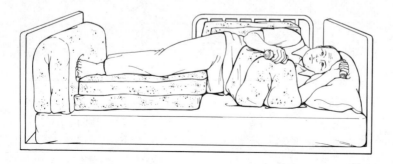

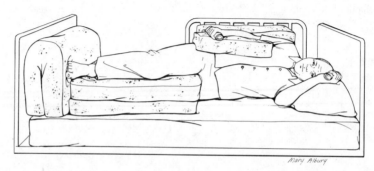

Figure 13–5 Basic side lying position with foot support, leg support, back support, hand roll and alternate arm positions.

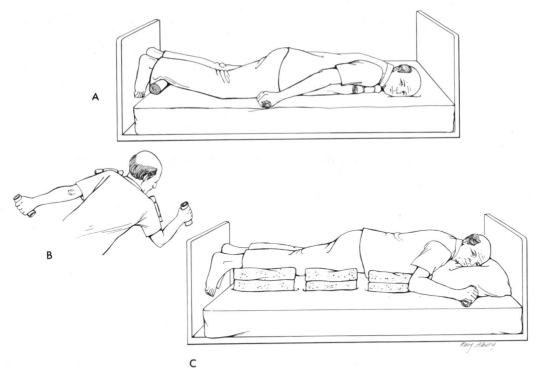

Figure 13–6 Prone positioning. *A,* Basic prone position with foot support, shoulder support, hand roll and no pillow. *B,* Alternate arm positions. *C,* Alternate bridge prone position with pillows.

usually positioned in a comfortable position on a pillow which is near the patient's head.

b. Extend the wrist and place a roll in the hand.

4. *Lower extremities*—Flex the top leg and bring it forward. Support it with two or more pillows so that there is no internal rotation of the hip. The lower leg can be straight with the spine. The top leg should never rest directly on the bottom leg, as this can cause pressure. A pillow can be used to prevent the foot from dropping. The hip can be pulled slightly backward to prevent the patient from rolling backwards.

PRONE POSITION (SEE FIG. 13–6)

The prone position is a particularly valuable position for patients who are chronically ill and for patients who have lower extremity amputations. It should not be used, however, without making sure that it is not contraindicated by the medical condition. The following technique is used to achieve the correct prone position:

1. *Head*—No pillow is used.
2. *Trunk*—Align the body so that the spine is straight. Use a flat pillow under the abdomen to protect the back.
3. *Upper extremities*
   a. Prevent the shoulders from rolling forward by using shoulder rolls lengthwise under each shoulder.

    b. Place the arms with the elbows either in flexion or extension depending on the patient's preferences and needs.

    c. Extend the wrists and place the rolls in each hand.

4. *Lower extremities*—Place the feet in the space between the mattress and the footboard. The feet fall into an acceptable position. If there is pressure on the foot or toes from the bedboard or from the frame of the spring or bed, place a small pillow or roll under the ankles.

TURNING THE PATIENT FROM ONE POSITION TO ANOTHER

    When the patient turns from front to back to side and so forth, personnel must pay attention to the same basic considerations:

1. *Head*—Lower the headrest, remove any pillows and turn the head in the direction of the turn.
2. *Upper extremities*—Place arms over the chest (at the side if the patient is turning to the prone position).
3. *Lower extremities*—Cross ankles in the direction of the turn.
4. *Trunk*—Move to the side of the bed opposite from the direction of the turn to allow space for the turn. Place the palm of one hand of the attendant on the shoulder and the palm of the other hand on the hip and gently turn. *Use two persons if necessary.*

COMPLICATING FACTORS

    The presence of conditions such as edema, tissue damage, pain and fractures can limit the length of time to be spent in each position and the variety of positions that can be used. Several conditions affect the positioning procedures in particular. They are contractures, spasticity and edema.

    When contractures are present, procedure adaptation is usually necessary. By positioning and supporting the extremity at the limit of its range of motion, further loss of motion will be avoided. The procedures for achieving a correct position must be modified to allow for limitations in joint motion. Any procedure intended to increase joint motion must be ordered by the physician or under the guidance of a physical therapist.

    When spasticity is present, positioning procedures should be done slowly and carefully, allowing the muscle contraction to relax. Once the extremity has been moved through its complete range of motion, it is then positioned. Positioning must be checked frequently whenever spasticity is present. If straps and sandbags are used, they must be recommended by the physician. Padding should always be used with such devices in order to reduce pressure.

    Because edema obstructs the free flow of blood and lymph, nutrition to the skin is therefore reduced and the skin becomes more susceptible to breakdown. Cleanliness is somewhat more difficult, since swollen tissue is tender and it is sometimes difficult to separate fingers and toes.

    Persons with loss of function, loss of sensation and poor circulation, and persons who are inactive have an increased tendency to develop edema, especially of the hands and feet, whether walking, sitting or lying in bed. The physician is likely to order measures to minimize edema, such as diuretics, exercise, external support of the tissues and positioning to assist circulation from the area. Positioning of the lower extremities might include elevating the legs on a pillow; however, prolonged use of pillows may be inadvisable because of the danger of hip and knee flexion contractures. The physician may order elevation of the foot of the bed as an alternative. If this cannot be done mechanically, the bed may be placed on blocks under the legs at the foot of the bed. Whatever method is used, it must insure a safe and stable bed.

For the patient who is up in a chair, a footstool or another chair can be used to elevate the legs. For those who use a wheelchair, an elevating leg rest can be obtained. For positioning the upper extremities, the arm can be elevated on a pillow in bed. If the patient is up and around, a sling can be used to support the forearm and hand. When the patient is sitting, a pillow can be placed in his lap to elevate the arm whether he is in an armchair or a wheel chair. An arm tray can be attached to a wheelchair to support the hand and arm.

PROTECTION FROM OTHER SOURCES OF PRESSURE AND IRRITATION

There are many sources of pressure that can cause pressure sores other than the patient's position per se. It seems appropriate to consider these at this time. The patient's clothing can cause edema or tissue damage if it restricts circulation. Seams and wrinkles in either clothing or bed linen may also cause pressure. Items in pockets of trousers and slacks should be carefully checked if the patient lacks sensation. Shoes that are too tight or have heavy seams may cause excessive pressure. We have all had blisters or other foot injuries from shoes that were either new or improperly fitted. If the person lacks sensation, he will be unable to feel any discomfort from pressure. Even though a pair of shoes, a brace, a splint or a corset fits initially, with use it may become misaligned, or the patient may have gained or lost weight which causes a change in the fit. Therefore, appliances should be evaluated and re-adjusted about every six to nine months. Just because something fits once does not mean that it will always fit!

A cast can also cause pressure sores. The nurse must, therefore, be alert to any complaint about how a cast feels, and she should observe the condition of the skin at the edges of the cast. Any abnormal condition or unusual odor should be reported to the physician so that corrective action can be taken. If a cast is used as a positioning splint, the edges should be covered so that they are smooth. During a cast change, it is always vital to examine the skin very carefully to make sure that pressure sores are not impending or in existence.

Splints, corsets, braces, and prostheses can cause discomfort and redness as well as pressure sores. Whenever redness occurs, the appliance should be re-evaluated by the physician and modified for a better fit. Even when equipment fits properly, padding may be needed to prevent pressure, but such padding must not alter the alignment or support of the apparatus or apparel.

Bandaging of an extremity should be firm but not so tight that circulation is restricted, and wrapping should always be in a spiral rather than a circular direction. If excessive wrinkling of a bandage occurs on movement, the bandage should be removed and re-applied.

The skin can be damaged in other ways, such as by friction, bumping, cuts or extremes in temperature. The nurse can help minimize friction by several very important methods. Whenever a patient is moved or lifted in bed, the pa-

Injury	Situation	Precaution
Bumping	Moving from bed to wheelchair.	Remove footrest from wheelchair. Watch position of legs and feet.
	Getting foot caught under wheelchair when spasticity causes foot to slip off footrest.	Use strap around footrest and patient's calves or place a panel between uprights behind calves.
Cuts	Preparing food	Use safe techniques in cutting. Stabilize item to be cut. Use a sharp knife.
Burns	Bathing	Check water temperature with normal extremity or thermometer, or have someone else check it. Repair dripping faucets.
	Touching hot pipes	Wrap pipes with insulating material.
	Ironing or cooking	Wear oven mit or mits. Use a wheeled cart for transporting warm items.
Frostbite	Riding in a car in cold weather or attending outdoor sports activities.	Dress warmly. Use a hot water bottle or handwarmer on top of mittens or boots.
Irritation	Wet or soiled bedding and clothing	Change immediately so that skin is clean and dry.

tient's skin should not come directly in contact with the bed linen. If a skin area is red or sensitive, very soft washcloths and towels should be used for cleansing. When drying the skin, it is better to pat rather than rub. Restraints often cause skin breakdown from friction. Padding, therefore, should always be used under leather restraints and for any patient who is restless or has spasticity.

Cuts, burns, frostbite and bumps must be avoided for any person. It is particularly important, however, to avoid them for persons who lack sensation or function and persons who have spasticity or reduced circulation. Careful handling of body parts is particularly important for these persons because their tissues are more easily traumatized in the first place, and healing is slower because of lack of sensation, circulation and muscle function. The chart at the top of this page suggests measures in which problems can be avoided or at least minimized.

TREATMENT OF DECUBITUS ULCERS

While nursing care should be primarily focused on prevention of bedsores, special care is required when a patient's skin does break down. Besides pressure, there are other causes of decubitus ulcers over which the nurse may have little control. They include such things as the use of certain drugs, poor circulation, poor nutrition, dehydration and the general debilitation that may accompany some diseases.

A bedsore may have four stages. Stage I is manifested by a reddened area that does not disappear when pressure is removed for 30 minutes. All of the measures suggested in this chapter may prevent further development. Stage II is demonstrated by superficial skin breakdown. The skin should be kept clean and exposed to air and light at this stage. In Stage III, both the dermis and the epidermis are involved, and during Stage IV, there is destruction and death of tissue of both muscle and bone.

There are literally hundreds of ways of treating decubitus ulcers, and successful results have been reported for a majority of them. The following list of treatments, mainly for Stages III and IV, are not necessarily recommended, but they have been reported successful in the literature and by word of mouth.

Antibiotics	Nilevar
A & D ointment	Phisohex
Bismuth and bourbon paste	Polyethelene foam mesh cushion
Brine (saturated salt solution)	Saline packs
Elase ointment or solution	Sugar and glycerine
Gold leaf	Surgical debridement
Hydrogen peroxide	Tincture of benzoin
Hyperbaric oxygen and	Ultraviolet light
miniature hyperbaric oxygen	Water beds
Karaya vegetable gum powder	Whirlpool bath

There are many other treatments, but they all have three things in common: (1) removing pressure from the affected area, (2) scrupulous aseptic technique and (3) maintenance of the patient's nutrition and hydration. It takes between seven days and three months to heal a bedsore, depending on the tissue involved and the general condition of the patient. It is important to serve a high protein diet and provide ample hydration throughout treatment. Vitamin and iron supplements are usually recommended also. In addition, a variety of equipment can be used to hasten the healing process.

SUPPLIES AND EQUIPMENT USED FOR SKIN CARE AND POSITIONING

It is important for the nurse to know the major kinds of supplies and equipment that will help her to care for her patient's skin and positioning needs. Many items listed in this section are available from national hospital supply companies such as the American Hospital Supply and Abbey Rents. Resources for purchase of items that are more difficult to locate are given. The list, however, is by no means complete.

BEDS

A bed should have a sturdy frame and be firm enough to support the patient's body. A high bed makes it possible for the nurse to care for patients with less strain; a low bed enables the patient to transfer more easily. Ideally, a bed should be adjustable for both height and position, have a metal tray rather than springs to hold the mattress, and allow space for the heels between the end of the mattress and the foot of the bed. Such beds are available from most of the companies manufacturing hospital beds. It is sometimes possible to change the height of beds which are not adjustable for height. The following methods may be helpful:

To lower a bed:

- Remove the casters. This can lower a bed three to five inches.

- Saw the legs off to the desired height. Use gliders on the ends to protect the floor.

To raise a bed:

- Place a wooden block under each leg. Make certain that the bed is stable by having each bed leg fit securely in the block. (Coffee cans filled with sand can be used as substitutes for blocks.)

- Place entire bed on a platform.

- Add another mattress.

When a weak, heavy or severely disabled patient is moving in and out of bed, the bed must be completely stable. A sliding bed can endanger both the patient and the nurse. A bed can be stabilized by the use of locked casters on all four wheels. The greatest stability is accomplished by the removal of casters which are replaced with gliders with caps to protect the floor.

The *water bed* or *air bed* may be used for persons who have pressure sores or burns. They are especially effective during the period of healing. For purposes of good skin care, turning is usually unnecessary when a water or air bed is used. However, attention to range of motion is essential to prevent contractures.

Turning frames are often used in the acute and convalescent stages of severe accidents and when turning is difficult. It is important to remember, however, that re-positioning of the extremities is essential even when a frame is used.

Some resources for purchases of special bed equipment used for positioning are:

Air Bed	*Turning Frames*
Milton Roy Company PO Box 12169 St. Petersburg, Florida 33733	Stryker Corporation 420 Alcott Street Kalamazoo, Michigan 49001
Water Bed	Chick Orthopedic 821 75th Avenue Oakland, California 94621
Jobst Institute, Inc. Box 653 Toledo, Ohio 43601	

What is known as the poor man's water bed, the "Ted Williams," a 37 by 86 inch air mattress, can be filled with water. It is available from Sears Roebuck and Co.

BEDBOARDS

A bedboard consists of one or more boards placed between the spring and the mattress to provide support for the mattress, which in turn helps to maintain body alignment. Some newer hospital beds now have a metal panel which substitutes for the bed spring. This not only provides excellent mattress support but is easily cleaned. Slatted bedboards, which have the advantage of being flexible, are also available.

Some suggested sources for slatted bedboards are:

Harco Corporation   Orthopedic Equipment Co., Inc.
1407 Park Street   Bourbon, Indiana 46504
Hartford, Connecticut

MATTRESSES

The mattress promotes good posture, comfort and rest by supporting the body properly. Support must be firm enough to allow ease of movement in bed, to facilitate transfers and to prevent sagging of body segments; it should not be so firm that it causes pressure over bony prominences.

Even a firm mattress may not be beneficial if there is sagging where the heaviest part of the body (the buttocks) rests. This is prevented by using a bedboard or a bed without springs.

It is recommended that a mattress have the following features: be firm and provide uniform support, be usable on both sides, be easy to keep clean and have a cover that is non-allergenic, waterproof, odorproof and stainproof.

A foam rubber mattress in a firm density (34 lbs. compression ratio) with a plastic cover meets these recommendations. For the patient who cannot tolerate a mattress this firm, a medium density (28 lbs. compression ratio) foam mattress is satisfactory.

In order to provide heel space (for the supine position) and toe space (for the prone position), the mattress can be pushed to the head of the bed or be made a few inches shorter in order to allow three- or four-inch blocks between the foot of the bed and the mattress.

An alternating pressure mattress is sometimes ordered by the physician for a patient who is susceptible to or may already have skin breakdown. This is actually a pad with longitudinal cells that fill and empty at intervals and is placed on top of the regular mattress. A pin hole can damage this item and lessen its therapeutic effect. It should be considered as a supplement to rather than a substitute for regular change of position according to the patient's skin tolerance and careful observation of pressure points.

Alternating pressure mattress may be obtained from:

R. D. Grant
10 Riner Street
Stamford, Connecticut 06901

FOOT SUPORTS

Foot supports (see Fig. 13–7) are used to maintain the feet in a functional position (at a right angle to the legs to prevent the development of foot drop).

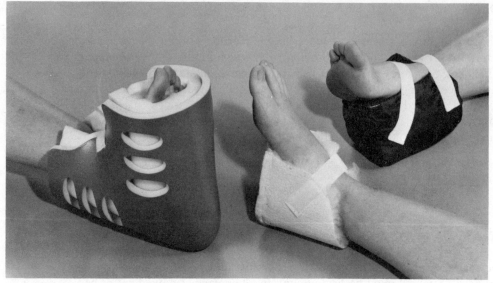

Figure 13–7   Soft foot supports. (Courtesy Stryker Corporation, Kalamazoo, Michigan.)

This can be accomplished by using a foot board, a footguard, or an aluminum gutter splint, padded with a thin layer of foam rubber to prevent skin breakdown, to support the foot. When a footboard is used, it should be stable and have a smooth finish. It should extend at least two inches above the patient's toes. Padding may add to the patient's comfort.

Other nursing measures can be helpful. Keeping the bed clothes off the feet by draping them over the foot of the bed or bedboard is one method. The use of a foot or body cradle is another.

Equipment of this type can be obtained from:

J. T. Posey Company
39 South Altadena Drive
Pasadena, California 91107

Vern S. Ryan, Inc.
2565 Stone Valley Road
Danville, California 94526

HEAD AND NECK SUPPORTS

If a patient is not able to keep his head erect in the upright position, support is needed. A high-back chair will provide adequate support in some cases. Additional support can be obtained through use of a neck collar or a head halter unit; the latter is attached to an overhead frame on the chair or wheelchair.

SHOULDER SUPPORTS

Rolls and cushions used under the shoulders in the prone position straighten the shoulders, promote comfort and make breathing easier. Shoulder rolls can be made by folding a bath towel lengthwise. It is then rolled loosely and secured with masking tape. Shoulder cushions can be made by placing a block of sponge rubber (about five inches by nine inches by two inches) in a rolled bath towel.

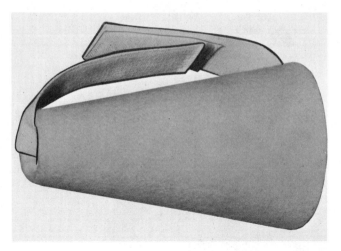

Figure 13–8 Palm cone. (Courtesy J. T. Posey Company, Pasadena, California.)

TROCHANTER SUPPORTS

A trochanter roll is placed under the hip to prevent external rotation of the hips in the supine position. A trochanter roll is made of a soft, smooth material (e.g., cotton blanket or thin mattress pad). Fold it lengthwise so it is 12 to 14 inches in width, and roll to a thickness of four or five inches. The roll is toward the underside to prevent unrolling when in position.

HAND AND WRIST SUPPORTS

Supports may be needed to maintain the hand and wrist in a functional position. The size of the patient's hand and the severity of contractures determine the desired circumference of the roll. The basic hand roll is made with two washcloths. Place one cloth on top of the other, fold in half, roll loosely and secure with masking type.

If this roll will not stay in place, one can place it in a narrow piece of stockinette which wraps across the back of the hand. The ends can be sewed or taped together. A palm cone may also be used (see Figs. 13–8 and 13–9).

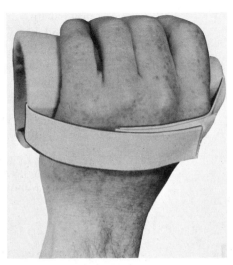

Figure 13–9 Palm cone in place for left hand. (Courtesy J. T. Posey Company, Pasadena, California.)

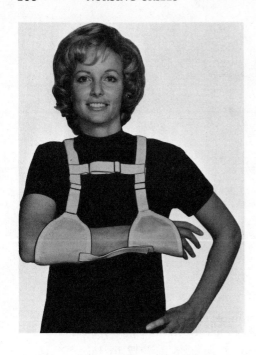

Figure 13–10   Ortho sling. (Courtesy J. T. Posey Company, Pasadena, California.)

The palmar positioning splint prevents wrist flexion and keeps the fingers in extension with the thumb in the position of opposition. Maintenance of finger extension is desirable when finger flexion tightness or spasticity is developing. It is often used for stroke patients. This device has the advantage of providing support for a specified period and is used only when ordered by a physician.

SLINGS

The purpose of a sling is to support the arm in a functional position in case of shoulder pain or edema of the wrist or hand, or when a cast is present. The hand is either level with or slightly higher than the elbow. See Figure 13–10 for one type of sling.

Several precautions must be considered when a sling is used. The position of the arm needs to be changed at intervals and the sling should be removed periodically to prevent discomfort and tightness. The stroke patient should wear a sling on the affected arm when walking to prevent subluxation or partial dislocation of the shoulder. If a sling has a knot or a buckle, it should not press on the collarbone or a vertebra.

Adjustable slings may be obtained from:

J. T. Posey Company
39 South Altadena Drive
Pasadena, California 91107

Textal Company
510 First Avenue North
Minneapolis, Minnesota 55403

Metro Surgical Company
128 South 10th Street
Minneapolis, Minnesota 55403

SANDBAGS

Sandbags are used as aids in positioning the trunk and extremities, as weights on equipment and as resistance for exercises. For the latter purpose, sandbags are generally ordered by the physician. When loss of sensation exists, they are not recommended.

STRAPS

Straps are used for support and safety when balance is poor, when involuntary movement occurs or when there is lack of muscle function. Straps are also used to maintain a joint area in a specific position; if this involves stretching, the physician's permission is needed.

CUSHIONS AND PADS

Cushions and pads are used to provide a soft surface and distribute body weight, thereby promoting comfort and helping to prevent skin breakdown. Cushions can also be used to free an area from pressure. Materials used include foam rubber, polyurethane, various other synthetics, gel, air and water. Many new materials are constantly being introduced (see Fig. 13–11).

Foam rubber, polyfoam, sheepskin, synthetic fiber, water and gel pads can be used under and around bony prominences for protection. If the pad has a cover, usually a washable plastic, it is important that seams are positioned so that they will not cause pressure. If the pad is made of a synthetic fiber or sheepskin, careful washing will prolong its life and usefulness.

Sheepskin and synthetic fiber padding should be washed with a soap for delicate fabrics in lukewarm water. After thorough rinsing, the pad should be rolled in a bath towel to remove excess moisture. It should then be draped over a rack to dry, but any direct heat should be avoided since it causes matting and stiffen-

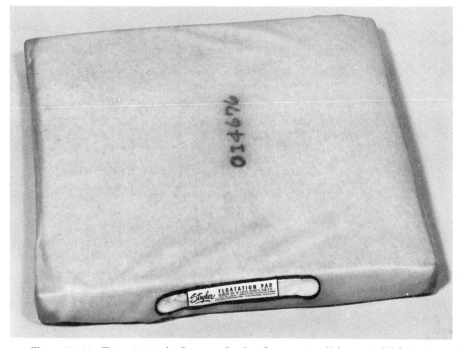

Figure 13–11   Floatation pad. (Courtesy Stryker Corporation, Kalamazoo, Michigan.)

ing. In the case of sheepskin, a small amount of mineral oil should be rubbed into the leather side while the sheepskin is still wet. This will help to keep the material soft and pliable.

When the patient is in bed, pressure on the ankle, knee or elbow can be relieved by suspension of the area between two pieces of two-inch foam rubber. Heel, ankle and elbow protection can also be provided by cutting a depression or opening in a piece of foam rubber to fit over the area. The foam can be held in place by an elasticized bandage. Doughnuts are not recommended for these areas, as they tend to reduce circulation to the area by increased pressure.

For the trochanter or sacrum, large pieces of four-inch foam rubber are usually needed. The thickness will depend on the size and weight of the person. Small pieces of foam rubber may be used between the thighs or calves, to prevent pressure when the knees and ankles are against each other.

Sources of the supplies just discussed include:

Everest & Jennings   Stryker Corporation
1803 Pontius Avenue   420 Alcott Street
Los Angeles, California 90025   Kalamazoo, Michigan 49001

SUMMARY

One of the major nursing responsibilities is prevention of complications. This chapter has dealt primarily with the prevention of contractures and pressure sores. The initiation of proper positioning techniques and turning schedules, the use of appropriately selected equipment and constant vigilance are essential to the patient's welfare in the hospital and in his home.

REFERENCES

Artificial fat prevents bed sores. *Journal of the American Medical Association Medical News,* *45*:197, 1966.
Carney, G.: The aging skin. *American Journal of Nursing, 63*:110, 1963.
Coles, Catherine H., and Bergstrom, Doris A.: *Basic Positioning Procedures.* Rehabilitative Nursing Techniques #701. Minneapolis, Sister Kenny Institute, 1971.
Foss, G.: The how-to's of bed positioning. *Nursing '72, 2*:14, August, 1972.
Gaul, A. L., et al.: Hyperbaric oxygen therapy. *American Journal of Nursing, 5*:892, May, 1972.
Gordon, Janet E.: Circolectric beds. *Nursing '77,7*:42, February, 1977.
Hagerman, C., and Moore, V.: Handbook of bed positions and guide to electrically operated beds. *Nursing '72, 2*:19, March, 1972.
Harmon, Vera, and Steele, Shirley: *Nursing Care of the Skin.* New York, Appleton-Century-Crofts, 1975.
Harvin, J. S., and Hargest, T. S.: The air-fluidized bed: a new concept in the treatment of decubitus ulcers. *Nursing Clinics of North America, 5*:181, 1970.
How to negotiate the ups and downs, ins and outs of body alignment. *Nursing '74, 4*:46, October, 1974.
Kosiak, Michael: Decubitus ulcers. *In* Krusen, F. H., et al.: *Handbook of Physical Medicine and Rehabilitation.* 2nd Ed. Philadelphia, W. B. Saunders Co., 1971.
Larson, C., and Gould, M.: *Orthopedic Nursing.* St. Louis, C. V. Mosby Co., 1974.
Merlino, A. F.: Decubitus ulcers, cause, prevention and treatment. *Geriatrics,* March, 1969, pp. 119–123.
Miller, M., and Sachs, M.: *About Bedsores.* Philadelphia, J. B. Lippincott Co., 1974.
Montagna, William: The skin. *Scientific American, 212*:56, 1965.
Pfaudler, Marjorie: Flotation, displacement, and decubitus ulcers. *American Journal of Nursing, 68*:2351, 1968.
Roach, L. B.: Skin changes in dark skin. *Nursing '72, 2*:19, November, 1972.

Rubin, C. F., et al.: Auditing the decubitus ulcer problem. *American Journal of Nursing, 10*:1820, October, 1974.

Schlappner, O., and Shelley, W.: Polyethylene mesh. *JAMA, 223*:430, January 22, 1973.

Shafer, Kathleen, et al.: *Medical Surgical Nursing.* 6th Ed. St. Louis, C. V. Mosby Co., 1975.

Spence, W. R., et al.: Gel support for prevention of decubitus ulcers. *Archives of Physical Medicine, 48*:283, 1967.

Sverdlik, S. S., and Chantraine, A.: A spongy cushion over hypersensitive areas of the skin to increase threshold to pain. *Archives of Physical Medicine and Rehabilitation, 45*:430, 1964.

Torelli, Michael: Topical hyperbaric oxygen for decubitus ulcers. *American Journal of Nursing, 3*:494, March, 1973.

Wallace, Gladys, and Hayter, Jean: Karaya for chronic skin ulcers. *American Journal of Nursing, 6*:1094, June, 1974.

Chapter 14

RANGE OF MOTION EXERCISES

Therapeutic exercise is defined by Frederic J. Kottke as "the prescription of bodily movement to correct an impairment, improve musculoskeletal function or maintain a state of well-being." Exercise has both a local and a general effect on the physiology of the body, particularly the musculoskeletal, nervous, circulatory and endocrine systems. The specific exercise to be done will vary with the person's goal and may range from reducing a flexion contracture of the hip to the general conditioning of the body done by an athlete. An exercise program is therefore designed to meet an individual person's needs and is implemented only after a medical evaluation.

Basically, exercise may be prescribed for five reasons: (1) to increase or maintain mobility of joints and soft tissues, (2) to improve neuromuscular coordination, (3) to develop muscular strength (the maximum tension that can be exerted during a contraction), (4) to develop muscular endurance (the ability to carry on an activity over a prolonged period of time) and (5) to promote physical relaxation. Of these purposes, the nurse will be responsible for only one with any frequency; namely, to increase or maintain mobility of joints and soft tissues. The so-called *range of motion exercises* (ROM) that accomplish this may even be inititated by the nurse.

When the nurse does range of motion exercises, her primary aim is to preserve the patient's present range of motion, thereby preventing deformity and further loss of motion. In considering this aim, one must distinguish between the responsibility and goal of the nurse and those of the physical therapist. The physical therapist's primary role concerns evaluation and restoration of function, while the nurse's primary responsibility is related to the maintenance of present function and prevention of further deterioration. This distinction is vital. In practice, this means that the nurse *maintains* the patient's range of motion, while the therapist works toward *increasing* the patient's range of motion.

How does the nurse know when the limit of a joint's range is reached? She must stop a movement if the patient experiences pain or when further movement requires force. The limit of the extent to which she moves each joint will vary with a single patient as well as among different patients.

Range of motion exercising is one of the various nursing skills used as a preventive measure. It helps to prevent contractures and to maintain joint integrity and mobility. Other preventive measures, of course, include proper body alignment, change of position, adequate support to various parts of the body and the use of equipment to prevent pressure. Range of motion exercises can also be used to identify tight muscles and joints when performed during a bath, while positioning and while performing other activities.

Not everyone has the same range of motion for a particular joint. Individual range is influenced by genetic makeup, developmental pattern, the presence or absence of disease and the amount and kind of physical activity in which the person engages. Diseases and conditions that limit range of motion include arthritis, muscle abnormalities, spasticity, contractures and rigidity. Persons who are inactive or who have immobilized joints over a period of time will also lose range of motion unless a plan to prevent that loss is implemented and used regularly.

Each patient will try to attain optimal functioning in his daily routine. In order to achieve this goal, a plan for regular range of motion exercises is essential. Such a plan need not be rigid. It can be based on the patient's individual needs and capabilities and carried out within his daily schedule.

A patient's primary aim is to be able to perform his own activities of daily living (ADL's). Therefore, being able to do full range of motion may not be required, as ADL's can be done without having full range of motion. Because of this, upper extremity exercises are often neglected when ADL's can be performed. However, the patient may have other goals that will require a greater range, and thus it is important to engage in upper extremity exercises.

The range of motion of a particular joint is the extent to which it is capable of being moved without pain or undue force. This range, together with the strength, coordination and endurance of surrounding muscles, determines to what extent a body part can be utilized in physical activity. When the muscles surrounding a joint contract and thus shorten, they will produce motion in one direction. When the same muscle lengthens, it allows motion in the opposite direction.

Under normal circumstances, motion of a joint is an active process. In other words, movement is initiated and produced by the individual. When a patient is unable to do this, an assistant will be required. In this event, all movements should be slow, smooth and rhythmic and should always be stopped whenever there is any sign of fatigue. If a person is to continue range of motion exercises at home, it is important that the family be taught how to assist whenever the person cannot exercise properly on his own.

DEFINITION OF TERMS

Before going further, it will be helpful to review the most frequently used terms related to range of motion. Referring to Figure 14–1, study the following terms in relation to the possible movements of each joint.

General Terms:

Range of motion—the extent to which a joint is capable of being moved.
   Active—range of motion performed by the patient without assistance.
   Active assistive—range of motion performed by the patient with the help of an assistant or a device.
   Passive—range of motion done by an assistant when the patient cannot move himself.
   Flexion—bend.

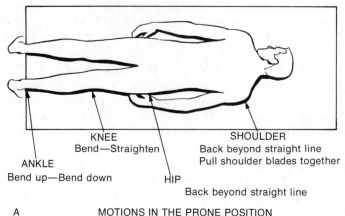

KNEE
Bend—Straighten

ANKLE
Bend up—Bend down

HIP
Back beyond straight line

SHOULDER
Back beyond straight line
Pull shoulder blades together

A   MOTIONS IN THE PRONE POSITION

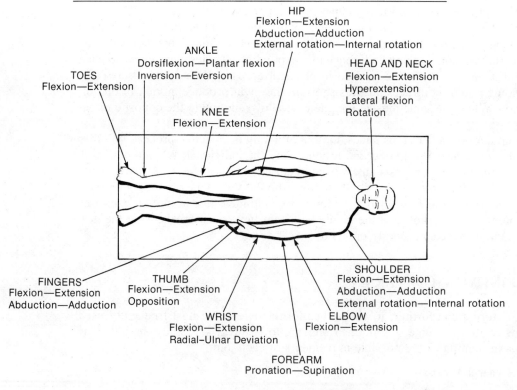

HIP
Flexion—Extension
Abduction—Adduction
External rotation—Internal rotation

ANKLE
Dorsiflexion—Plantar flexion
Inversion—Eversion

TOES
Flexion—Extension

KNEE
Flexion—Extension

HEAD AND NECK
Flexion—Extension
Hyperextension
Lateral flexion
Rotation

FINGERS
Flexion—Extension
Abduction—Adduction

THUMB
Flexion—Extension
Opposition

WRIST
Flexion—Extension
Radial–Ulnar Deviation

FOREARM
Pronation—Supination

ELBOW
Flexion—Extension

SHOULDER
Flexion—Extension
Abduction—Adduction
External rotation—Internal rotation

B   MOTIONS IN THE SUPINE POSITION

Figure 14–1   Motion of joints.

Extension — straighten.
Hyperextension — move back beyond straight line.
Abduction — move away from side.
Adduction — return to side.
Internal rotation — roll in.
External rotation — roll out.

Terms Related to the Upper Extremity:

Pronation — palm down.
Supination — palm up.
Ulnar deviation — move hand in direction of little finger.
Radial deviation — move hand in direction of thumb.
Opposition — move thumb toward little finger.

Terms Related to Foot Motions:

Dorsiflexion — bend foot up.
Plantar flexion — bend foot down.
Inversion — turn foot in.
Eversion — turn foot out.

Figure 14–2 illustrates and describes these functional motions of the joints of the body.

INDIVIDUALIZING RANGE OF MOTION EXERCISES

Range of motion programs are planned to meet the individual needs of each patient. The maximum range of one person is not and need not be the same as that for another. The objective is to maintain or achieve the degree of motion necessary to perform one's daily activities and is, therefore, a functional objective. As a result, the goals of an aged woman will usually not be the same as those of an active young man. In most instances the patient will have uninvolved joints that can be used as a guide for the normal range of motion to be achieved in the involved joints.

If a patient has had a right mastectomy, the nurse will teach the patient to begin to use her right arm and shoulder as soon as the healing process begins. Gradual increase in use will, of course, be guided by the physician's instructions. If the patient has had a stroke, it is just as important for him to exercise his paralyzed extremities as it is his uninvolved extremities. As in other preventive measures, it is just as important to prevent uninvolved parts from deteriorating as it is to prevent further deterioration of already involved parts. Whether the nurse works in a hospital, a nursing home or a rehabilitation center, or helps the patient in his own home, this is a key to keeping the patient as active and as independent as possible.

Range of motion exercises should become an ongoing procedure, beginning as soon as medically permissible whenever there is physical inactivity. The physician, with the assistance of other members of the health team (such as the nurse, physical therapist and occupational therapist) sets functional goals for each patient. These persons and the patient then work together toward those goals.

The same patient may require both passive and active exercises. For example, he may need passive exercises of the lower extremities but be able to ac-

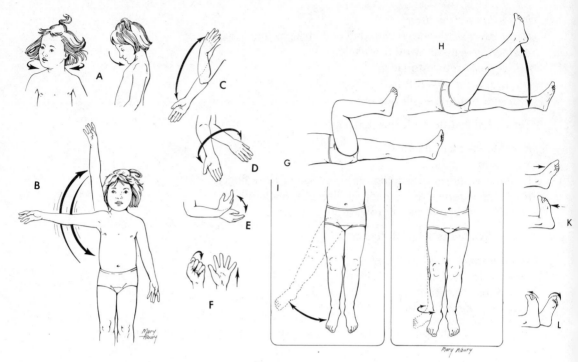

Figure 14–2 Functional joint motions. *A*, Head rotation and flexion. *B*, Shoulder abduction and adduction. *C*, Elbow flexion and extension. *D*, Forearm supination and pronation. *E*, Wrist flexion and extension. *F*, Finger flexion and extension with adduction. *G*, Knee flexion and extension. *H*, Hip flexion and extension. *I*, Hip abduction and adduction. *J*, Hip internal and external rotation. *K*, Ankle plantar flexion and dorsiflexion. *L*, Ankle inversion and eversion.

tively exercise his upper extremities. Another person may progress from passive, through active assistive, to active motions as joint range increases and the muscles become stronger. Some active assistive and active exercises utilize devices. Some devices (such as pulleys for reciprocal motion) are therapeutic, while others merely add variety and interest to an exercise program.

Some patients enjoy doing exercises in a group. If a patient dislikes exercise sessions, he may progress faster with group exercise, since socialization tends to increase some persons' motivations. When exercise is viewed as recreation, it is often more acceptable to the patient. The nurse can help to find the most acceptable time and method for her patients.

CONDITIONS INFLUENCING MUSCLE CONTROL

There are four conditions which frequently accompany the disease process of patients requiring range of motion exercise. The nurse must understand these conditions and adjust the exercise program accordingly.

A *contracture* is a shortening and thickening of connective tissue and results in limited joint motion. It occurs when range of motion has not been done frequently enough. If a contracture exists, any forced movement must be especially avoided, because pain and injury can easily occur.

Spasticity occurs when there are sudden, involuntary muscle contractions (hypertonus). This often occurs in patients with central nervous system damage. It is felt as either resistance or assistance during range of motion. The muscle may contract and release several times during one motion. You may lessen or avoid spasticity by performing the motion slowly. If resistance is felt during an exercise motion, the nurse should stop the movement, wait, and when the patient feels the muscle relax, resume the motion.

Clonus is spasticity in which contraction and relaxation of muscles alternate in rapid succession. It also occurs in patients with central nervous system damage. It is common in the ankle, and occasionally in the fingers and wrist. It can be triggered by a quick, forceful change in position. Re-starting the exercise motion very slowly and exerting a firm, sustained pressure will usually control the clonus.

Rigidity is a cogwheel-like movement that makes rapid motions difficult and is frequently found in patients with extrapyramidal dysfunction. By moving against the pressure of the rigidity, the nurse can slowly continue the exercise motion.

CRITERIA FOR SELECTING AN EXERCISE METHOD

Whenever a nurse plans a range of motion program, she will find that a physical therapy consultant can provide valuable suggestions. If a consultant is not available, the nurse can select an exercise method based on various criteria.

- Does the patient have any medical condition (such as inflammatory disease, infection or edema) that affects joint motion and that may, therefore, contraindicate range of motion exercises? (If so, the patient's physician must approve any exercise plan.)

- Does the patient have osteoporosis, making the need for gentle handling mandatory?

- What causes the limitation of his range of motion?

- Do you know the prognosis of these limitations?

- Is there spasticity, contracture or decreased sensation?

- What is the patient's present range of motion in the affected and unaffected joints?

- In what areas does the patient have voluntary muscle control?

- What activities can the patient do?

- What activities is the patient unable to do?

- What activities does the patient do with difficulty?

- What is the patient's fatigue tolerance during activities and exercises?

GUIDELINES FOR PERFORMANCE

- Know why you do range of motion exercises.

- Be sure that the patient, the family or anyone else involved understands what you are doing and why.

- Always use proper body mechanics to conserve energy and to avoid unnecessary strain.

- Make sure the patient is in good body alignment during exercises.

- When handling a patient's extremity, hold it at the joint if the patient has muscle pain. Grasp it above or below the joint if the patient has joint pain. Never place your hands on a pressure sore or incision. Use a firm but gentle hold.

- Note the patient's needs, especially those of an infant, a mentally incompetent person, an unconscious patient or someone with a sensory loss.

- Perform motions smoothly, slowly and rhythmically.

- If head and neck exercises cause dizziness, do only one exercise each time, or if necessary, discontinue them.

- Never exceed the patient's existing range of motion, and never force movements. Stop the movement whenever pain is felt.

- Repeat each motion three times for passive range of motion. Active assistive or active exercises can usually be planned into the patient's daily routine.

- Be sure that restrictive clothing is removed before exercising.

- Report to the physician any increase in limitation of movement or any deformity.

EXERCISES

PASSIVE

The patient's condition determines which motions need emphasis and which ones do not. In general, it is important to emphasize any motion that the patient does not use. For example, if an arm is held close to the body, it is important to work on shoulder abduction, not adduction. In addition, if a person frequently moves a joint throughout the day, passive exercises are less likely necessary. The following section, Figures 14–3 through 14–16, illustrates passive range of motion exercises performed on the supine and prone patient.

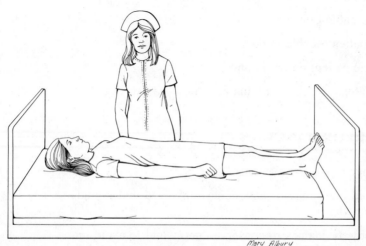

Figure 14–3 Proper supine position. Patient is lying straight on the back and is positioned on the side of the bed nearest the assistant, with space around the head and feet. There is no pillow under the head, heels are together and arms are at the sides.

Mary Albury

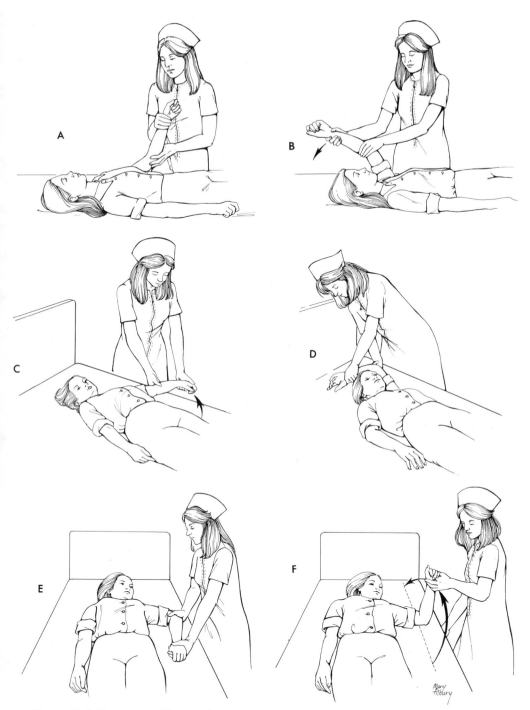

Figure 14–4   Passive shoulder exercises—supine.

A, Lift the arm straight up toward the ceiling.

B, Continue toward the head of the bed until tightness or pain occurs. Then return the arm to the side.

C, Bring the arm out to the side, turn the palm up, then continue the motion toward the head.

D, Bend the elbow to avoid the headboard. Place one hand on the patient's shoulder if it tends to "hike" up toward the ear.

E, Take the arm out to the side at the shoulder and bend the forearm to a right angle. Keeping this position, bring the arm down until the palm touches the bed.

F, Then bring the forearm up, so that the back of the hand touches the bed.

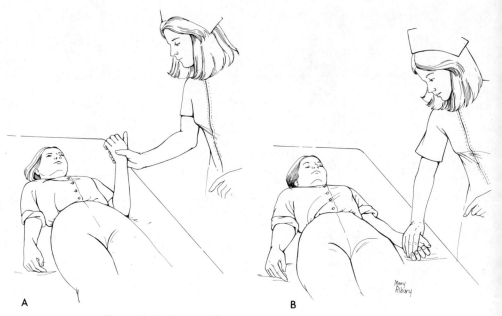

A   B

Figure 14–5   Passive elbow exercise—supine.
A, Bend the elbow, bringing the fingers toward the shoulder.
B, Then straighten the elbow completely.

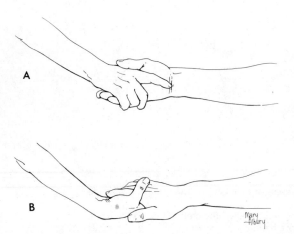

A

B

Figure 14–6   Passive forearm motions—supine.
Grasp the patient's hand as if to shake hands,
support the wrist and turn the palm up (A) and down
(B). Hold the upper arm with the other hand so
motion takes place in the forearm, not the shoulder.

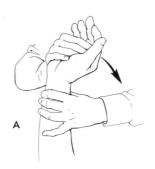
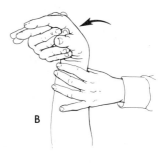

Figure 14–7   Passive wrist exercise—supine.

A, Supporting the forearm, bend the wrist backward.

B, Straighten it and bend the wrist forward.

C, Move the hand toward the thumb side.

D, Move the hand toward the little finger side. This motion can be omitted if the wrist assumes this position when relaxed.

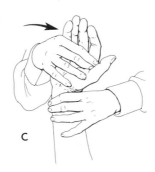
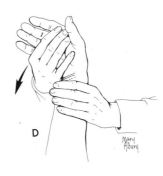

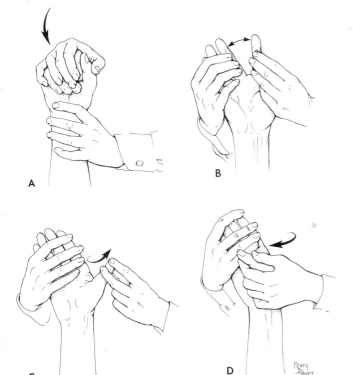

Figure 14–8   Passive finger and thumb exercise—supine.

A, Supporting the wrist, bend and straighten the thumb and fingers at all joints. For the hemiplegic hand, only extend the joints.

B, Move the thumb and each finger, in turn, away from the adjacent finger and then back.

C, Bring the thumb outward in a circling motion.

D, End with the thumb toward the little finger.

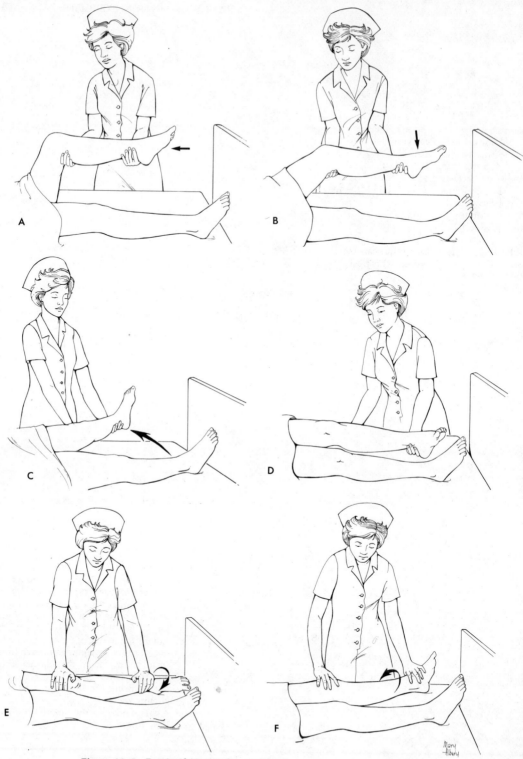

Figure 14–9 Passive hip exercise—supine.

A, Bend the knee and raise it toward the chin.

B, Lower the leg.

C, Take the leg out to the side.

D, Return leg and cross it over the opposite leg. CAUTION: Do not cause pain. Keep the leg close to the bed, but avoid dragging it on the bed.

E, Resting the leg on the bed, roll it inward.

F, Roll the leg outward. This motion may be omitted, since the leg usually assumes this position when the person is supine.

182

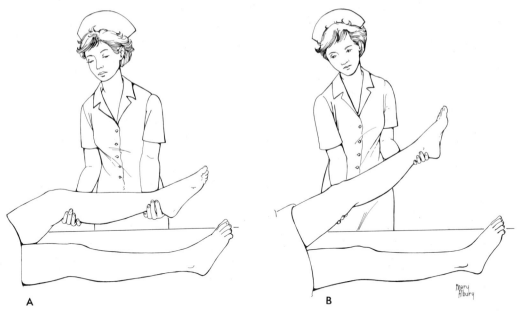

Figure 14–10 Passive knee exercise—supine.
A, Raise the leg and bend it.
B, Straighten it.

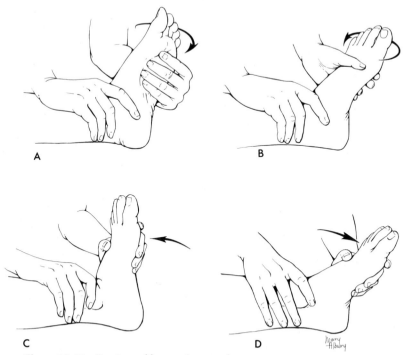

Figure 14–11 Passive ankle exercise—supine.
A, Support the leg and turn the foot outward (toward little toe).
B, Turn the foot inward (toward big toe).
C, Bend the foot up and backward. CAUTION: Do not force. Being able to achieve a right angle of the ankle joint is sufficient for standing; slightly more range is needed for walking.
D, It is rarely necessary to bend the foot down (foot drop), since the force of gravity and the weight of bedclothes encourage this position.

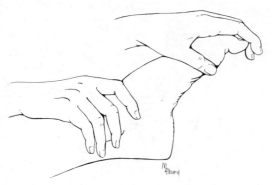

Figure 14–12 Passive toe motions—supine. Supporting the ankle, bend (curl) and straighten the toes.

Figure 14–13 Proper prone position. When the patient is lying prone, the toes should be over the mattress. If this is impossible, place a small roll under the ankles to prevent pressure on the toes and feet. CAUTION: If the prone position is restricted medically, most prone exercises can be done in the side lying position (see Chapter 13).

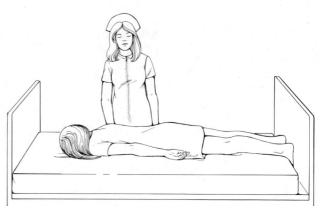

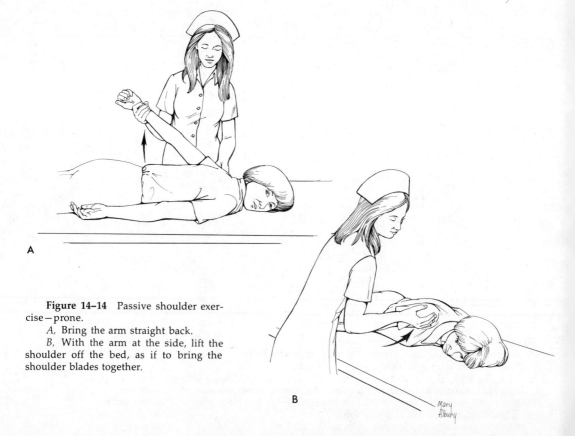

A

Figure 14–14 Passive shoulder exercise—prone.

A, Bring the arm straight back.

B, With the arm at the side, lift the shoulder off the bed, as if to bring the shoulder blades together.

B

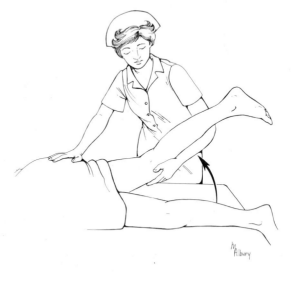

Figure 14–15 Passive hip exercise—prone. With hand pressure on the buttocks to prevent the hip from lifting off the bed, raise and lower the leg. This exercise helps to achieve optimal hip mobility.

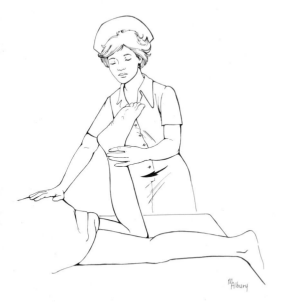

Figure 14–16 Passive knee exercise—prone. Bend the knee, taking the heel toward the buttocks. CAUTION: Do not push beyond the point of resistance.

ACTIVE ASSISTIVE

When the patient actively does a *part* of the motion, an exercise is called active assistive. Range of motion can be performed by the patient with assistance if functional ability exists. Assistance may either come from his own normal extremity (self-assistive) or from devices such as pulleys. Use of devices often makes the exercise easier and more interesting for the patient.

A reciprocal pulley can be purchased as an assembled set, or it can be assembled by the family. It consists of a length of smooth rope threaded through one or two pulleys. These may be mounted in a doorway or on a ceiling. The rope must be long enough to allow one of the patient's arms to hang halfway down his side when the other is over his head.

The patient may slip a fabric cuff over his involved wrist and hook it to one end of the rope. Or he may wear a mitt or glove which is strapped to a handle attached to the rope. With his normal hand he grasps a handle at the other end of the rope.

Figure 14–17 shows a self assistive exercise of the shoulder joint. Figure 14–18 shows an assistive exercise of the shoulder using a reciprocal pulley.

ACTIVE

Active exercises are those in which motions are performed without assistance (or without resistance from an outside force). They can be done individually or in groups. Since routine daily activity encompasses a wide range of movements, an exercise plan generally is not needed unless activity is limited. We maintain some range of motion by walking and by performing daily tasks such as washing dishes, sorting laundry, dressing, bathing and eating, as well as by a host of recreational activities.

When it is necessary to maintain an optimal range of motion because of a curtailed daily routine, the patient may actively perform the exercises described under passive range of motion (Figs. 14–3 through 14–16) or functional motions (Fig. 14–2). The nurse instructs the patient in the motions. The patient can then exercise while standing, sitting or lying down, although the lower extremities should not be exercised in the sitting position.

ISOMETRIC EXERCISE

While this chapter has been concerned with maintaining mobility of joints and soft tissues by appropriately planned range of motion exercises, a few comments on isometric exercise seem imperative. The purpose of isometric exercise is to improve the strength of a muscle group.

Isometric exercises do not involve joint motion, a change of muscle length or any external muscular movement. More positively stated, isometric exercises *set* muscles, create a tension and make muscles contract against an immovable object. They are useful when joint movement is contraindicated and usually involve hand-grip, quadriceps-setting, abdominal-setting and gluteal-setting. According to Müller, the most effective way of increasing muscle strength is to set (contract maximally) the muscle for six seconds and then rest it for two seconds. This is to be done five times daily.

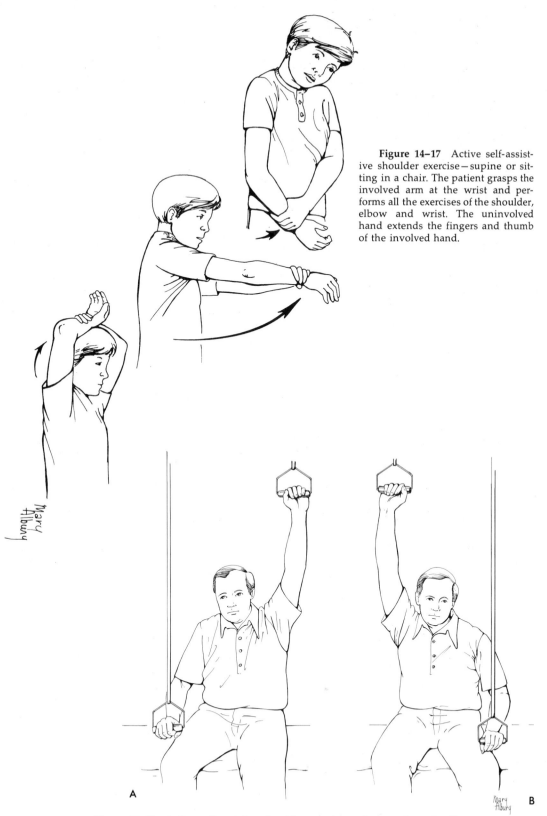

Figure 14–17 Active self-assistive shoulder exercise — supine or sitting in a chair. The patient grasps the involved arm at the wrist and performs all the exercises of the shoulder, elbow and wrist. The uninvolved hand extends the fingers and thumb of the involved hand.

Figure 14–18 Active self-assistive shoulder exercises using a reciprocal pully.

A, As the patient pulls down with the normal hand, the involved hand is brought up over the head.

B, As the normal arm raises, the other will automatically return to the side.

187

Isometric exercises place little demand on the cardiovascular system if the breath is not held during the contraction. They should not, however, be recommended to persons with cardiovascular disease without a specific medical order. They are recommended for postsurgical and orthopedic patients as well as other inactive persons.

SUMMARY

Range of motion exercise is one of the most vital preventive techniques available to the nurse. Assessment of the person's goals, incapacities and potential losses from inactivity forms the basis for early implementation of a range of motion exercise program.

REFERENCES

Brower, P., and Hicks, D.: Maintaining muscle function in patients on bed rest. *American Journal of Nursing, 72*:1250, 1972.

Ciuca, R., et al.: Range of motion exercises, active and passive: a handbook. *Nursing, '73, 3*:24, December, 1973.

DeLorme, T. L., and Watkins, A. L.: *Progressive Resistance Exercise.* New York, Appleton-Century-Crofts, 1951, pp. 113–115.

Foss, G.: Postmastectomy exercises. *Nursing '74, 4*:23, June, 1974.

Guttmann, Sir Ludwig: Spinal shock and reflex behavior in man. *Paraplegia, 8*:100, 1970.

Kamenetz, H. L.: *Exercises for the Elderly.* Chicago, Armour Pharmaceutical Company, 1971.

Kottke, F. J.: Therapeutic Exercise. *In* Krusen, F. H., et al.: *Handbook of Physical Medicine and Rehabilitation.* 2nd Ed. Philadelphia, W. B. Saunders Co., 1971.

Lavin, Mary Ann: Bed exercises of acute cardiac patients. *American Journal of Nursing, 73*:1226, July, 1973.

Müller, E. A.: Influence of training and of inactivity on muscle strength. *Archives of Physical Medicine, 51*:449, August, 1970.

Smith, D. W., and Germain, C. P.: *Care of the Adult Patient.* 4th Ed. Philadelphia, J. B. Lippincott Co., 1975.

Toohey, Patricia, and Larson, Corrine: *Range of Motion Exercises: Key to Joint Mobility.* Minneapolis. Sister Kenny Institute, 1968.

Chapter 15

TRANSFER TECHNIQUES*

Progressive mobilization is a term used to identify the many activities and steps that are taken by the patient to gain independence. It begins on the day of admission with a plan of care that comprises preventive, maintenance and restorative measures. For instance, correct bed positioning prevents problems associated with contractures. Bed activities, range of motion exercises and self-care skills help to maintain abilities and prevent further impairment. All of these measures will permit the fastest possible progression of mobility. Once a person is able to get out of bed, special steps for transfer planning are then developed.

The word *transfer* has a specific meaning to anyone working at a rehabilitation center, but to personnel working in a general hospital, the term either has little meaning or is considered applicable to a rehabilitation center only. As a result, patients in acute-care hospitals are moved about from bed to chair, to commode, to wheelchair and back to bed without the benefit of the knowledge, skill and equipment that could make such movements both easier and more comfortable for patients and personnel alike.

Transfer refers to the movement of a patient from one surface to another; that is, from bed to wheelchair, wheelchair to toilet, wheelchair to car and so forth. The transfer is considered active if the patient contributes to the procedure both mentally and physically, even though some help from an assistant may be required. If the patient is severely disabled and must be moved by an assistant or by mechanical means, it is called a passive transfer.

There are two basic types of transfer techniques—sitting and standing. Certain principles and knowledge can help personnel and patients to perform both the sitting and the standing transfer with minimal strain and maximal independence, whether the setting be the hospital, the home or the nursing home.

As soon as the medical condition permits, the patient must be provided with the opportunity of getting out of bed. Physical activity will not only improve joint motion, increase strength, promote circulation, relieve pressure on the skin and improve the function of the urinary and respiratory systems, but it will also be of benefit psychologically by offering increased social activity, mental stimulation and environmental change. (See Chapter 5 for a detailed discussion of the adverse effects of bed rest.)

For a majority of patients, the selection of a proper transfer technique is the

*The material in this chapter was adapted from *Transfer for Patients With Acute and Chronic Conditions* by Sandra J. Jurkovich and Patricia Flaherty, Minneapolis, Sister Kenny Institute, 1970. Assessment table reprinted with permission.

responsibility of the nurse. If a patient has a disability that includes trunk instability or an ambulation problem or both, a physical therapist will usually select the technique and, in many cases, teach it. Even in this instance, however, the nurse must know the technique and use it, so that the patient learns a consistent method from both professional disciplines. The role of the physician in transfers varies greatly between institutions and usually depends on the patient's condition, the role of paramedical personnel and the specialty and degree of participation of the individual doctor.

A TRANSFER PLAN

Assessment of functional ability will determine the selection of a technique. For the majority of acutely ill patients, this can be done rather quickly. For a disabled person it is more complicated because of the severity and complexity of physical problems and the amount of teaching necessary. In either case, the nurse needs to know what factors determine the method of transfer and the extent of planning that may be required. A nurse, physical therapist or physician may be responsible for developing the transfer plan. If the nurse must assume the responsibility, she will need a physical therapist consultant for many of her patients.

ASSESSMENT AND DEVELOPMENT OF ABILITIES

Assessment of the patient's ability and the extent of his weakness is essential before a transfer plan is initiated. Evaluation is a continuing process, since the patient's physical status will change, and modifications in transfer technique will be necessary. Considerations in assessment are:
1. Physiological condition
2. Mobility
3. Strength
4. Balance
5. Comprehension
6. Motivation

Once an assessment of these factors has been made, activities can be planned to help the patient develop the ability to transfer. The following table shows the interrelatedness of functional problems and development of ability in order to guide the nurse's judgment and action. See Table 15–1 for the relationships of these factors.

SELECTION OF TRANSFER METHOD

Depending upon the assessment of the patient's physical abilities, one of the two basic types of transfers (standing or sitting) is selected.

Standing Transfers.   A standing transfer requires that the patient can fully or partially bear weight on one or both legs. Your assessment along with the patient's diagnosis gives an indication whether this ability exists. Persons with hemiplegia, a fractured leg, a fractured hip, unilateral amputation or generalized weakness usually have enough strength of one or both lower extremities to bear weight and can therefore perform a standing transfer. The ability and degree of

TABLE 15–1   ASSESSMENT TABLE

ASSESSMENT OF ABILITIES	DEVELOPMENT OF ABILITIES

Physiological Condition

Physiological condition can be partially assessed by observing the patient's physical reaction to increased activity. If a patient has been in bed or on a turning frame for any length of time, postural hypotension must be considered. The circulatory system, having adapted to the reclining position, cannot readily adjust to the upright position. Such signs as nausea, dizziness or fainting will occur if the patient sits up or stands up too quickly.

Elevating the patient gradually will facilitate the adjustment of the circulatory system. Place the bed in a reverse Trendelenburg position or elevate the patient to a semi-reclining position for several short periods during the day. Start at a low level of elevation and increase only as indicated by the patient's tolerance of each level. Immediately lower him to a flat position if signs of fainting or shock are evident. An abdominal binder and elastic stockings are sometimes applied to aid circulation through the abdomen and lower extremities, thus improving the patient's tolerance of the upright position.

Mobility

Note any limitation of joint motion which may interfere with or alter the transfer. For example, if the hip joints have limited motion, the patient may not be able to bend forward in a sitting position.

Joint mobility is maintained through movement. Range of motion exercises and frequent changes of position should be used to provide movement of the joints of weak or paralyzed extremities. Daily activity and active movement should in most cases sufficiently maintain joint mobility of non-affected extremities.

Strength and Endurance

The patient's diagnosis may indicate his areas of greatest weakness. The extent of the weakness may be determined by observing his ability to use his arms and legs in such activities as moving up and down in bed, rolling over and sitting up.

Performance may be limited by fatigue. Some patients will become too fatigued to complete an activity. Others may perform better in the morning than in the afternoon. Determing the amount of activity a patient can tolerate is essential for transfer learning.

Transfers will be easier if the patient's strength is maintained through daily activity. Encourage your patient to feed himself, carry out his personal hygiene activities and change and shift his position in bed. If he is too weak to perform these tasks independently, provide him with the necessary assistance. Assistive devices may increase independence for example, side rails are an aid to rolling over and sitting up.

To develop sufficient upper extremity strength for transfers requiring extensive use of both arms, the patient should do pushups (in the sitting position) against a firm mattress. Blocks, books or trowels may be used to raise the level and increase the effectiveness of the exercises. Pushups on the wheelchair armrests should also be encouraged.

If a patient's endurance is poor, plan periods of rest between scheduled activities. If his endurance is so limited that he cannot complete an activity, have him participate in only one phase of the activity until he improves.

Table continued on following page.

TABLE 15–1   *Continued.*

ASSESSMENT OF ABILITIES	DEVELOPMENT OF ABILITIES
Balance	
Observe the patient's posture and ability to balance while sitting. Determine whether he needs to use his arms for support to keep from falling. Note any tendency to fall or lean to one side. This same tendency will probably be evident when you attempt the transfer with him. Look for any spasticity which may cause a sudden loss of balance.	If your patient has any difficulty with balance while sitting still, he will have even greater difficulty with balance when he transfers. Practicing balance while seated at the edge of the bed will help him develop this skill.
	Stand in front of him to provide support and protection as he attempts to balance without assistance and without supporting himself with his arms.
	Quick movements often trigger spasticity. Therefore, a patient with spasticity should carry out his activities slowly to avoid sudden spastic reactions. If a spastic contraction occurs, he should wait until it has relaxed before proceeding with the transfer.
Comprehension	
Determine whether the patient can follow verbal instructions. If comprehension seems poor, check to see if he has difficulty hearing or seeing. Find out whether he will follow short simple commands or gestures. Note any signs of confusion or forgetfulness.	Understanding is essential to learning. If a patient has difficulty with comprehension, it is especially important to establish a consistent procedure and to use simple directions. Whenever possible, teach transfers at times when the patient needs to transfer. This will help him to understand the purpose of the activity. Regardless of the patient's ability to comprehend, all personnel should teach the same transfer technique. Variations confuse a patient and delay his learning.
	To promote better learning when comprehension is diminished:
	•Teach one step at a time.
	•Use short commands. ("Lock the brakes." "Push down." "Sit up.")
	•Repeat the same instruction often.
	•Use gestures or demonstration.
	•Be patient. Give him plenty of time to respond to a command.
	•Give praise, even for trying.
Motivation	
Observe the patient's reaction to the progression of activities. Is he eager and willing? Or does he avoid activity by giving numerous complaints and excuses?	You can increase the patient's awareness of the value of the activity you are encouraging. It may be helpful to provide him with the opportunity to observe others performing transfers. Praise and encouragement may give him courage to make further efforts. If the patient is fearful, allow him to express his fears and give him moral support. If pain prohibits a patient from participating in the activity, it may be necessary to administer a medication for pain before he attempts to transfer.

independence for a standing transfer also depends on the amount of arm strength and the ability to maintain balance.

Sitting Transfers.   The patient with paralysis or amputation of both lower extremities must use a sitting transfer. The sitting transfer is also used for patients who are incapable of assisting with the transfer procedure. There are two positions commonly used in a sitting transfer: the short sitting position, and the long sitting position (see Fig. 15–1).

The long sitting position can be almost effortless if the hip and knee joints are flexible. For the quadriplegic, it can be more stable and avoids problems with sitting balance. If the hips and knees are less flexible, it is more difficult, since the patient is unable to lean far enough forward to maintain balance.

Transfers can be made laterally; occasionally forward or backward movement is preferred. Transfers may be accomplished more easily by paying attention to specific pieces of equipment. For instance, firm stable surfaces are important. A soft innerspring mattress makes it extremely difficult for transfer because physical effort is dissipated into the mattress and is not available for movement. A firm mattress with a bedboard between the spring and the mattress will make greater stability possible and maximize the effect of effort. In addition, the casters should be removed from the bed and replaced with flat gliders, to keep the bed from sliding during the transfer if the casters cannot be locked securely.

The type of wheelchair is essential also: it should be one of sturdy construction, fit the patient's body and provide adequate back and arm support. Brakes are essential for safety and stability and must always be applied during any transfer procedures. The wheelchair with swinging detachable footrests and, in some cases, detachable armrests will also permit the patient to move more easily from surface to surface as well as reduce the distance between the transfer areas. (See Chapter 16 for further details on the purposes of wheelchair features.)

The use of short side rails on the bed will often assist the patient to transfer. The side rail can be grasped when turning or sitting up in bed, as well as used to steady the body while sitting. Some patients can turn by merely grasping the side of the mattress. Some use a rope to pull themselves to a sitting position (see Fig.

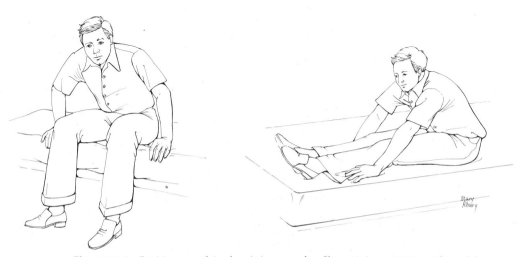

Figure 15–1 Positions used in the sitting transfer. Short sitting position (*left*) and long sitting position (*right*).

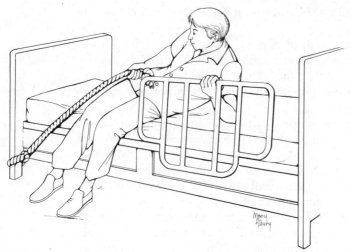

Figure 15–2 Patient may use a rope to come to a sitting position.

15–2). Properly positioned grab bars in the bathroom at the toilet, shower and bathtub are also important for ease of transfer.

Two basic considerations are fundamental to all transfers. First, the levels of the two surfaces between which the transfer will be made should be the same height. If the toilet is lower than the wheelchair, an elevated toilet seat may be needed. If the patient is transferring to a high surface, he might use a cushion in his wheelchair to equalize the height. Second, the ease of the transfer will be enhanced by having the smallest possible distance between the two surfaces. Many transfer problems are solved by correcting these two situations.

PROCEDURES

ASSISTING THE PATIENT TO TRANSFER

The inabilities and abilities that are identified at the time of assessment will determine the amount and kind of assistance required by a patient during a transfer. Refer to Table 15–1 again. The patient should only be given the assistance that he actually needs. The principal guideline for assistance is to provide safety and protection during the transfer. In the case of an especially obese patient, two persons might be required.

The following basic concepts will help personnel to transfer patients who require more than maintenance of stability:

1. *Stand as close to the patient as possible.* This means standing in front of the patient to assist with a sitting transfer. For standing transfers that require extensive assistance, stand in front of the patient so that you can provide both support and protection. If only minimal assistance is needed in the standing transfer, you may stand at the side, preferably at the weaker side.

2. *Stand with a broad base of support.* In other words, your feet should be kept apart, with one foot slightly ahead of the other. This will improve your balance and let you shift your weight more easily when moving.

3. *Assist the patient at the waist* rather than pulling his arms or shoulders. The use of the belt of the man's pants or a transfer belt allows a good grip without causing the patient pain.

4. *Bend your hips and knees, keeping your back straight,* as described in Chapter 12, while actually assisting the patient to move from one surface to another.

5. *Make sure that the patient can see* the surface to which he is transferring.

6. *Always move your body in the direction in which the transfer is taking place.*

7. *Make sure the patient is wearing shoes* (and a brace if this has been prescribed) in order to prevent possible slipping, foot injury or turning an ankle.

8. If the patient is learning to do an independent transfer, it is important that you *teach the procedure step by step.*

STANDING TRANSFERS

Unassisted Standing Transfers (See Fig. 15–3). When a patient is going to transfer without an assistant, the bed should be lowered so that the patient's feet touch the floor when he sits on the edge of the bed. By using the side rail, the patient can then slide to the edge of the bed. By placing the feet back (slightly under the bed) and slightly apart, with the stronger foot behind the other foot, the patient can bend forward and stand up by pushing down on the bed, the side rail or the nearest armrest. Once standing, he can reach for the far armrest of the chair. If it is a wheelchair, the wheels are of course locked. He then pivots his body to the front of the seat, bends forward slightly and lowers himself to the sitting position by holding onto the arms of the chair.

Assisted Standing Transfer (See Fig. 15–4). When the nurse uses a transfer belt around the patient's waist, she stands directly in front of the patient with her feet slightly apart. She bends her hips and knees to the level of the patient and assists the patient by pulling him to the standing position by grasping the belt at the waist from underneath. If the patient has weakness at the knee, she can brace her knee against the patient's weak knee in order to stabilize it. Once the patient is in a standing position, she can assist him to pivot. Again, the patient leans forward and gently lowers himself into the chair.

Transferring the Hemiplegic Patient. Before the hemiplegic person can learn to transfer from bed to wheelchair, he must learn to sit up in bed by himself and to get up and out of bed. It is recommended that the hemiplegic learn to transfer toward his uninvolved side.

The patient begins the procedure by lying in bed and placing the normal foot under the knee of the involved leg. The involved hand can rest on the abdomen. Next, the patient moves the foot down to underneath the involved ankle and then lifts both legs toward the edge of the bed. He turns over, faces the side rail, grasps it and then pulls himself to a sitting position. Next, see that the wheelchair is placed at about a 60 degree angle facing the foot of the bed. The nurse then assists the patient by using the transfer belt and, if necessary, bracing the patient's weak side with her knee, always making sure that the patient can see in the direction of the transfer. Review Figure 15–4 for the basic steps.

SITTING TRANSFERS

The sitting transfer has additional basic elements that are applicable to every patient.

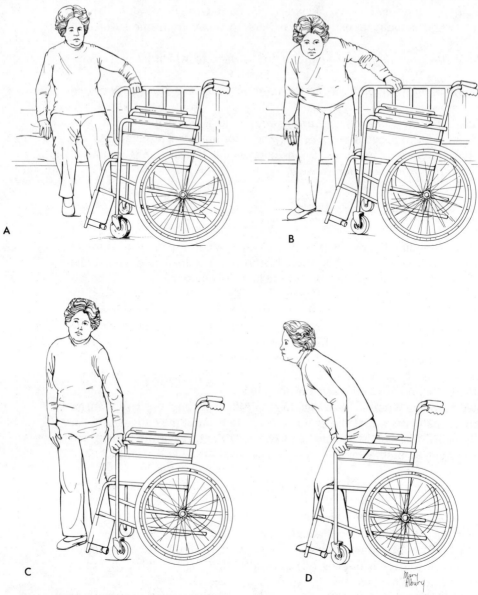

Figure 15–3 Unassisted standing transfer.
A, Leaning forward and doing short push-ups, the hips are angled toward the transfer surface.
B, Pushing on the bed and the short side rail, the patient comes to a standing position.
C, Grasping the armrest, the patient then turns with back to seat.
D, Grasping both armrests, the patient then sits down.

1. *The patient should wear a transfer belt around the waist if he needs assistance.*

2. The wheelchair should be positioned at a 45 degree angle to the opposite surface if the armrests are not removable. If the armrests are removable, the chair may be positioned directly parallel to the opposite surface.

3. *Brakes must be locked.*

4. *Footrests should be moved away* in most cases.

5. *If a sliding board is used, it must rest securely on both surfaces*—the sur-

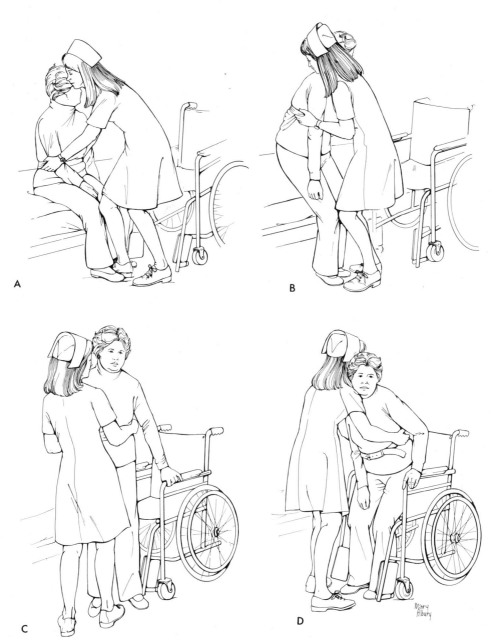

Figure 15–4 Assisted standing transfer.

A, The assistant bends hips and knees to the level of the patient, grasps the transfer belt from underneath and moves the patient to the edge of the bed.

B, The assistant's knees support the patient's knees while the patient comes to a standing position.

C, Still supporting the knees, the assistant pivots the patient around into a slightly lateral position.

D, Continuing to brace the knees and using the transfer belt, the assistant lowers the patient into the chair.

face to which the patient is transferring and the surface from which the patient is transferring.

Starting the Sitting Transfer.   If the patient is in bed, he must first come to a sitting position in order to do a sitting transfer. Patients who have control of their legs as well as some arm strength may simply roll over to the edge of the bed, lower their legs and come to a sitting position.

If the patient is a paraplegic, he begins the procedure from a supine position. He can come to a sitting position by pulling himself up by using an overbed trapeze unit or a rope attached to the foot or sides of the bed. If there is neither a rope nor a trapeze, he can push himself up by using his arms alternately. Once he is partially sitting, he straightens his arms by leaning forward and placing the palm of one hand on the bed; he raises up further and does the same thing with his other hand. He then moves his legs to the edge of the bed with one hand while supporting himself with the other. He moves first one leg and then the other until his feet are on the floor (see Fig. 15–5).

Unassisted Sitting Transfer.   In the unassisted sitting transfer, the patient brings himself to a sitting position at the edge of the bed. He leans forward and by doing short pushups, shifts his hips so that they are angled toward the surface to which he is going to transfer. As he leans forward, he does another series of pushups to lift himself onto the other surface (chair, toilet, and so forth). He adjusts the position of his legs as he shifts. He then replaces the armrest on his wheelchair and brings himself to a proper sitting position.

Assisted Sitting Transfer.   In the assisted sitting transfer, the patient wears a transfer belt and comes to the edge of the bed as in the unassisted transfer. The assistant bends her hips and knees to lower herself to the level of the patient. She grips the transfer belt from underneath and assists the person to angle

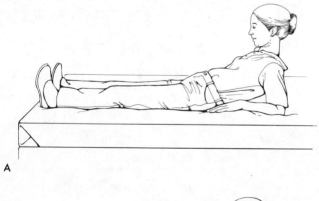

A

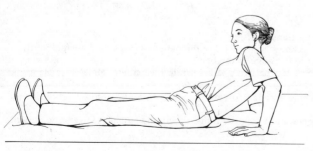

B

Figure 15–5 A person with paraplegia coming to a sitting position.

A, Raise upper trunk and rest on elbows.

B, Alternately push up with arms.

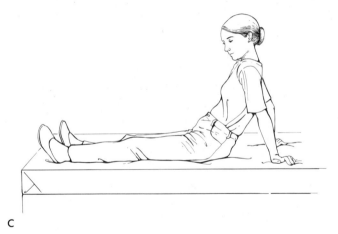

C

Figure 15–5 *Continued.*

C, Once the sitting position is achieved, lean forward.

D, Come to side of bed and move each leg to the floor with the hands.

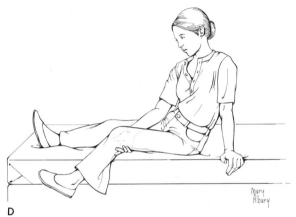

D

toward the chair. As the patient moves from one surface to another, she supports the patient's knees with her own knees. Using the transfer belt she is able to lift the buttocks up and onto the other surface. Throughout the transfer, the patient leans forward in order to maintain trunk balance. Once in the chair, she may have to help to position the patient by pushing her knees against his. This is done while he leans his trunk forward or does a pushup. She can also move him back into the chair by standing behind the chair and using the transfer belt.

Using a Sliding Board to Transfer (See Fig. 15–6). When a sliding board is used, one side is placed under the patient's buttocks and the other half is on the surface to which the transfer is to be made. By doing pushups with the hands to shift the buttocks, the patient slides across the sliding board to the other surface. If assistance is needed, the patient wears a transfer belt, and the assistant again supports his knees with her own. If balance is poor, the patient may lean forward so that his trunk will be supported by the nurse's shoulder. This transfer can be made easily and safely in this manner.

The Long Sitting Transfer (See Fig. 15–7). For the transfer in the long sitting positon, the patient comes to the sitting position as described by pushing up on his arms alternately until he is sitting up in bed. A longer sliding board bridges the bed and the wheelchair. The wheelchair is brought to the edge of the bed, and

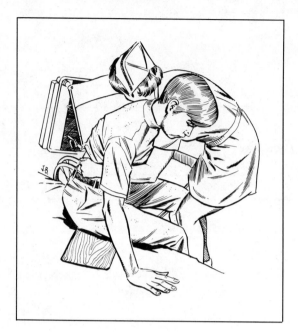

Figure 15–6 Assisting with a sitting transfer using a sliding board.

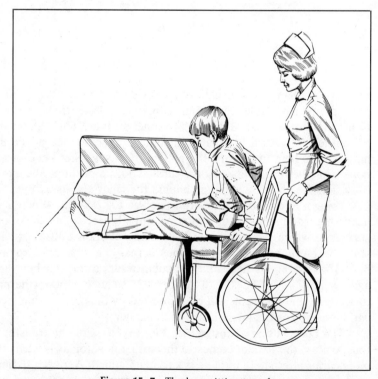

Figure 15–7 The long sitting transfer.

the patient merely does seated pushups to a position in front of the board and then slides backward into the chair.

SPECIAL TRANSFERS

Car Transfer.   The transfer to and from the car is simpler if the front seat of the car is used. The window of the car door can be rolled down and the car door can be used as a base of support just as the side rail of the bed was used. The wheelchair should be brought to the car, as close as possible and angled slightly. If the patient stands to transfer, he uses the door for support, pivots and sits down. The patient should sit down sideways and then swing both legs into the car. When getting out of the car, the patient should turn and his legs should be brought outside the car before he attempts to stand, pivot and get into the wheelchair. If the patient sits to transfer, a longer sliding board (28 or 32 inches long) expedites the move greatly.

Toilet Transfer.   The toilet transfer may vary because of the limited space and arrangement of most bathrooms. The wheelchair, however, should be positioned as close to the toilet seat as possible. Grab bars should be available in order to have safe support during the transfer. Since the standard toilet is only 16 inches high, a raised toilet seat (pp. 82 and 83) may be required to make the transfer surfaces the same height. In some instances, the patient might have to transfer toward his weaker side when moving to or from the toilet. In this case, greater assistance may be needed. If he stands, he can loosen his clothes once out of the wheelchair. He may need assistance in loosening his clothing and in securing them after he has used the toilet. The hand rail should be grasped at all times throughout the transfer. If he sits to transfer, a removable armrest is most

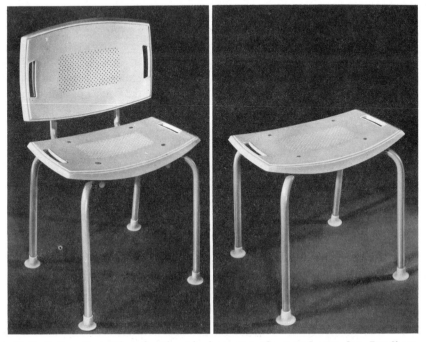

Figure 15–8   Bath seats—with and without back support. (Courtesy Lumex, Inc., Bay Shore, New York.)

advantageous. Some persons with paresis prefer to transfer straight forward onto the toilet, thus straddling the bowl.

Tub Transfers.   A patient may transfer directly into the bathtub from a wheelchair if he has good arm strength and good trunk balance. This is possible for a paraplegic. The tub should always have non-abrasive, non-slip tape, and securely installed railings are essential. Another method is to have the patient transfer to a chair or a tub bench inside the tub (see Fig. 15–8). It is recommended that the tub be filled prior to the transfer to avoid burns. However, if the tub is filled after the transfer, turn the cold water on first, and off last.

Showers.   One of the simplest ways of bathing is the shower. Shower seats which can simply be rolled into a shower (if there is no step at the threshold) are available. Be sure that brakes are secured during the shower. If there are no brakes, plastic-covered sandbags can be used to secure the chair during the transfer.

SUMMARY

A knowledge of the basic principles of a comfortable and safe transfer is essential for the nurse working in any setting. It will lessen fatigue and prevent back strain for the nurse. It will help the patient by reducing pain and discomfort from improper assistance and improper use of the body.

For the nurse working with chronic disability, basic principles will be used along with special equipment and the consultation services of a physical therapist. In these cases, a more thorough and intensive plan will be necessary along with careful patient and family teaching.

Suggested Sources for Equipment Used for Transfers

The following list of sources for equipment used for transfer is by no means complete. The nurse can receive her greatest assistance from local hospital equipment and supply companies. Another invaluable resource nationally, Abbey Rents & Sells, can be found under "Hospital Equipment and Supplies" in the Yellow Pages of your telephone book.

Sliding Boards

Hausman Industries
130 Union St.
Northvale, New Jersey 07647

Metro Surgical Company
128 S. 10th Street
Minneapolis, Minnesota 55403

Transfer and Safety Belts

Buffalo Weaving and Belting Co.
260 Chandler Street
Buffalo, New York 14207

Redicare
3047 Hennepin Avenue
Minneapolis, Minnesota 55408

Short Side Rails

Orthopedic Equipment Co., Inc.
Bourbon, Indiana 46504

Hill Rom Company, Inc.
Highway 46
Batesville, Indiana 47006

Beam-Matic Hospital Supply Inc.
25–11 49th Street
Long Island City, New York

Elevated Toilet Seats

Sears, Roebuck & Co.

Lumex, Inc.
100 Spence Street
Bayshore, New York 11706

Commode Chairs

Duxe Products
Medical Specialties
P.O. Box 1192
Cincinnati, Ohio 43201

E. F. Brewer Company
P.O. Box 711
Butler, Wisconsin 53007

Everest & Jennings
1803 Pontius Avenue
Los Angeles, California 90025

Tub Seats

Brearly Company
2107 Kishwaukee Street
Rockford, Illinois 61125

Lumex Inc.
100 Spence Street
Bay Shore, New York 11706

Shower Seats

Everest & Jennings
1803 Pontius Avenue
Los Angeles, California 90025

Lumex, Inc.
100 Spence Street
Bayshore, New York 11706

Hand-Rails

National Steel Products Company
1111 North Formosa Avenue
Los Angeles, California 90046

Charles Parker Company
50 Hanover Street
Meriden, Connecticut 06450

Invacare Corporation
1200 Taylor Avenue
Elyria, Ohio 44035

REFERENCES

Ellis, Rosemary: After-stroke sitting problems. *American Journal of Nursing, 73*:1898, November, 1973.

Flaherty, Patricia, and Jurkovich, Sandra: *Transfers for Patients with Acute and Chronic Conditions.* Minneapolis, Sister Kenny Institute, 1970.

Fowles, B. H.: *Syllabus of Rehabilitation Methods and Techniques.* Cleveland, Stratford Press Co., 1963.

How to Do a Swivel-Bar Transfer from Bed to Wheelchair. Downey, California, Rancho Los Amigos Hospital, Physical Therapy Department (undated).

Jordan, H., and Kavchak, M.: Transfer techniques. *Nursing '73, 3*:19, March, 1973.

Kern, F., and Poole, L.: Transfer techniques. *Nursing '72, 2*:25, July, 1972.

Krusen, Frank H., et al.: *Handbook of Physical Medicine and Rehabilitation.* 2nd Ed. Philadelphia, W. B. Saunders Co., 1971, Chapter 17.

Lawton, Edith Buchwald: *Activities of Daily Living for Physical Rehabilitation.* New York, McGraw-Hill Book Co., 1963, Chapter 3.

Rusk, H. A.: *Rehabilitation Medicine.* 3rd Ed. St. Louis, C. V. Mosby Co., 1971.

Chapter 16

GETTING ABOUT*

One of the most essential aspects of a physical rehabilitation program is to help the patient become mobile. The method of getting about will obviously be determined by the patient's disability. In an acute condition such as a fractured leg, the patient will be able to move about in his home, socially and in his job fairly quickly. For the chronically disabled person, the goal may be the same, although it will naturally take a great deal longer to achieve.

When a patient can work, travel, visit with friends, or go to the theater or concerts, his disability handicaps him to a minimal degree. The matter of learning to get from place to place needs special consideration whether the person will require a cane, crutches, leg braces or a wheelchair. Regardless of the assistance needed, the goal is to be able to get about.

AMBULATION

Some persons get around less and with greater difficulty because of foot discomfort. Pain from such minor problems as corns, calluses and bunions are often minimized or overlooked entirely. The nurse must be cognizant of this possibility and secure the care of a podiatrist whenever indicated. Foot discomfort may also be related to improper fit of shoe or need for repair of heels and soles.

Generally speaking, gait training is not the responsibility of the nurse if the patient is severely handicapped, nor is it usually her responsibility in a large metropolitan institution. This, of course, leaves a great many nurses who must either supervise or in some way be responsible for teaching crutch walking to the less severely or temporarily disabled person. This occurs in small institutions which do not have the benefit of a physical therapist, and in large institutions where the physical therapist works mainly with severely disabled persons. In the latter case, the physician may assume the responsibility of evaluating the patient's needs, determining the type of equipment that will be required and prescribing whatever gait training the patient must learn. Even when a physical therapist is available, the nurse still has a responsibility to have at least a basic knowledge of the various gait patterns and equipment that patients use to get about. The nurse

---

*The section on crutch walking is adapted from *Ambulation: A Manual for Nurses* by Lois Sorenson and Patricia Ulrich, Minneapolis, Sister Kenny Institute, 1966. The section on wheelchairs is adapted from *Wheelchair Selection—More than Choosing a Chair with Wheels* by Beverly Fahland, Minneapolis, Sister Kenny Institute, 1967.

will be asked questions about these matters by both patients and families and therefore needs to know the fundamental principles of ambulation.

CANES

The simplest and most uncomplicated walking aid is the cane. It is primarily used to assist in the area of balance. While its main purpose is not for weight bearing, it can somewhat lessen the weight-bearing strain on an involved limb. It assists balance by widening the base of support and therefore offers a sense of security to a patient who has a fear of falling.

The cane should be approximately as long as the distance between the patient's greater trochanter and the floor. Because individual arms vary in length, measurement can also be determined by observation. The proper cane length allows the patient to stand with his elbow just slightly flexed (about 30 degrees) when the cane rests on the floor about six inches to the side of the foot (see Fig. 16–1). Comfort is an important factor in determining the length of the cane. It is vital that the cane have a safe suction crutch tip. This prevents the cane from slipping by providing a secure hold on the floor.

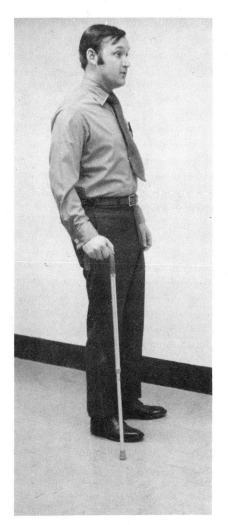

Figure 16–1 Proper cane length: elbow is flexed 30 degrees when cane rests on floor 6 inches to the side of the foot.

A cane is always held in the hand opposite the affected limb. It is advanced when the involved limb is advanced. When the cane is moved forward, it should remain close to the body, so that the person is not leaning out toward the cane. It should move only as far as the involved foot, so that the cane is never ahead of the toe of the involved foot when it is advanced.

When the hemiplegic person first begins to learn to walk, he should always hold on to a stable surface such as the end of a bed, a counter or a sink. There may be a tendency to fall toward the weaker side, and this support lessens the fear of falling. When helping the person to stand properly, the nurse can assist by pressing her knee or hand against the weakened knee until there is enough knee control to stand and ultimately attempt to use a cane. These persons need a great deal of encouragement as progress is very slow and in some instances ambulation may not be ultimately possible. In addition, repetitive teaching may be necessary because of the hemiplegic person's problem with communications (described in Chapter 7).

In addition to the regular straight cane, there are three-point and four-point canes. The quad cane varies in width of base and type of hand grip (see Fig. 16–2). Patients with balance problems may not be able to progress to a single-end cane. Although the quad cane is more cumbersome, it may be needed for independence. These canes help the elderly person who needs assistance with balance by providing a broader base of support and sense of security on the street or in the grocery store, as well as within the home. If stairs are used with any frequency, be sure that the cane fits on a stair.

Safety measures are essential. Loose rugs, slippery floors, waterspots on the floor and various obstacles must be avoided to prevent falls. Good lighting is also essential.

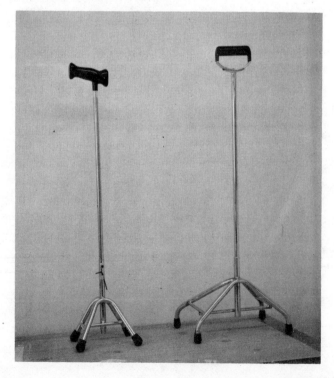

Figure 16–2 Narrow-based quad cane with pistol grip and wide-based quad cane with regular handle. (Courtesy Everest and Jennings Co., Los Angeles, California.)

WALKERS

A walker provides a wide base of support. It also gives a sense of security because it seems to provide support on all sides and therefore lessens the fear of falling. Many older persons prefer walkers rather than crutches because they feel more secure. The height of a walker should be about the same as the length of the cane. In other words, the patient is measured from the greater trochanter straight to the floor, or the walker is adjusted to enable standing with the feet between the rear legs of the walker, with the elbows flexed about 20 to 30 degrees.

There are two basic types of walkers. One is the pick up walker and the other is the rolling walker. In addition, there are many variations such as large hand grips for arthritics, stair climbing attachments for the pick up walker and padded seats and axillary rests for the rolling walker.

The Rolling Walker. The rolling walker, which usually has a seat, should be used judiciously. In addition to the height of the walker, the height of the seat must be considered. The seat height must allow for proper sitting posture, as described in Chapter 12. Because the walker rolls, it can cause a person to lose his balance when standing. It is bulky to carry upstairs, fairly expensive and can cause falls if the patient forgets to put down the seat before sitting. A hand brake is available and is recommended. The rolling walker is, however, used for persons with low physical endurance, for persons who are unable to lift a pick up walker and for persons who can propel themselves with their legs while sitting. The latter is sometimes recommended after hip surgery, before a person can bear weight on the affected side, to help maintain circulation and muscle strength of the lower extremities. When patients are slightly confused, however, caution must be used, since they may attempt to stand and walk.

When the rolling walker is used, the seat should be upright while the patient is walking, to prevent it from impeding the person's legs. The patient takes one or two steps, then pushes it forward. If the walker does not have a brake, it is important that the walker always be backed against a wall for stabilization when the patient sits down or gets up.

The Pick Up Walker (See Fig. 16–3). The pick up walker, sometimes called a walkerette or walking aid, is used for persons who are too unstable to use crutches and need more assistance than that provided by a quad cane. It is also used for non-weight-bearing geriatric patients. A walker, however, does not encourage the development of independent balance, and it encourages an abnormal gait pattern. Its use is determined by the patient's needs and abilities.

Two gait patterns may be used with a walker. The patient can either advance the walker and then step with each leg, using the arms for support, or he may advance the walker and the weaker leg together and then step with the other foot. The first gait is weight bearing, and the second is partial or no-weight bearing.

The patient should learn certain pointers when using a walking aid. When getting in or out of a chair, the walker should be backed up against the chair and the arms of the chair, *not the walker,* should be used for support. When walking, the weaker leg steps forward first and the strong leg swings past the weak leg, so that even steps are taken. The walker should be put down so that all four legs land on the floor simultaneously. The patient should be encouraged to look up while walking. Since there is a slight tencency to fall backwards when picking up the walker, the patient should be instructed to keep his weight forward and use his arms to lift the walker rather than bending and straightening the body.

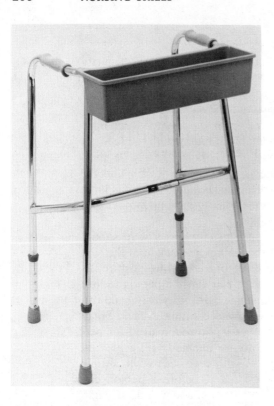

Figure 16–3   Pick up walker.

CRUTCHES

By far the most complicated walking aid is the crutch. When severely disabled persons are learning to walk with crutches, it is essential that it be done under the guidance of the physical therapist and physician. There are, however, many persons who are taught crutch walking by nursing personnel. A better understanding of how to measure crutches, general guidelines on crutch walking and posture and knowledge of basic gait patterns will be helpful to the nurse whether she works in an institution, at a clinic or in the home.

Preparation For Crutch Walking.   Whenever a patient walks with crutches, gait should be as nearly normal as possible. The person who has been ill or disabled over a long period of time cannot simply get up and learn to walk with crutches. The reasons for this are of course related to the physiological changes resulting from immobility. Preparation for crutch walking actually should begin as early as possible and continue throughout the illness by maintaining muscle strength and joint range of motion. Assuming that this was done during the illness, the first step is to develop muscle strength of the back, chest, arms and shoulders. Next, the patient begins to learn sitting balance, which was also basic to learning to transfer. Physical preparation is done through muscle setting exercises (alternately contracting and relaxing a muscle), isometric exercises (in which a muscle is contracted and held against resistance for 10 to 15 seconds) and active exercises to develop both sitting and standing balance and ability. Pushups, both in the prone position and in the sitting position, the use of a trapeze on the bed and other prescribed exercises help to achieve these goals.

Once the patient has physical strength and sitting balance, the third preparatory step is to learn to acquire good standing balance. This is obviously crucial to walking, whether or not it is done with crutches, canes, leg braces and so forth. Fourth, the person will learn how to shift his body weight with crutches. Finally, he will work toward the ultimate goal—that of training in a specific gait.

Looking at this sequence of necessary abilities, one can readily see that a patient may begin to learn crutch walking at any one of these levels of preparation, depending on his physical strength and ability. The person who has been in good health and fractures a leg will enter the program on the fifth level (learning a specific gait), whereas a chronically ill or severely disabled person may enter at the first level (developing muscle strength).

Measuring For Crutches.   There are three basic ways to measure for crutches. If it is possible, the most accurate way is the standing measurement. Have the patient stand, with shoes on, in a natural posture against a wall. Mark the point where an imaginary line at the end of the big toe crosses an imaginary line from the outside of the foot. Using a tape measure, measure two inches away from that point, then six inches forward (Fig. 16–4). Mark this point and then measure from it to two inches below the axilla. This distance will be the length of the crutch.

The second way of measuring for crutches is in bed. Have the patient lie straight in bed and measure from the axilla to six to eight inches away from the heel. If the patient is not measured for crutches, you can merely subtract 16 inches from the patient's height.

Besides the crutch length, it is important to determine the proper placement of the handbar. The palms of the hand—not the axilla—should bear the weight of the patient. The wrist should be slightly hyperextended and the elbow flexed about 30 degrees. When the height of the handbar allows this arm position, it is correctly placed. This measurement can be taken in bed as well as in the standing position. Under ordinary circumstances the handbar does not have to be changed unless the leg of a crutch is altered more than two or three inches. Generally, a person should be able to lift his body weight on his hands, leaving the feet free from the floor.

Gait Pattern for Crutches.   Whenever a patient learns to walk with crutches, awareness of good posture becomes crucial. The basic standing crutch posture is

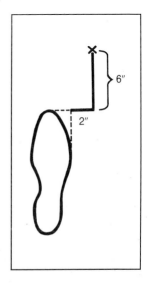

Figure 16–4   Point on floor to begin crutch measurement.

one in which the head is held high, the pelvis is slightly forward over the feet and the crutches are about four inches to the side and four inches to the front of each foot to allow the hips to pass between the crutches comfortably. This provides a broad standing base. The patient's weight should be on the palms of the hands, with wrists extended and the elbows slightly flexed. The crutches are also held close to the chest to provide lateral stability. This brings the top of the crutch (the axillary bar) to about two inches below the axilla. With this posture, the possibility of crutch paralysis due to pressure on the radial nerve in the axilla is eliminated. The patient should understand the possibility of this problem so that he refrains from getting into the habit of leaning on the axillary bar of the crutch.

There are a variety of gait patterns for patients who use crutches and canes. Each pattern differs in speed, safety and the amount of energy that is required. The gait to be used is generally ordered by the physician. Both the patient and the family should understand the gait pattern used when the patient needs assistance to walk. In this way the patient will have assistance when a professional person is not nearby for supervision.

THE FOUR-POINT GAIT (SEE FIG. 16–5). Persons who lack coordination or balance, persons with muscle weakness and persons who are afraid of falling are usually taught the four-point gait pattern. In order to perform this pattern, the person must have enough muscle power in the arms to hold the handgrip and lift the crutch and be able to keep the elbow fairly straight. The person must also have enough muscle power in the legs to move either foot forward and to straighten the knee. Some persons may require muscle strengthening from a physical therapist before they are able to do this gait pattern, which is considered to be the safest and most stable.

With the weight of the body on both legs and both crutches, the patient first shifts his weight to both legs and one crutch and then moves the other crutch forward to a distance slightly less than that of a normal step. Next, he shifts his weight onto one leg and both crutches and moves the other leg forward. These two movements are repeated to advance the other side.

Pattern: One crutch forward, the opposite leg advanced, the other crutch forward, the opposite leg advanced.

THE TWO-POINT GAIT PATTERN (SEE FIG. 16–6). The two-point gait is faster than the four-point gait, but it requires better balance because there are only two points of weight bearing. It closely resembles normal walking. With the weight of the body on both legs and both crutches, the patient first shifts his weight to one leg and the opposite crutch. He then moves the other leg and the other crutch forward. The two movements are repeated to advance the other side.

Pattern: One leg and the opposite crutch advance together. Repeat with other crutch and leg.

THE THREE-POINT GAIT PATTERN (SEE FIG. 16–7). The three-point pattern is a non-weight-bearing gait, used by patients with normal use of both arms, the trunk and one leg. Orthopedic patients and persons with unilateral amputation before a prosthesis fitting use this gait. The crutches act as the weight-bearing surface during half of the gait. Therefore, the patient's arms must be strong enough to support the entire body weight when the leg is advanced. The patient begins with the weight of the body on the normal leg and both crutches, standing with the pelvis forward and bending at the ankle rather than at the hips to maintain balance. He then shifts his weight to the normal leg and moves both crutches ahead four to six inches. Next, the weight of the body shifts onto the

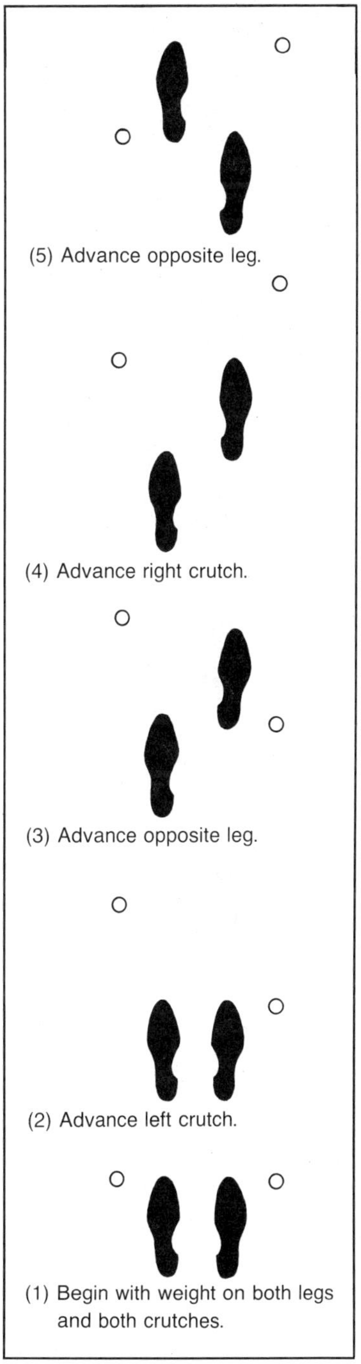

(5) Advance opposite leg.

(4) Advance right crutch.

(3) Advance opposite leg.

(2) Advance left crutch.

(1) Begin with weight on both legs
and both crutches.

Figure 16–5   Four-point gait pattern.

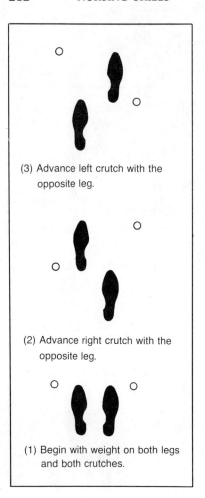

(3) Advance left crutch with the opposite leg.

(2) Advance right crutch with the opposite leg.

(1) Begin with weight on both legs and both crutches.

Figure 16–6   Two-point gait pattern.

Figure 16–7   Three-point gait pattern.

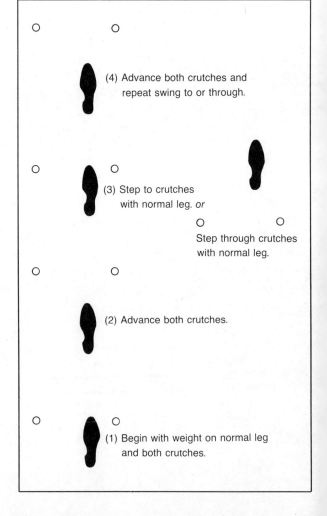

(4) Advance both crutches and repeat swing to or through.

(3) Step to crutches with normal leg. *or*

Step through crutches with normal leg.

(2) Advance both crutches.

(1) Begin with weight on normal leg and both crutches.

crutches and the person steps ahead with the normal leg. The foot lands just behind the crutches (the toes about even with the crutches). This is called a swing-to or step-to pattern.

Once the patient has mastered this, he may be able to master stepping through the crutches (his foot lands ahead of the crutches). This is called a swing-through or step-through pattern.

Pattern: Both crutches advanced. With normal leg he steps to or through the crutches.

Using Stairs. Generally speaking, the key to using stairs is to have the strong leg do all the work. In order to accomplish this, "the good foot goes up and the bad goes down." In other words, the sequence for going upstairs is (1) good foot goes up, (2) the crutches go to the same step and (3) the bad foot joins them. Going downstairs, the order is (1) the crutches go down, (2) the bad foot goes down to the same step and (3) the good foot joins them.

When a patient is first learning stair walking, it is wise to have him wear a belt and to stand behind him with your hand on one shoulder. This is always done going upstairs. Going downstairs, the nurse is often told to stand in front of the patient; however, some persons feel it is better to stand behind the patient. When this is done, the nurse stands behind, holds the patient's belt with one hand and uses her other hand to hold the patient's shoulder or the hand rail. With this method, the nurse not only does not obstruct the patient's view but she can control his balance more easily with one hand on his shoulder and the other at his waist. She can also easily break any fall by pulling the patient back against her as she comes to a sitting position on the stair. The helper must, of course, be alert to the need for a second helper for obese or very dependent patients.

General Nursing Responsibilities for Patients Using Crutches. Even if the nurse does not teach the gait pattern, she will frequently be with the patient when he uses crutches. She therefore can help him to use the crutches properly and be able to assist intelligently if she applies some basic knowledge.

First of all, the nurse has a basic responsibility for her patient's safety. Floors should be without loose rugs, unwaxed, and without wet spots, flower petals, or other slippery substances. She should impress her patient with the importance of good crutch care, emphasizing the replacement of worn or damaged crutch tips.

She must also observe the patient for proper walking posture. The patient should not look down, slouch at the shoulders or stoop. If the three-point gait is used, the nurse should make sure that the involved extremity does not flex at the knee and hip any more than is necessary to keep the foot from hitting the floor. Patients who use crutches sometimes develop foot drop because they walk merely on the balls of their feet. They must be reminded to strike the floor first with the heel, then with the ball of the foot (a heel strike).

When a nurse or family member must assist a person to walk, certain measures will make the task both easier and safer. First of all, a transfer or walking belt (see Chapter 15) should be worn by the patient. The assistant should stand to the side and slightly in back of the patient. If the patient is weaker on one side, the assistant stands on that side and helps the patient by holding the belt with an underhand grip, neither pushing nor pulling on the belt. If the patient falters or tips, the assistant can help him to recover his balance by merely holding the belt firmly and placing his other hand on the patient's shoulder. Should the patient's legs give out, additional help can be given if the assistant widens his own base of support and stands close to the patient. A last alternative is to allow the patient to slide to the floor gently.

BRACES

Another type of walking aid that is individually fitted is a brace. Braces are often used with some other walking aid such as a cane or crutches. Some patients may use a wheelchair for most travel but be able to walk to a limited extent. The ability to use braces enables an individual to enter places where a wheelchair cannot go, makes stepping up to and down from curbs easier and prevents problems with some stairs. In addition, ambulation, even for short periods of time, is excellent exercise and increases circulation, nutritional processes and bone strength. Sometimes daily ambulation even has a beneficial effect on spasticity.

A brace may either permit or restrict movement. Its main purpose is to promote normalcy either posturally or functionally. The nurse cannot be expected to learn all about bracing. She can, however, be observant regarding the following:

1. Is the brace giving support and yet comfortable?
2. Does the patient check his skin after each use of the brace?
3. Is the brace bent or worn? Are screws loose or missing?
4. Has the person grown in height or weight since the brace was prescribed?
5. Are locks clean and do they move freely?
6. Is the leather cleaned regularly with mild soap and water, saddle soap or a good leather cleaner?

WHEN A WHEELCHAIR IS USED TO GET ABOUT

When a person's condition requires the use of a wheelchair to get about, an individually prescribed chair is a must. In the vast majority of instances, a properly prescribed wheelchair can mean independence because it can then be maneuvered by the patient rather than by personnel. The prescription for a wheelchair is analogous to buying the proper shoe size. The wrong size may not only be uncomfortable but may also actually impede walking.

The most important considerations in determining an appropriate wheelchair are patient height and weight, safety, diagnosis, prognosis, transfer technique, mode of propulsion, living habits and cost. A special wheelchair feature can be selected to assist the patient in each of these matters, which are discussed in greater detail in the following section. A rehabilitation nurse, physical therapist or occupational therapist can easily learn to prescribe a wheelchair capably. When a physician is experienced and knowledgeable in this area, he will of course be consulted prior to any investment on the part of the patient.

There are hundreds of possible combinations of wheelchair features available. Wheelchair manufacturers distribute excellent catalogues describing the features and dimensions of their particular brand of chair. Because wheelchairs are fitted to patients, not patients to wheelchairs, rehabilitation facilities usually have chairs of different sizes with various special features such as reclining backs and detachable armrests and footrests. In this way, the patient and the staff have an opportunity to evaluate what wheelchair features best serve an individual. When an institution does not have a variety of chairs, a wheelchair sales representative can arrange to loan or rent a chair with individually selected features for a brief period of time. Because a wheelchair is costly, it is vital that it serve the person optimally, but it is also essential that useless deluxe features be eliminated.

WHAT FEATURES ARE NECESSARY?

Certain wheelchair features can be viewed as requirements for most handicapped persons, while other features are more individualized. Brakes, large wheels in the rear, removable footrests, and eight-inch front casters along with durability and ease of propulsion and folding can be considered essential, not luxury, features for persons who use a wheelchair regularly. The following individual considerations are also essential.

The Patient's Height and Weight. Wheelchairs come in three main sizes: (1) standard adult, (2) intermediate or junior, for small adults and older children and (3) children's, which is ideal up to about six years of age. A growing chair has an adjustable feature for children during the period of rapid growth between the ages of six and twelve years.

On occasion, a custom size chair is necessary. When you select wheelchair size, there are four critical dimensions: (1) seat width and depth, (2) height of seat from the floor, (3) back height and (4) height of armrests. When footrests are adjustable, they can be set at the ideal distance from the popliteal fossa to the heel to achieve proper sitting posture to provide lower extremity support (see Chapter 12). When the patient's height and weight are appropriate to the dimensions of the wheelchair, it can be said to fit. Once the proper size is found, there are other considerations.

Safety. The next consideration relates to safety. Brakes are required on all chairs mainly because it is unsafe to do any kind of a transfer without them. A second important safety measure is the seat belt. This can be attached at the hips, waist or chest according to the physical and mental problems of a patient.

A unique safety problem occurs when a person has had a unilateral but more especially an above the knee bilateral lower extremity amputation. Since 64 per cent of our body weight is distributed in the head and upper trunk and 36 per cent in the lower extremities (18 per cent in each leg), bilateral lower extremity amputation results in a higher center of gravity. It actually shifts the center of gravity from the pelvis to the chest. With a decreased counterweight in front, a chair has a tendency to tip backwards. Therefore, the chair must have more posteriorly placed rear wheels to prevent tipping and to provide stability (see Fig. 16–8). When such a chair is not available, weights (10 lbs. or more) can be placed on each footrest of a regular wheelchair to compensate for the change in the center of gravity.

If a person has had a below the knee amputation, the knee requires support to prevent knee flexion contracture during the period of pre-prosthetic walking. This can be accomplished by using a padded board with a knee extension or an elevating leg rest.

A not uncommon incident for a person who lives in a wheelchair is that of falling forward out of the chair while attempting to pick up something from the floor. If the person has the ability to reach to the floor, a fall can be prevented by

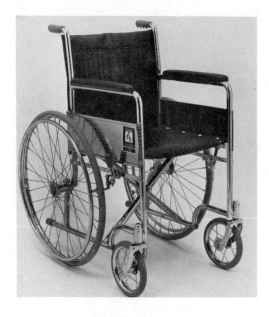

Figure 16–8   Amputee chair. Rear axle is set back 2 inches to compensate for the altered center of gravity of a person who has had a bilateral lower extremity amputation. (Courtesy Everest and Jennings Co., Los Angeles, California.)

using the safety function of the front caster wheels. When a wheelchair stops after having been moved forward, the front casters are pointing backward. When a wheelchair stops after having been moved backward, the front casters are pointing forward. If a person leans forward with the wheels in this position, the chair does not tip forward. A person should, therefore, learn to go beyond the object he wishes to pick up, and then back up to it in order to get the front casters in a safe position for picking the object from the floor (see Fig. 16–9).

Diagnosis and Prognosis.   Not only the patient's diagnosis but also his prognosis should be carefully considered in selecting the proper wheelchair. For example, future trunk weakness can be anticipated in progressive muscular dystrophy. Therefore, a semi-reclining back might be essential to prevent the purchase of two chairs. Trunk weakness may be compensated for by the use of a semi-reclining or reclining back or by adding back height. Head extensions can be attached to the back of a chair when the patient has neck weakness. A semi-reclining chair is also used during the early stages of a rehabilitation program if someone has postural hypotension due to prolonged bed rest.

Elevating legrests are important when someone has a leg cast or dependent edema (see Fig. 16–10). Toe loops on the foot pedals will hold down a spastic foot, while heel loops on the pedals will support a weak or spastic foot.

Most patients are more comfortable when they use a seat cushion. When there is sensory loss, a cushion is essential. It may be made of four-inch foam rubber, and horseshoe shaped. Cushions may also be filled with water, resin, gel or air. Seat boards used under cushions can improve lower extremity posture. (See end of Chapter 15 for list of resources.)

Transfer Technique.   It has already been stated that brakes are necessary for all transfers. In addition, the transfer technique dictates the types of armrests and footrests that are necessary. If someone does an anterior sitting transfer, sliding out of the front of the wheelchair, swinging detachable footrests will allow closer placement of the chair to the bed, car, toilet and so forth. A lateral sitting transfer, whether it is done with or without a sliding board, requires detachable arms plus a swinging detachable footrest (see Fig. 16–11). If footrests are a problem for a standing transfer, a simple detachable footrest may be all that

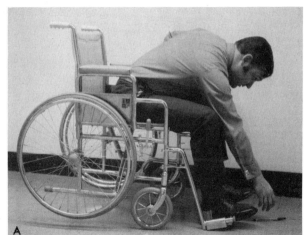

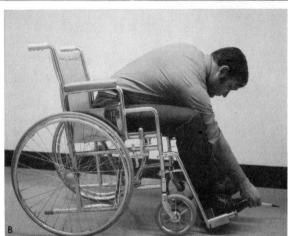

Figure 16–9   Position of front casters can have a safety function if patient has the ability to reach the floor. *A,* Unsafe—the chair tips (footrests touching floor) when front casters face backward. *B,* Safe—the chair is steady when front casters face forward.

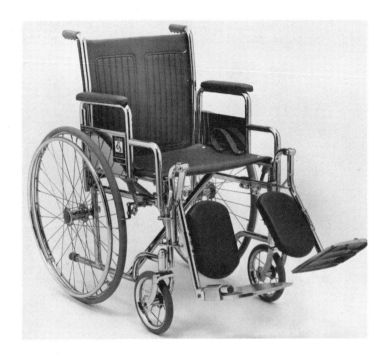

Figure 16–10 Wheelchair with elevating legrests. (Courtesy Everest and Jennings, Los Angeles, California.)

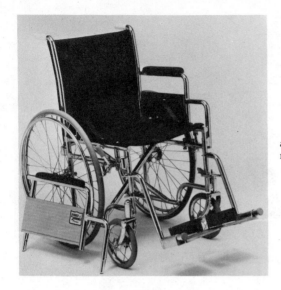

Figure 16–11 Wheelchair with removable armrests and swing back footrests. (Courtesy Everest and Jennings, Los Angeles, California.)

is necessary. If a person lacks finger dexterity and cannot swing the footrest, a release that can swing footrests with the top of the wrist is manufactured (see Fig. 16–12).

PROPULSION TECHNIQUES.   The mode of self-propulsion will influence footrest and hand rim selection. A hemiplegic patient will learn to propel his chair with the normal arm and leg. This requires removal of the footrest on the uninvolved side. A lightweight chair may be best for an arthritic or for a person with weak muscles. A lightweight chair, however, does not hold up well if the person weighs over 160 pounds.

There are one-arm drive chairs. These have a double handrim on the side. The smaller inner rim controls the opposite wheel.

When the patient has a poor grasp, as in quadriplegia or arthritis of the hands, a hand rim with vertical projections will improve the ability to propel the chair (see Fig. 16–13). Vertical rather than horizontal projections are preferred because they do not widen the chair. Battery powered wheelchairs are available.

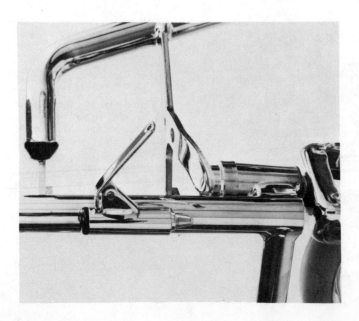

Figure 16–12 Quad release makes it possible for a person without finger dexterity to swing footrests by using the wrist. (Courtesy Everest and Jennings, Los Angeles, California.)

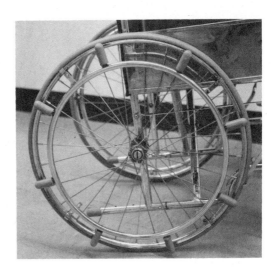

Figure 16–13 Vertical hand projections for persons with poor hand grasp.

They are operated by a control stick which does not require hand dexterity. These chairs are more costly and heavy, but add independence to the severely disabled.

Living Habits.   It is important to know the design of the house. Doorways must be measured to make sure that a wheelchair can pass. A doorway can often be widened adequately by simply removing the inner molding. In some instances a small adult can be fitted with a junior size chair, which is usually about two inches narrower than adult size chairs.

Other room dimensions for wheelchair living are important. In order to turn a chair around, a space five feet by five feet is necessary. Mirrors, cupboards, light switches, wall telephones and other such items must be lowered to be usable for wheelchair living. Steps can be replaced by ramps which should rise no more than one inch in height for every one foot of ramp length.

Various other features are available. Pneumatic tires are available for the person who travels on soft or uneven ground. Desk arms or adjustable armrests can be selected by individuals who work closely at low desks and tables (see Fig. 16–14). A lap board can be placed over the arms of the chair when armrests are not adjustable.

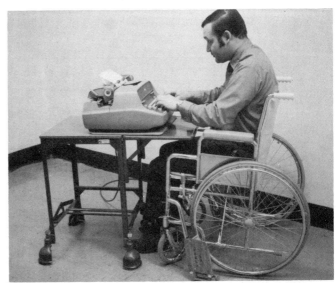

Figure 16–14 Desk arms on wheelchair to allow proximity to a work surface.

TABLE 16–1 STANDARD ADULT MULTI-PURPOSE WHEELCHAIRS*

Legend: ● standard ○ available in this model or series

STANDARD ADULT MULTI-PURPOSE WHEELCHAIRS		Colson Classic 1471-H-275	Colson Champion 1221-S-275	ECM Arrow 712-LR	ECM Arrow 632-LR	Everest & Jennings Premier 8-AU250-774	Everest & Jennings Universal U8A 250-764	Gendron-Diemer Monarch 7810-54-62	Gendron-Diemer New Yorker 6408-62	Gendron-Diemer Regency 5810-54-62	Invacare Rolls Custom 318-24	Invacare V.I.P. 1-24	Theradyne Standard 820-13	Theradyne Health Care 620-13
SPECIFICATIONS	Approx. weight	51	51	52	47	52	58	61	55	66	45	41	55	59
	seat width (in.)	18	18	17	17	18	18	18	16½	18	18	18	18	19
	overall width (in.)	26¾	26¾	25	25	26¼	26¼	25	24½	24½	26	26	25	25½
	folded width	12	12	10	10	11½	11½	11	11	12	10½	10½	11	11
	size modification (custom seat & back)	○				○		○			○		○	
FRONT CASTERS	5 inch			●										
	8 inch	●	●		●	●	●	●	●	●	●	●	●	●
SEAT	solid	○	●	○	○	○	○				●		○	○
	hammock (sling)	●	○	●	●	●	●	●	●	●	●	●	●	●
	upholstery options	●	○	○	○	○	○	○	○	○	○	○	○	○
BRAKES	lever	●	●					○	○	○	○			
	toggle	○	○	●	●	●	●	●	●	●	●	●	●	●
HEADREST	extension available	○	○			○	○	○	○	○	○	○	○	○
ARM STYLES	removable full-length	●	●	●	●	●	●	●	●	●	●	●	●	●
	removable desk-type	●	○	○	○	○	○	○	○	○	○	○	○	○
	adjustable height	●				○	○				○		○	○
	retractable	○				○		○						
FOOT & LEG RESTS	folding footrest	●	●	●	●	●	●	●	●	●	●	●		●
	adjustable height	○	○	●	●	●	●	○	●	●	●	●	●	●
	elevated legrest	●	●	●	●	●	●	●	●	●	●	●	●	●
	swing/detach. legrest	●	●	○	○	●	●	●	●	●	●		●	●
COST	recent approximation	366	344	192	204	425	324	337	260	252	304	292	241	284

● standard   ○ available in this model or series

In addition, table legs may be a barrier, requiring footrests which can be swung aside or detached.

Cost. A good basic chair with features that are individually selected for specific patient needs is a worthwhile investment. Tricky unnecessary features are an expensive luxury. Careful handling and a regular maintenance routine as recommended by the manufacturer will prolong the life of the chair.

See Table 16–1 for a listing of wheelchair dimensions and features. Also see Table 16–2 for a guide to wheelchair selection in relation to a person's diagnosis and disability.

TABLE 16–2 A GUIDE TO WHEELCHAIR SELECTION ACCORDING TO DISABILITY*

A GUIDE TO WHEELCHAIR SELECTION ACCORDING TO DISABILITY (● = Preferred, ◐ = Alternate Choice)

Category	Feature	Hemiplegia	Paraplegia	Quadraplegia	Cerebral Palsy	Arthritis	Bilateral Amputation
TYPE	Standard	●	●	●	●	●	
	Motorized			◐			
	Special	◐			◐		●
HANDRIMS	Standard	●	●	●	●	●	●
	One-arm Drive	◐		◐			
	Pegs or Knobs			◐	◐	◐	
BRAKES	Toggle	◐	◐	●	●	●	◐
	Lever	◐	●		◐		●
	Brake extension	●		◐		◐	
	Special	◐		◐			
BACK	Fixed	●	●		●	●	●
	Reclining			●	◐	◐	
	Head extension	◐	◐	●	◐	◐	◐
ARMRESTS	Fixed	●			●	●	●
	Removable		●	●	◐	◐	
FOOT & LEGRESTS	Swing-detachable	●	●	●	●	●	●
	Elevating legrest	◐	◐	◐	◐	◐	
	Heel loops	●	●	●	●	●	
	Toe loops		◐	◐	◐	◐	

● Preferred   ◐ Alternate Choice

*Reprinted with permission from the November 1973 issue of *Nursing '73.* Copyright © 1973 by Intermed Communications, Inc., Jenkintown, Pennsylvania 19046.

WHEELCHAIR PRESCRIPTION

Name _Mark Allen_ _____ Date Ordered ___ 7 / 11 / 77 _____

Address _Abbott - Park Industries_ _____

To Whom Billed _____ Dealer _____

Brand Name _____ Model _____

Size: Adult __✓__ Junior _____ Large child _____ Small child _____ Special _____

Type: Fixed back __✓__ Added height _____ Semireclining _____ Full reclining _____ Amputee _____

Brakes: Lever __✓__ Toggle _____

Detachable Footrests: Lift off _____ Button _____ Swinging __✓__ Elevating _____

Footplates: Regular _____ Large __✓__

Heel Loops: Right __✓__ Left __✓__

Armrests: Padded __✓__ Fixed _____ Removable __✓__ regular _____ adjustable __✓__ desk _____ _____

Wheels—24": 28 spokes _____ 36 spokes __✓__

Tires—24": Regular _____ Air-filled 1¾" __✓__ 1¼" _____

Axle: Regular _____ Heavy duty __✓__

Handrims: Regular __✓__ Vertical projections (number) _____ Other _____

Front Casters: 8" regular _____ 8" semipneumatic _____

Cushion: Seat: 2"___ 3"___ 4"___ Horseshoe __✓__ Measurement _____
   Covered with protective material _____
Back: 1"___ 2"___   Measurement _____
   Covered with protective material _____

Color of Upholstery: _Brown_ _____

Ordered by _R. C. Morris_ _____ M. D.

Figure 16–15   Wheelchair Prescription form. (Courtesy Sister Kenny Institute, Minneapolis, Minnesota.)

THE WHEELCHAIR PRESCRIPTION

Institutions, agencies and wheelchair manufacturers recommend the use of a wheelchair prescription form to assess and order a wheelchair with individually ordered features. This provides an organized way of relating each aspect of a chair to an individual. (Figure 16–15 shows the typical items of information required.) Remember that this should be done only after the patient has had successful experience using the type of chair that is being ordered.

MULTIPLE USE CHAIRS FOR INSTITUTIONS

Before completing our discussion of wheelchairs, it might be helpful to suggest some guidelines for purchasers of chairs that are to be used by patients with a variety of conditions. This means getting versatility with the dollar.

Most hospitals use chairs to transport weak and nondisabled patients to and from various departments such as x-ray, admitting, physical therapy and so forth. A folding chair with brakes, a luggage rack and footrests can be used by a majority of patients. Most hospitals find that a quality chair saves dollars in terms of numbers of years of use. The chair should be washable, and a planned preventive maintenance program as recommended by the manufacturer will prolong the life of a chair.

Beyond this, an institution must look at its special needs. Orthopedic areas and emergency areas will need to have chairs with reclining backs and elevating legrests. A rehabilitation center and extended care facility serving patients with a variety of disabilities require at least one chair with removable armrests and removable footrests as well as brakes. Removable features allow for exchange of parts and chair versatility. Such parts, of course, must be made by the same manufacturer.

To reduce the amount of time nursing personnel may spend searching for the right wheelchair, most nurses agree that a majority of chairs should have removable armrests and swing-away legrests. Extra sets of armrests and legrests may reduce the actual number of chairs needed. This allows versatility at a minimal cost. In addition, long-term care facilities need to be cautioned against the purchase of any chair that fosters dependence on personnel or increases social isolation. The purpose of a wheelchair is to gain independence, not to restrict activity. This point is particularly applicable to geriatric patients.

SUMMARY

An essential aim of any rehabilitation program is to enable the patient to return to as many normal activities as possible. In order to do this, a new way of getting about may have to be learned. It may require using a wheelchair or merely a cane. It may involve a temporary or a permanent disability. It may occur in an institution or in a home. It is up to the nurse to have basic information on safety, fit of assistive equipment, posture and gait, especially when physical therapy consultation is not available.

REFERENCES

Beaumont, Estelle: Wheelchairs. *Nursing '73, 3*:48, November, 1973.
Bergstrom, D. A.: Report on a conference for wheelchair manufacturers. *Bulletin of Prosthetics Research,* Spring, 1965, pp. 60–89.

Cicenia, E. F., et al.: Maintenance and minor repairs of the wheelchair. *American Journal of Physical Medicine. 35*:206, 1956.

Deaver, G. C., and Brown, M. E.: The challenge of crutches. *Archives of Physical Medicine,* Vol. 26, 1945: Methods of crutch walking, pp. 397–403; Crutch walking: muscular demands and preparation, pp. 515–525; Standard crutch gaits and how to teach them, pp. 525–573; Prescribing crutches for orthopedic disabilities, pp. 747–56.

Decencio, Dominic V., et al.: Verticality perception and ambulation in hemiplegia. *Archives of Physical Medicine and Rehabilitation, 51*:105, 1970.

Fahland, B. B.: *Wheelchair Selection—More than Choosing a Chair with Wheels.* Minneapolis, Sister Kenny Institute, 1967.

Fowles, B. H.: Evaluation and selecton of wheelchairs. *Physical Therapy Review, 39*:525, 1959.

Frost, Alma: *Handbook for Paraplegics and Quadriplegics.* Chicago, The National Paraplegia Foundation, 1964.

Gilbert, Arlene: *You Can Do It from a Wheelchair.* New Rochelle, New York, Arlington House Publishers, 1973.

Hildebrandt, G.: Energy costs of propelling the wheelchair at various speeds: cardiac response and effect on steering accuracy. *Archives of Physical Medicine and Rehabilitation, 51*:131, 1970.

Jordan, Helen, and Cypres, Robert: All-around care for the leg amputee. *Nursing '74, 4*:51, 1974.

Kamenetz, H. L.: *The Wheelchair Book.* Springfield, Illinois, Charles C Thomas, 1969.

Kamenetz, Herman: Wheelchairs for hemiplegics. *In* Licht, Sidney (Ed.): *Stroke and Its Rehabilitation.* Baltimore, Waverly Press, 1975.

Larson, C. B., and Gould, M.: *Orthopedic Nursing.* 8th Ed. St. Louis, C. V. Mosby Co., 1974.

Lee, Mathew H. M., et al.: *Wheelchair Prescription.* Public Health Service Publication #1666 (undated). Superintendent of Documents, Washington, D.C. 20402.

Lowman, Edward, and Klinger, Judith: *Aids to Independent Living.* New York, McGraw-Hill Book Co., 1969.

Olson, V. L., and Cantey, J. B.: *Care of Your Wheelchair.* Spain Rehabilitation Center, University of Alabama in Birmingham, April, 1973.

Peizer, E., et al.: Bioengineering methods of wheelchair evaluation. *Bulletin of Prosthetics Research,* Spring, 1964.

Ranalls, John: Crutches and walkers. *Nursing '72, 2*:21, November, 1972.

Rusk, Howard: *Rehabilitation Medicine.* 3rd Ed. St. Louis, C. V. Mosby Co., 1971.

Snyder, L. H.: Living environments, geriatric wheelchairs and older persons' rehabilitation. *Journal of Gerontological Nursing, 1*:17, November/December, 1975.

Sorenson, Lois, and Ulrich, Patricia: *Ambulation: A Manual for Nurses.* Minneapolis, Sister Kenny Institute, 1966.

Spiegler, J. H., and Goldberg, M. J.: The wheelchair as a permanent mode of mobility. A detailed guide to prescription. *American Journal of Physical Medicine,* Vols. 47 and 48. Part I: December, 1968, pp. 315–316; Part II: February, 1969, pp. 25–37.

Chapter 17

SELF-CARE OF THE PERSON

Recent attention has been directed to the so-called "sick role," which may be summarized in terms of three basic elements. During an illness, a person is (1) exempt from normal social role activities, such as those of breadwinner and parent, (2) exempt from personal responsibility, because "pulling oneself together" cannot alter a physical ailment and (3) usually obliged to want to get well and to seek professional help. This pretty much describes patients in the acute-care setting. Once the illness has subsided, most persons almost automatically return to their previous roles.

When a person enters into a rehabilitation program, however, he must begin to shed the "sick role" in spite of the continuing effects of the illness. Two things may interfere with this transition. First, the attitude and conduct of professional staff may not encourage or allow this to happen. Second, sometimes the desire to get well (or to become more independent) is in conflict with the patient or his family. Only knowledge of each patient and family as well as awareness of our own behavior can help us to understand when conflicts do actually exist. Chapter 4 deals with the psychological aspects of disability in greater detail. For this chapter, a few examples of role conflict between nurse and patient will suffice to highlight the devastating effects this can have on patients.

One of the most frustrating experiences for a disabled person is to be admitted to a hospital for treatment of an acute disease. In many instances, the patient is suddenly treated as being as helpless as the disability makes him, rather than as independent as his ability allows. When a person wants to be independent but is not allowed to by staff, lack of knowledge on the part of the staff may be the cause. Lack of knowledge, however, should not cause so much embarrassment that the nurse makes her patient unnecessarily dependent. Every nurse cannot possibly be expected to be expert in the care of all conditions. The acute-care nurse may not know how to use adaptive equipment or do a sliding board transfer, but she must remember that the patient does! This is true of most aspects of care of a chronically disabled person. A good history and assessment of the patient *with* the patient is the basis for bridging this dilemma.

At the other extreme, the already rehabilitated person may become acutely ill and become as helpless as the non-disabled during an acute illness with acute distress. For example, a dentist, a polio victim who has virtually no ability to use his upper extremities, both teaches and conducts research in his field. His car has been adapted so that he can steer with his lower extremities He feeds himself using a rocker feeder. He is married, has a family and engages in the same everyday activities as you and I. When this man became acutely ill with pneumonia, he had a temperature of 105° and was admitted to the hospital. He was too weak to even handle his rocker feeder and needed to be fed. An overzealous nurse told him he should try to feed himself so he could learn to be independent! While an acute illness is not necessarily debilitating, an evaluation of its effect is necessary before we try to rehabilitate in such inappropriate situations.

In the rehabilitation setting, an expression of the nurse's comprehension of and desire to fulfill the philosophy of rehabilitation is her acceptance of the responsibility for teaching self-care activities. When the spirit of rehabilitation is fully practiced, the nurse will capitalize on a person's function, no matter how minimal, in order to promote the dignity and pride that come from as much independence as possible. Depending on the work setting, the nurse may or may not receive appropriate guidance from an occupational therapist in the area of self-care.

DEFINITIONS

Before discussing nursing responsibilities related to self-care activities, it will be helpful to discuss the terms we will use. There is often confusion between the terms self-care, activities of daily living (usually referred to as ADL's) and functional activities. Definitions, everyday usage of terms and even the scope of self-care vary in different parts of the country and from institution to institution.

Functional independence is a broad term which refers to all of the activities which permit a patient to be independent in living. It includes (1) bed activities such as turning, rolling over, moving upward, downward, backward and forward and coming to a sitting position and moving in that position; (2) transfers to and from bed, tub, shower, toilet, car and so forth; (3) propelling a wheelchair; (4) ambulation with the help of walkers, canes, crutches and braces; (5) activities that require hand dexterity, such as handling the telephone and money and using light switches; (6) personal care including personal hygiene, self-care at the toilet, dressing and eating; (7) homemaking; (8) avocational activities; and (9) vocational activities. The ability to perform a given activity may require exercise as well as the use of certain mechanical aids to make the required movements.

The terms *activities of daily living* and *self-care* are sometimes used interchangeably. They may imply as wide a range of activities as functional activities, but are usually used to describe a narrower range of functions. There is still another variance—the use of the term self-care to mean only dressing, personal hygiene and eating.

This chapter deals primarily with the latter: eating, dressing, and personal hygiene. For our purposes we will consider them as three functional activities which are personal in nature.

PERSONAL SELF-CARE ACTIVITIES

Personal self-care activities are concerned with three major areas. The first includes personal hygiene activities, which encompass bathing, general skin care, nail care, oral hygiene, grooming (shaving, combing hair and putting on makeup) and the ability to attend to one's bowel and bladder needs. Suggestions for the latter were made in Chapter 8. The second area of activity is dressing, and the third is eating. Before determining the ability of a patient to perform in these three areas, one must first identify functional abilities which will be capitalized.

The major problems that are likely to be encountered will be contracture, pain, paralysis, lack of one or more extremities, general weakness, lack of coordination or lack of sensation. Some persons will have the physical ability to perform a task, but they will be impeded by perceptual problems. The severely paralyzed person will require a finger flexion splint activated by wrist action in order to achieve prehension. Others will have multiple problems. Knowing the diagnosis as well as knowing what that diagnosis means in terms of functional ability will help to determine not only what a patient can do but how it will be done. If it takes a woman 20 minutes to put on her lipstick, it is usually far better for her to do it than to let her sit for 20 minutes waiting for the nurse to come and do it. When a person has a severe disability, the nurse must provide every opportunity for pride and self-esteem that come from as many successes and as much independence as possible.

A major responsibility of the nurse in the general hospital is to introduce the concept of rehabilitation very early in the patient's illness. Indeed, it is usually found that the earlier rehabilitation activities begin, the greater the success of the ultimate rehabilitation program. This means realistic goals. If a patient has virtually no hand function but can put on her own makeup, we must talk about abilities and tasks that can be performed in spite of the permanent nature of the problem. Not only can the acute-care nurse assist the patient to understand what rehabilitation will be about, but she can also assist the family to understand what some of the goals may be.

Once the patient begins to realize that he will be able to do things for himself, it is important to have him learn slowly and in keeping with his newly developed muscle strength and ability to use adaptive devices. This must also be in keeping with his psychological state and his learning ability, and within his frustration tolerance. Prevention of contractures and pressure sores of course is never delayed. At one rehabilitation center, where spinal cord injuries come as early as the second week after the injury, there is no attempt to totally rehabilitate the patient during the first admission. Rehabilitation is started and the patient is sent home; he returns to the center about six months later to complete a rehabilitation program. The reason for this is to allow the psyche to "catch up" to the reality of the physical problem. In other words, readiness takes time and must be considered in all teaching and rehabilitation. Chapter 10 discussed problems related to teaching and learning in greater detail.

The learning of self-care techniques must be projected to the patient's home. Some rehabilitation nurses visit the home during hospitalization to observe the kinds of problems that the patient may encounter before going home for the first trial weekend. When this is not possible, especially when patients come from out of town, the family can draw pictures of room design, measure doorways and count the number of stairs up to the house. Continuity of care must be concerned with all functional activities and was discussed in more detail in Chapter 11.

The number of assistive devices for dressing, eating and personal hygiene are innumerable and cannot possibly be listed in detail. This chapter, therefore, will only attempt to describe some major kinds of problems that the nurse is most likely to encounter and to suggest some of the most frequently used types of self-help devices. Further resources are suggested in the list of references at the end of the chapter.

Whether the nurse is in a public health agency, a clinic or an institution, she will do well to check with local suppliers and with physical therapy and occupational therapy consultants for specific patients. Self-help devices are often very individualized. The role of the occupational therapist is to prepare the patient to use his hands, to select and adapt appropriate assistive devices and to teach him necessary techniques. The nurse should seek consultant help whenever available, as it may mean the difference between dependence and inactivity and independence and function. In some instances, usually for the less disabled, the nurse will teach the technique and select appropriate assistive devices.

EATING

Loss of hand grasp, coordination and range of motion are the usual reasons for a patient's inability to feed himself. There are many adaptive devices that aid in solving this problem. They include long handles for a patient who cannot get his hand to his mouth (such as the arthritic patient) and a handle which has a large circumference for persons with a weak grasp. Another type of extension handle is the joint handle, which bends. There are also built up and swivel handled utensils, kniforks (a combination knife and fork), sporks (a combination spoon and fork) and others. A small strap with a pocket for an eating utensil can be attached around the hand for the patient with virtually no hand grasp. Drinking liquids can be expedited with a cup with a large handle, a special glass holder which slips over the hand or the use of a drinking straw. If the patient has coordination problems, the use of unbreakable and weighted dishes and glasses is recommended. Stabilization may be achieved by using a plate guard or a suction cup, or by placing a wet washcloth under the plate (see Fig. 17–1).

The patient should be brought to a dining table as soon as possible in order to encourage socialization and to promote the feeling of health rather than disease. If he must eat in bed, he should be made comfortable and have a table that makes it as easy as possible for him to feed himself. A person may always have to have someone cut up his meat and butter his bread, and he may always have to eat with a spoon, but he still can feed himself. Many patients, however, begin with a spoon and gradually learn to use a knife and fork. When a person feels ready to eat in public or at the home of friends, he may need to bring special equipment along. A small, attractive plastic bag can be used to carry the utensils and adaptive devices that may be needed.

DRESSING

Dressing with Quadriplegia.   In many instances, a quadriplegic person can learn to dress himself partially and, in some cases, totally. Both the technique and the equipment, however, must be individualized because of variances in level of injury, muscle strength, range of motion and sitting balance. There are several contraindications to teaching a quadriplegic person to dress himself. They include uncontrollable muscle spasms of the lower extremities, persistent pain in the neck or trunk while dressing, instability of the spine at the site of injury and pressure sores or a tendency to skin breakdown from the rolling or scooting motions necessary to transfers. Because of the complexity of individualizing quadriplegic dressing, the consultation of an occupational therapist is essential.

Dressing the Upper Trunk with One Hand.   Persons who have the use of both hands and arms generally have no problem dressing the upper trunk. If the

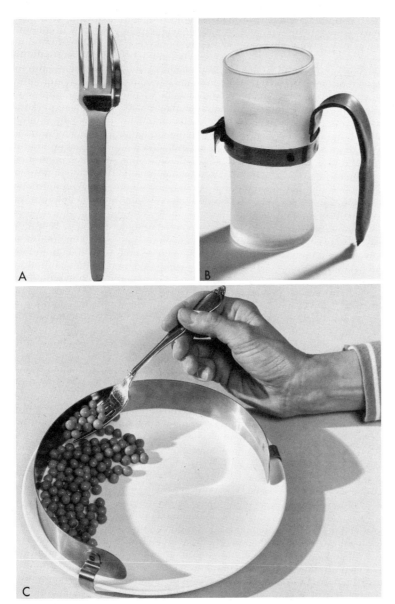

Figure 17–1   Commonly used devices for eating: *A,* Knifork. *B,* Glass holder. *C,* Plate guard.

person has only one functional upper extremity (someone who has hemiplegia, a fractured arm, or possibly an upper extremity amputation) certain dressing techniques will have to be learned.

For women, a difficult problem is the brassiere. The simplest answer is to wear a front-opening brassiere. A regular model can be worn if it is hooked in front and turned around, and if it has stretch straps. Some persons prefer a brassiere that is stretchy and without any fastenings. This can merely be slipped over the head. A regular brassiere can be adapted. It is kept hooked in back, the front is cut and a Velcro strip and ring are inserted so that it can be handled with one hand.

For both men and women, a pullover shirt is a common piece of clothing.

For the man it may be a T-shirt; for the woman it may be a pullover sweater or a dress. In either case, the procedure is as illustrated in Figure 17–2.

The other type of upper trunk clothing is the front-opening garment, such as a jacket, sweater, dress or coat. Buying clothing a size larger will prevent stress and tearing in putting these garments on. The procedure to be followed is shown in Figure 17–3.

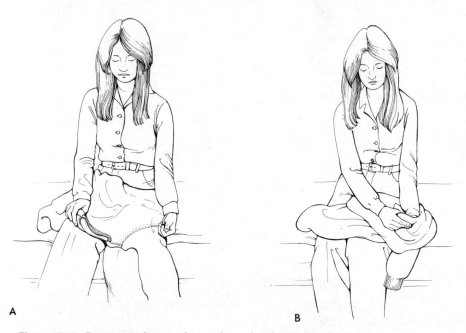

A

B

Figure 17–2 Putting on slipover shirt with one hand.

A, Place the shirt on the lap with the back of the shirt on top.

B, With the strong hand, gather the shirt up to the sleeve (on the weak side) and then place the weak hand in the arm hole.

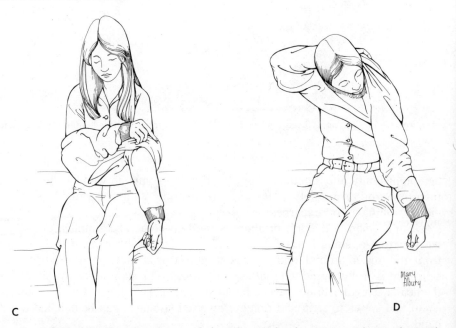

C

D

C, Put the strong hand in the other arm hole and work the sleeve onto each arm alternately until the sleeves are above the elbows.

D, Bring the shirt over the head and pull it down.

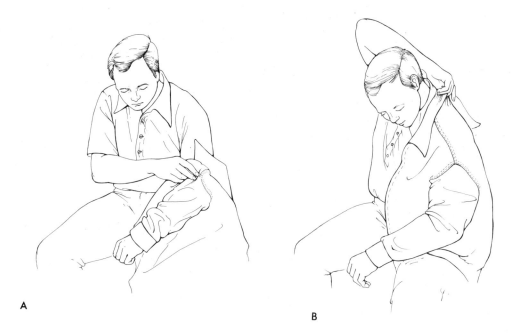

A

B

Figure 17–3 Putting on front-opening jacket with one hand.
A, Pull the sleeve up over the affected arm to the shoulder.
B, Reach for the neckline at the back, slide hand around the collar and bring the other side of the shirt around over the shoulder.

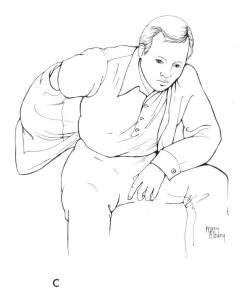

C

C, Reach back and place the strong arm in the other sleeve.

The key to both procedures is to remember to dress the weaker arm first and to undress the strong arm first.

Lower Trunk Dressing. The person who has problems with the lower extremities can learn to dress fairly easily if he has the use of both hands, sitting balance, adequate range of motion and no uncontrollable spasticity. Such a person can sit up and dress the lower extremities by bending each leg to bring the foot close enough to place the foot and leg into the trousers. If the patient is in a cast and is unable to bend his legs, assistance in pulling the pants up over the feet and lower legs will be necessary, or a device may be used. Naturally, if the patient has no use of his hands he will require a device and should be allowed to do as much as possible. With the use of both hands it is usually easier to dress in bed and then raise the hips to pull the skirt down or the pants up to the waist.

If the person has the use of only one hand and has good sitting balance, dressing may be easier to perform while sitting on the edge of the bed. If the patient is a hemiplegic, the affected leg should be dressed first while it is crossed over the good leg. Once the pants are pulled up over that leg, the good leg can then be dressed. Next, the patient can stand to pull the trousers up and fasten them (see Fig. 17–4).

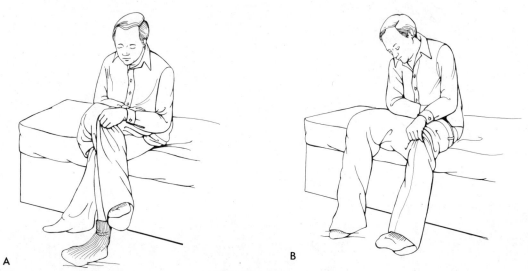

A   B

Figure 17–4 Putting on trousers with one hand.
A, Cross the involved leg and dress it first.
B, Uncross legs and dress the uninvolved leg next.

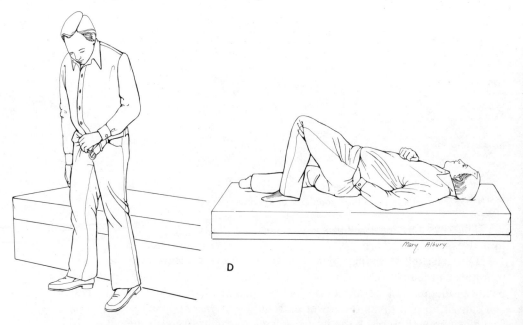

C   D

C, Put on shoes before standing to pull up trousers, bringing the uninvolved side up first.
D, If standing balance is poor, lie down to pull trousers up with the palm of the hand down.

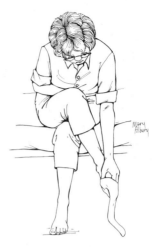

Figure 17-5 Putting sock on with one hand.

If a patient with only one good extremity does not have good standing balance, he should dress in the supine position on the bed. While raising the hips, the pants are pulled up. It is usually better to place the hand palm toward the bed to get a better grip on the waist of the trousers.

Pants should always be full enough to go over any brace or cast that might be worn. The double-knit slack is ideal because it stretches while it is being put on but returns to an attractive size afterwards. Zippered legs or Velcro openings on pants are an alternative if a person is unable to handle regular pants. A clothespin on the end of a stick can be useful in putting on shorts or pants. By hooking the clothespin to the pants, they can be pulled up by the stick.

Putting on Shoes and Stockings.   If the woman desires to wear hosiery, it is usually possible. Pantyhose may be used if the patient has enough hand dexterity. There are garter adapters which help to pull on regular hosiery if a garter belt or a girdle is worn.

For the one-handed person, it is easier to put on socks than hosiery. The sock can simply be folded inside out with the toe indented, put over the toes and worked up over the foot and ankle. Another method is to spread the cuff with the thumb and forefinger, bring it over the toes and pull it over the foot until it is smooth (see Fig. 17-5).

It is important that a good supporting shoe be worn. This often requires a shoe with at least a three- or four-hole lace, although some loafers do come up higher and have fair support. Placing a shoe aid in the back of the shoe will enable the foot to slip into the shoe easily. The patient may be able to learn how to tie the shoe with one hand by using a special technique, or a shoemaker may put on a zipper or other kind of closing. For the person who must tie his shoes with one hand, the top two eyelets of the shoe can be replaced on each side with hooks. The shoelace is then laced through the bottom eyelets and tied to the appropriate length. When the shoes are put on or taken off, the person merely hooks or unhooks the lace.

When the patient has use of both upper extremities, shoes and stockings can be put on in bed. Sitting on the edge of the bed and using a long-handled shoe horn will help the person who cannot reach down to put on the shoe (see Fig. 17-6A).

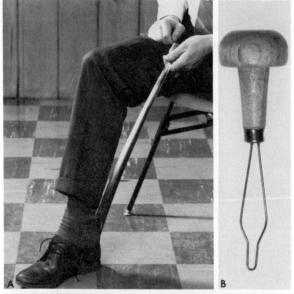

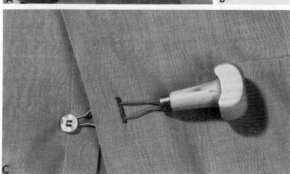

Figure 17–6 Commonly used devices for dressing. *A,* Long-handled shoe horn. *B,* Button hook. *C,* Button hook in use.

Underclothing. For the woman, a slip may be a problem. This can be made easier by the use of a half slip or pettipants or by placing a zipper up the front of the slip.

Girdles and corsets can also be a problem; however, they are used less commonly and some persons find they can get along without them. If a person prefers to wear one, it is wise to use a corset which has a front zipper for ease of dressing.

When the patient is incontinent, underclothing should naturally be water repellent as described in Chapter 8. In this case, outer clothing should be washable and preferably not require ironing.

Problems with Fastening. Even though the patient may successfully put on his clothes, he may not be able to handle zippers, buttons and hooks. The type of fastening, therefore, also determines the amount of independence that a patient may have. For instance, buttonholes may be made slightly larger. Large buttons are easier to handle than small ones. Buttons may be sewed on with elastic so that they can be pulled through more easily. Clothing without buttons such as pullovers may be desirable. The use of button hooks may enable a person to fasten clothing (see Fig. 17–6*B* and *C*). A pre-tied necktie with a clip that can merely be clipped onto the collar simplifies dressing and increases the amount of independence of a man who has only one hand or one very weak hand.

Velcro is an indispensable item. It is not only washable but it also comes in various colors and widths and can be used on coats, shirts, underclothes and so forth. It can be used in the fly of pants, on coat openings and on any number of other articles and makes for ease in fastening clothes.

Jewelry.   An important part of dressing for the female patient is the use of jewelry. This enhances her appearance and increases general morale. A necklace can be put over the head with one hand if the patient does not have hand dexterity to enable her to handle a small clasp. A watch which has a snap bracelet or stretch band is handled by most patients. A ring may be worn, generally on the weaker hand by using the stronger hand to put it on. There should be caution in case of edema. Rings, unless adjustable, should not be worn on a finger that has a tendency toward edema. Nor should rings be worn on the involved arm of a hemiplegic person. Earrings are important. Many younger paraplegic and quadriplegic women have pierced ears, and pierced earrings are difficult to handle if hand dexterity is lacking. Assistance may not be required by the quadriplegic if snap earrings are worn. The woman may not consider herself dressed until she has put on her jewelry.

PERSONAL HYGIENE

Bathing.   Bathing is of little trouble for the person who has good to moderate use of his upper extremities. Persons can wash either sitting up in bed if they have good back support, or in a wheelchair at a sink.

When a tub is used, a bath lift may be the best way to accomplish bathing. A tub can also be used if the patient can learn a tub transfer as discussed in Chapter 15. Non-slip grab bars and non-slip tape are essential whenever a tub is used.

The use of a shower chair with good back support is probably one of the simplest ways for the patient to bathe at home. If the shower has a flush threshold, a drain, a non-skid base and a flexible shower handle, many patients can be moderately independent. If a shower chair is used, it should have caster locks, and they should be locked while bathing.

If the patient does not need to bathe completely every day, face, hands, underarms, and perineum should be washed daily. Daily use of an antiperspirant is also essential. If a person has a contracture, the skin surfaces in the tight area should always be bathed and dried thoroughly. For example, the axilla of the paralyzed arm and the hand of the hemiplegic should be thoroughly bathed daily. Instead of a washcloth, a sponge attached to a long handle or a bath mit is useful for patients who have problems with hand and arm function (see Fig. 17–7A). Range of motion is important since this can affect skin care by making it possible to bathe these areas properly. At the time of bathing, the skin should be observed for any reddened areas, which should remain pressure free to prevent impending pressure sores.

Fingernails need to be clean and filed short, and the cuticle should be cared for weekly. This is also true of the toenails. Many patients will require help in this area. The family or the nurse, therefore, may need to assist the patient in nail care.

For everyday hand care of the person with only one useful arm, the use of

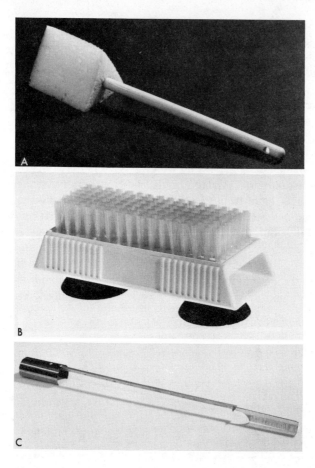

Figure 17-7 Commonly used devices for personal hygiene. *A*, Long-handled sponge for bathing. *B*, Hand brush on suction cups. *C*, Long-handled comb.

suction cups on a hand brush is most helpful (see Fig. 17-7*B*). In this way, the patient can wash his good hand without assistance.

Oral Hygiene.   Teeth should be properly brushed twice a day. Using an electric toothbrush allows many persons independence in this activity. However, this may have to be done by the nurse, an attendant, family member or by the person himself with an adaptive device.

If the patient has dentures and has a weak or paralyzed arm, have a denture brush attached to suction cups at the sink. The hemiplegic may be less aware of food in the affected side of his mouth and may need help or at least reminding to brush that side. The person with arthritis may require a toothbrush on a long, bent handle. Many quadriplegic patients and persons with degenerating neuromuscular diseases may need assistance with oral hygiene.

Grooming.   General morale and a sense of well-being and pride are increased with proper grooming. For the male patient, this means shaving. An electric razor is the safest and most useful if there is one hand that has function. Sometimes the patient may need to move his head as well as his hand in order to shave thoroughly. If a person cannot hold an electric razor, a regular razor can be attached to a long, bent handle, a shaver holder may be used or a hand splint may be needed. The hemiplegic person may need repeated reminding to shave on the paralyzed side which is so frequently neglected.

For women, the use of cosmetics is vital. One young quadriplegic woman who has virtually no hand function spends about 45 minutes each day putting on lipstick, powder and eye makeup. She is a stunning sight when she is through, and she says that this is one of the most important parts of her daily routine. She is proud that she can do this regardless of how long it takes, and she does it with great success.

Brushing and combing the hair is an important part of grooming for both sexes. A long-handled comb (see Fig. 17–7C), a simple short hairdo or long hair which can be easily combed back or recommended. Besides daily grooming, weekly or twice-weekly shampoos are essential depending on the amount of skin oil. Assistance is very often necessary for this activity.

MISCELLANEOUS ADL'S

It is generally not the responsibility of the nurse to recommend homemaking activities and recreational adaptations. However, the public health nurse, extended care nurse, the nursing home nurse and many others do not always have an occupational therapy consultant available. Therefore, it will help to suggest other kinds of adaptive equipment as well as recommend a few resources.

In the area of homemaking there are hundreds of energy-saving devices that can assist a disabled homemaker. The use of a light-weight iron and keeping an ironing board set up at a level which allows the person to sit are simple recommendations. Placing a mirror over the burners of a stove so that a woman in a wheelchair can see whether the water is boiling, using revolving shelves and providing wheelchair space at a sink are frequent kitchen adaptations. These are but a few of hundreds of possibilities.

There are many other miscellaneous kinds of equipment and devices. Here are just a few. The use of a remote TV and radio switch saves energy, since it prevents the patient from getting up and down to adjust station, channel and volume. There are pencil holders, so that the person with poor hand function can write with little or no finger dexterity. There are book holders which allow the quadriplegic to read, as well as a rubber tip stick to turn pages. Many patients can do a great deal with their mouth as evidenced by some of the outstanding artwork done by mouth painters. Prismatic glasses are available so that the patient can read in a recumbent position. There are cigarette holders, so that no one is needed to put a cigarette in and out of someone's mouth. Card holders are available so that the patient can play bridge and other card games. There are many items which allow a person to sew and embroider when it is seemingly impossible.

Very important innovations are the various kinds of telephone adaptations. The occupational therapist should be consulted for simple devices that can make phone use possible when a person cannot dial a phone or cannot handle a receiver. She may suggest that the telephone company be called. For example, there is a telephone which has a speaker with buttons that can be operated by a toe, finger or a stick, and no receiver is needed.

The important concept for the nurse is to know that most patients can do seemingly impossible things if they have the right kind of adaptive equipment. It is recommended that the nurse review the resources that are starred in the references at the end of this chapter when she has a problem. Once an analysis of the individual's problem is made, she will more than likely be able to find an aid for that patient. Naturally, whenever an occupational therapy consultant is available, this source of assistance is both appropriate and best.

SUMMARY

While the nurse assists the patient in all ADL's, it is usually her primary responsibility to teach her patients such activities as personal hygiene, eating and dressing. She is also responsible for teaching self-care in toilet activities, which was discussed in Chapter 8. Her teaching will be highly individualized because of the nature of the person's physical illness, age, mental comprehension and psychological reactions. It will also be highly individualized in terms of kinds of adaptive equipment. Her creativity and ingenuity will be challenged over and over again. The area of ADL's is basic to the functional approach to rehabilitation. If a patient has a functioning muscle, it is up to the rehabilitation team to find out how the function can be used maximally. When this concept is started in the acute hospital, patients and families are better prepared for a rehabilitation program.

REFERENCES

Ballantyne, Donna: Evaluating ADL at the bedside. *American Journal of Nursing, 66*:2440, 1966.

*Be Ok—Self-Help Aids. Catalog available from Fred Sammons, Inc., Box 32, Brookfield, Illinois 60513.

Bursten, Ben, and D'Esopo, Rose: The obligation to remain sick. *Archives of General Psychiatry, 12*: 402, 1965.

Chaney, Patricia: Ordeal. *Nursing '75, 5*:27, June, 1975.

Cookman, Helen, and Zimmerman, Muriel: *Functional Fashions for the Physically Handicapped*. Institute of Physical Medicine and Rehabilitation, New York University Medical Center, 1961.

*Fashion-ABLE, Rocky Hill, New Jersey 08553. (Catalog available.)

Frost, Alma: *Handbook for Paraplegics and Quadriplegics*. Chicago, The National Paraplegia Foundation, 1964.

Gilbert, Arlene: *You Can Do it From a Wheelchair*. New Rochelle, New York, Arlington-House Publishers, 1973.

*Gordon, E. E.: *Do It Yourself Again: Self-Help Devices for the Stroke Patient*. New York, American Heart Association, 1969.

Hasselkus, B., and Kiernat, J.: Independent living for the elderly. *American Journal of Occupational Therapy, 27*:181, 1973.

*Hodgeman, Karen, and Worpeha, Eleanor: *Adaptations and Techniques for the Disabled Homemaker*. Sister Kenny Institute, Minneapolis, Minnesota, 1973.

Klinger, J. L., Frieden, F. H., and Sullivan, R. A.: *Mealtime Manual for the Aged and Handicapped*. Institute of Rehabilitation Medicine, New York University Medical Center, 1970.

Kottke, F. J.: Training for functional independence. *In* Krusen, F. H., et al.: *Handbook of Physical Medicine and Rehabilitation*. 2nd Ed. Philadelphia, W. B. Saunders Co., 1971.

Lawton, Edith: *Activities of Daily Living for Rehabilitation*. New York, Blakiston Division, McGraw-Hill Book Co., 1963.

*Lowman, Edward, and Klinger, Judith: *Aids to Independent Living*. New York, McGraw-Hill Book Co., 1969.

*Meldahl, Harriet, and Wascoe, Joyce: *Ability—Not Disability*. A series of pamphlets on homemaking, shopping, cooking, cleaning, etc., for persons with arthritis, hemiplegia and low energy. Extension Folders 316, Nos. 1 through 12, University of Minnesota, Department of Information and Agricultural Journalism, 433 Coffey Hall, St. Paul, Minnesota, 55108, 1975.

Peszczynski, M.: The rehabilitation potential of the late adult patient. *American Journal of Nursing, 63*:111, 1963.

*Runge, Margaret: Self-dressing techniques for patients with spinal cord injury. *American Journal of Occupational Therapy, 21*:367, 1967.

---

*Recommended resources for the nurse.

Rusk, Howard: *Rehabilitation Medicine.* St. Louis, C. V. Mosby Co., 1971, Chapters 6, 9, 11.

*Sandler, Bernard: Training in homemaking activities. *In* Krusen, F. H., et al.: *Handbook of Physical Medicine and Rehabilitation.* 2nd Ed. Philadelphia, W. B. Saunders Co., 1971.

Self-Care for the Hemiplegic. #704, Minneapolis, American Rehabilitation Foundation, 1970.

Trigiano, L. L.: Independence is possible in quadriplegia. *American Journal of Nursing, 70*:2610, 1970.

Wheeler, Virginia Hart: *Planning Kitchens for Handicapped Homemakers.* Institute of Physical Medicine and Rehabilitation, New York University Medical Center, Rehabilitation Monograph XXVII.

*Recommended resources for the nurse.

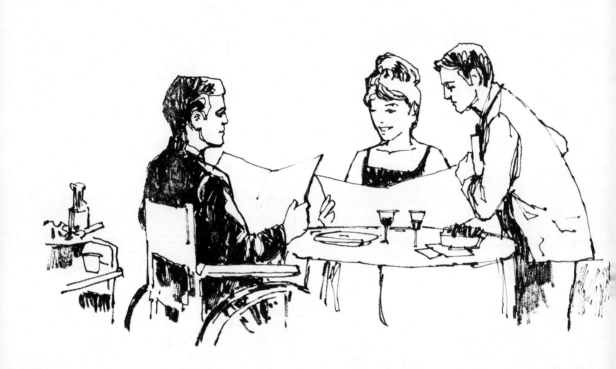

Unit IV

AFTER REHABILITATION—
AN ACTIVE FUTURE

Chapter 18

THE DISABLED IN THE COMMUNITY

Once a formal rehabilitation program has been completed and the patient has been discharged, what then? Survival is not enough. Quality of life is the ultimate goal, and it is sometimes difficult to achieve. When the disabled person returns to the community, he often must struggle with problems of segregation and isolation. The attitude of the public toward the disabled is frequently that of ignorance, apathy, suspicion and sometimes apprehension. These attitudes are reflected in major areas of a person's life, including housing, the use of public buildings, education, employment, transportation, travel and recreation.

For example, a large business may contribute generously to organizations serving the disabled, but be unwilling to employ the disabled. Local governments may have programs to teach the disabled new skills, but be unwilling to assure transportation systems or buildings that will permit the pursuit of those new skills. A majority of us will be fortunate enough to escape serious disability, but few will escape failing eyesight, diminished hearing and stiffened joints—natural outcomes of advancing years. It is estimated that 4000 men and women turn 65 years of age each day in the United States. Many persons may have multiple health problems such as poor vision and arthritis, diabetes and heart disease or osteoporosis and deafness. In addition, the disabled in our community include all the persons who have been injured in war and in industrial and auto accidents, and those whose problems result from congenital deformities, acute illness or other chronic diseases.

Those of us who are fortunate enough to have the ability to go up and down curbs, to enter buildings having heavy revolving doors, to get into telephone booths, to climb stairs and so forth take our activities for granted. Approximately 30 million Americans, however, cannot do these things because they are victims of unnecessary barriers in their community.

There are various ways in which each of us can become more sensitive to the problems of persons with a disability. We might imagine that we are blind for a day, deaf for a day or in a wheelchair for a day in order to identify some of the problems encountered by persons with such a disability. As more persons become aware of disability-related problems, the greater the chances are for community awareness. In spite of present problems, there have been many gains. A knowledge of community resources will assure the disabled person of being able to take advantage of these gains. General community information is available through the local community information and referral service. In addition, state and national resources may be located through some of the organizations named later in this chapter.

USE OF PUBLIC BUILDINGS

Many building requirements for the disabled can also be helpful to the general population. For example, non-slip floor coverings is a safety feature which can benefit all of us. Properly installed grab bars in bathrooms and railings in halls and stairs are used by everyone. A ramp is usually helpful to persons using bicycles, baby carriages and grocery carts. Sliding doors rather than hinged doors that are awkward are better for everyone. They not only prevent accidents but they assist all of us who carry bags of groceries and shopping items.

Some states have laws requiring certain building and remodeling codes to allow accessibility for the handicapped person. Federal legislation passed in 1968 stipulates that any federally funded building that is to be used by the general public in which disabled persons may work or live must be accessible. It will be many years, however, before the many inaccessible buildings are remodeled, and privately funded construction may or may not conform to these codes.

Architectural barriers may rule out a specific job, make it impossible to attend a class or deny someone the pleasure of attending a concert. Public bathrooms rarely allow wheelchair entrance. Drinking fountains are too high to use. Parking spaces need to be wide enough so that a wheelchair can be lifted out of a car and set up for a transfer from the car. Curbs and steps at building entrances are barriers. Tables in restaurants need to be high enough for a wheelchair to get under. While the 1968 legislation will ultimately change things, there are many steps and doors that make the church, the library, the public rest room, the shopping center, the grocery store, the theatre, the pay phone and the stadium inaccessible. Obtaining a birth certificate, a passport or voter registration card becomes a major problem. The disabled pay taxes, but they cannot obtain government services on an equal basis.

Sometimes the letter of the building code is met, but wheelchair accessibility is still not possible. I know of one hospital that is ramped from the sidewalk to the front door, but once inside the front door, there are six steps to the lobby. A brand-new sixteen story medical building has properly installed wide door bathroom cubicles with grab bars, but there is no way for a wheelchair to get to the wide door!

Besides the physical barrier, the feeling of self-esteem that comes from independence is certainly lost when a person must be carried upstairs or be given a urinal outside a rest room. Much humiliation and frustration stem from architectural barriers. In addition to the federal legislation of 1968, many state laws have changed, but some local building codes still do not have accessibility requirements. In a number of major cities, a guide to accessible buildings is available at the local office of the National Society for Crippled Children and Adults. Facilities that are wheelchair accessible are asked to display the symbol shown in Figure 18–1. This symbol is also used in the home to let firemen know that there is a disabled resident.

HOUSING

Whether the disabled person lives in a single dwelling or in multiple housing, certain physical adaptations are essential. (In addition to studying the following information, review Chapter 11 on discharge planning.) The American Standards

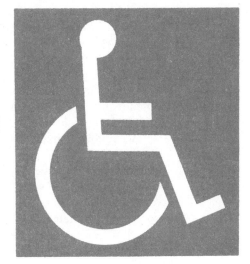

Figure 18-1 National logo indicating wheelchair accessibility to public buildings and parks.

Institute recommends the following specifications in any home occupied by a disabled person.

1. The lot on which a house is built should be graded so that it is level, and the house should be easy to enter.

2. Entrance ramps should rise one foot for each 12 feet of ramp, and be four feet wide. All ramps should have a non-slip surface, at least one hand rail and a flat platform five feet square at the top, so that a wheelchair can come to a full rest and turn at the door. In addition, there should be no less than a six-foot clearance at the bottom. Instead of a ramp, a lift over the stairs might be used (see Fig. 18-2).

3. If stairs are absolutely necessary, the height of each step should be no more than seven inches, and there should be no overhang on the steps. Hand rails should be extended 18 inches beyond the top and bottom steps. A stair lift may be appropriate in some instances (see Fig. 18-3).

4. All floors should be a non-slip surface with a common level.

5. Bathroom doors must be wide enough for a wheelchair to enter. Mirrors, shelves, towel bars and so forth should be placed within easy reach for persons in a wheelchair. Drain pipes and hot water pipes should be covered or protected, so that anyone without sensation will not burn himself.

6. Controls and switches for light, heat, ventilation, windows and so forth should be within easy reach of persons in a wheelchair.

Window height in a home is important. Windows should be low enough for a sitting person to see outdoors. It should be possible to open, close and wash windows with minimum effort. Pushbar handles and awning type windows are especially easy to operate. Some gear type handles are easy to operate also. Draw draperies are preferred to window shades because the latter tend to snap out of reach, and venetian blinds are awkward to open and close.

Non-skid floors made of asphalt or vinyl tile prevent slipping. If floors must be waxed, a non-slip wax must be used. Carpeting on floors makes the propulsion of the wheelchair more difficult, and can cause accidents with canes and crutches if the carpeting is loose. In all instances, the carpet should be nailed or glued down and throw rugs should be removed. Most persons using a wheelchair prefer no carpeting.

Light switches and fuse boxes should be placed about 36 inches from the floor. Wall switches can be made to control all light fixtures to avoid using lamp controls. A very helpful system for the disabled is to have several master switches which control all the lights in the house. Convenient placements of a master switch are in the bedroom, kitchen and living room. Electric outlets should be about 18 inches from the floor, so that they can be easily used by someone in a wheelchair. A night light is important for the area between the bedroom and the bathroom.

A telephone should be at the bedside of any disabled individual. Should he need help or become sick, the phone is available. Additional telephone outlets in the home may be time saving. The use of telephone jacks makes a home telephone system more versatile. The local telephone company should always be consulted, since there are many remarkable adaptations for persons who have problems with their hands or with hearing or vision.

All doorways should be wide enough (36 inches is recommended) for easy passage of a wheelchair. In addition, approximately five square feet is required for the turning of a wheelchair. A car port should be at least one or two feet wider than the average 12 feet in order to allow extra space for transferring between car and wheelchair.

It is naturally easier to plan a home from scratch than it is to remodel a home. In either case, however, there are several resources. In some instances, a stair elevator or a wheelchair lift on the stairway makes it possible for a home to be used as it was originally planned. There are two organizations that have an of-

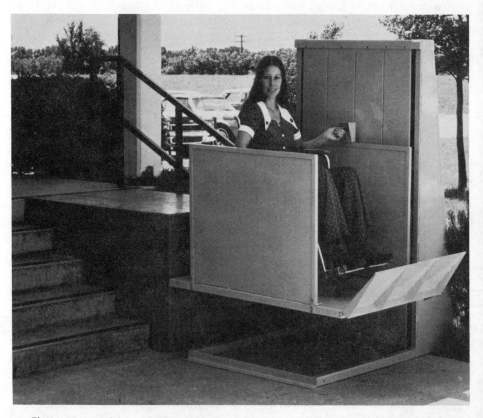

Figure 18–2 A lift to avoid steps to a porch, entry or elevated patio. (Courtesy American Stair-Glide Corporation, Grandview, Missouri.)

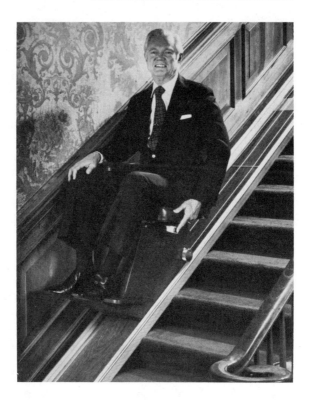

Figure 18–3 A motorized stairway lift. (Courtesy American Stair-Glide Corporation, Grandview, Missouri.)

fice in every state in the union. They are Abbey Rents and Everest and Jennings Inc. They can be called for rental and sale of home equipment. They would be knowledgeable about and could suggest other local organizations supplying equipment. The Functional Home for Easier Living located at the New York University Medical Center is a model home for the handicapped. The features of this house were planned for the person who uses a wheelchair. Whenever there is a problem with design, it is recommended that the individual be referred to the state chapter of the American Institute of Architects. It is important to ask to be referred to a firm or person who is conversant and familiar with designing for the disabled. In addition, by sending one dollar to Paralyzed Veterans of America, Inc., 3636 16th Street, NW, Washington, D.C. 20010, the monograph *Wheelchair Bathrooms* may be obtained. The same organization will send free on request an excellent *Bibliography on Paraplegia*. This includes a variety of resources.

EDUCATION

In some instances a person must change occupations after a disability in order to earn a living. A teacher may continue teaching; a manager may continue to manage, but a carpenter may have to change occupations. This requires education. The younger person who has not completed his education will naturally begin a new program or continue where he left off. In one study of mortality rates in paraplegia, it was found that the younger the injured person, the higher the survival rate. For many, this means a normal life span. The matter of education, therefore, is paramount.

Three major facets must be examined to determine the suitability of an educational program. What is a person's mental and physical ability? What are his interests? What is in keeping with his disability? In the discussion on discharge planning in Chapter 11, referral to the State Division of Vocational Rehabilitation was recommended as the first educational step in planning. Both financial aid and vocational counseling are available through this federally funded agency.

Once the person has selected an educational program, the next problem relates to the selection of the training center or college. Unfortunately, architectural barriers exist at most educational institutions. In some instances, certain buildings are accessible while others are not. Depending on the courses that the student requires, he may or may not be able to attend a particular college or university. *Mobility for Handicapped Students,* published by Rehabilitation Services Administration, Department of Health, Education and Welfare, Washington, D.C. 20201, lists educational facilities for persons with various types of disabilities.

While almost 200 colleges and universities have special features for a variety of disabilities, two that serve the disabled need particular mention. The first is the University of Illinois in Champaign. Mr. Timothy Nugent has spent a lifetime working with students in assisting them to overcome architectural barriers. He works with all kinds of disabilities and is also interested in recreation. He can assist blind persons with 14 different activities and wheelchair students with 22 activities. Mr. Nugent provides potential students with a special training program. Once they are able to perform certain tasks they are eligible to attend if they are otherwise qualified. Information about this program can be obtained by writing the Rehabilitation and Education Center, University of Illinois, Champaign, Illinois 61820.

The second is in Columbia, Missouri. The new buildings at the University of Missouri are accessible, and old buildings have been remodeled to be accessible for wheelchair patients. Ramped curbs, wide doorways, elevators and other adaptations were made through a special grant.

In addition to schools, certain organizations specialize in the training of disabled persons. Besides sheltered workshops, there are the Bulova School of Watchmaking in Woodside, Long Island; Abilities, Inc., in Long Island; and the Paraplegic Manufacturing Company in Bensenville, Illinois.

WORK

Work is central to the meaning of life to most individuals. Work occupies one-third of our time each day, and it is considered important to our mental well-being, as well as being obviously necessary for economic reasons. Vocational rehabilitation programs are not only beneficial to the individual who is handicapped, but it has proved to be economically beneficial to society. It reduces the number of disabled persons who must be supported by welfare funds. It increases the amount of tax revenue available by placing a greater number of persons in the work force. In some instances, it has even reduced the number of persons being cared for in state institutions, thus reducing the cost of tax-supported institutions.

To become totally self-supporting is just as much a goal for the disabled person as it is for other individuals. In many instances, the disabled can achieve this goal no matter how severe the disability. In some instances, however, this goal is only partially achievable, or a sheltered workshop may be advisable. Through assessment of the person's mental ability, his physical ability, his general interests and talents and, in some instances, through assessment in simulated work situations, a person will be provided with work alternatives. Training and education is obtained as indicated. An excellent resource is *How to Get Help If You Are Paralyzed,* which can be obtained from the National Paraplegic Foundation, 333 N. Michigan Avenue, Chicago, Illinois 60601.

Once again the problem of architectural barriers may loom up. Aside from actual job considerations, the disabled must ask many questions. Can he park his car and get to the building? Can he get through the front door? Is there an elevator? Can he use the rest room? Is he able to get to the cafeteria? The answers to those crucial questions are completely unrelated to the person's ability.

Employer attitude may also be a consideration. Many employers hold the false assumption that a disability will cause undependable attendance. Various studies have been made on the reliability, absenteeism, illness rate and turnover rate of disabled workers. In most instances it has been found that disabled persons are absent no more and usually fewer days than able-bodied persons. It is possible that they make exceptional efforts, knowing that the public is often quick to exaggerate problems and quick to criticize. In general, the disabled have been found to be exceptionally conscientious and reliable workers. In fact, some organizations have a special interest in hiring the disabled because they are aware of these facts. In some states, human rights legislation now prohibits discrimination in hiring practices of the disabled.

TRANSPORTATION AND TRAVEL

PUBLIC TRANSPORTATION

At the present time, the disabled person is unable to use many of our transportation systems. Bus steps are too high for the elderly person let alone for someone who has arthritis or is dependent on crutches. Buses are totally inaccessible to the wheelchair user. Persons with visual problems have an equally difficult time knowing what bus is approaching and whether they are standing at the correct bus stop. Only a few places in the country are presently attempting to provide transportation that could convey persons with mobility and visual problems. A most desirable feature for mass transportation is some type of hydraulic step that would lower and raise so that the person could enter a bus or train without using a step. A few cities are studying no-step buses and subways, and in a few instances buses with this feature are available at certain times of the day.

Until 1970, Maryland was the only state that required transportation terminals, such as bus or airport stations, to be included in its architectural barriers law. This does not mean that many new airport terminals are not accessible, but it does mean that the architect must be knowledgeable and the public must be vigilant during the planning stages of public transportation areas in order to build a barrier-free community.

THE DISABLED CAN DRIVE

Driving a car is a possible goal for many disabled persons. There are three facets that must be investigated. One is to adapt the car with appropriate equipment; the second, to obtain special training in the use of this equipment; and the third, to obtain licensure through a driving test. In some instances, car insurance is higher for the disabled person than it is for the nondisabled. A few companies charge the same rate whether special equipment is used or not.

There is a variety of adaptive equipment for automobiles. Some examples are right directional signals for the person with a left upper extremity amputation or left hemiplegia, a left gas pedal for a person with a right lower extremity amputation or right hemiplegia and hand controls for acceleration for someone with lower extremity paralysis. A hand control for brakes is also available. For those who do not have the use of their hands, special foot controls are available. When a person is severely handicapped, a special van can be purchased (see Fig. 18–4).

Special equipment can be located through training centers, car manufacturers and the State Department of Highways. Some Veterans Hospitals conduct a driver training program as well as assess persons for needed equipment. In addition to this, one can request *Vehicle Controls for Disabled Persons* from

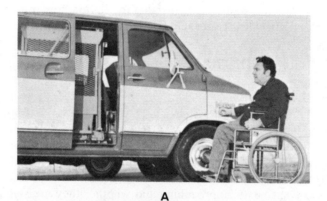

A

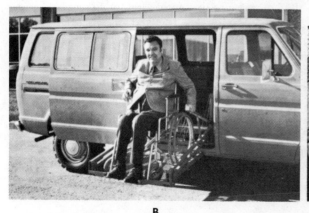

B

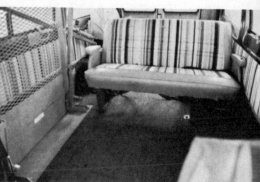

C

Figure 18–4 A lift designed for use in Chevrolet, Dodge and Ford vans. (Courtesy Para Lift Industries, Ltd., Calgary, Alberta, Canada.)

A, Door opens and lift comes to the ground by use of an outside key switch.

B, Automatic lift.

C, After entry the lift raises into the van and the door closes by an inside switch.

the American Automobile Association, 1712 G Street, N.W., Washington, D.C. 20006.

Driver's training in the use of special equipment can be obtained in all large metropolitan areas merely by looking in the yellow pages of the telephone book under Driver's Training. These people are often helpful in recommending names of companies with special driving equipment. The disabled person can obtain additional information from the State Department of Highways. It is well to remember, however, that not all employees of the highway department are familiar with regulations for and needs of the disabled driver. It may therefore be necessary for the family to persist until they talk to someone who has the proper information.

Once equipment has been selected and the person has gone through a training period, he is then ready to be tested. Driving tests are given just as they are to any other individual. However, it is important to set up an appointment time and to state that you will be taking the test with special equipment.

Once the test has been taken and insurance has been purchased, other aids are helpful. In Minnesota, a special highway flag is available to be used as a distress signal in the event of a mechanical breakdown or a flat tire. Some states use a windshield or bumper sticker to identify a car driven by a disabled person. In addition, the installation of a two-way car radio is invaluable in case of an emergency breakdown.

Some communities provide a special parking sticker or card, similar to that used by the press, which acts as a parking permit in specified no-parking areas. At work and at school, it is important to find and mark an appropriate parking space to allow for wheelchair transfers in and out of a car.

TRAVEL FOR PLEASURE

There is no reason why a disabled person cannot travel for pleasure provided that he thoroughly prepares himself for the trip. He will need to obtain certain information well in advance of a trip in order to make adequate plans and preparations. For example, early in 1971, a woman who requires a battery-operated pneumobelt to breathe when she is not in her respirator flew from California to Madrid and home again. A travel agency called Flying Wheels in Owatonna, Minnesota, specializes in planning trips for the disabled. They arranged this trip with the technical division of TWA, so that there were newly charged batteries at each stop of the 13-hour trip. They also arrange group tours, as does Wings on Wheels Tours in Lynnwood, Washington.

Generally speaking, there are three "musts" for any air traveler who uses a wheelchair or some other piece of equipment that could cause delay. First, call ahead of time, describe the nature of the problem and state if a wheelchair is needed and whether you will need help on boarding. Second, come approximately 40 minutes ahead of flight time, so that the handling of the wheelchair or other necessary equipment can take place before the peak period of activity. This helps to assure receiving adequate care. Third, the disabled person should always arrange to have someone meet him.

Most travel agencies do not know or understand the problems of the disabled. They are unfamiliar with the problems and are therefore unable to make plans to avoid them. The Moss Rehabilitation Hospital in Philadelphia has recently started the Moss Travel Information Center which provides free service to the handicapped and to travel agencies who serve the handicapped. Their information includes hotel, restaurant, transportation and entertainment information in Africa, the Orient and Europe. Other available travel information may be obtained from the following sources:

The Wheelchair Traveler, prepared by Douglass Annand, 169 Woodland Hill, California 91364. This book provides hotel and motel information.

National Park Guide for the Handicapped, prepared by the Superintendent of Documents, Stock No. 2405–0286, Washington, D.C. 20402. This booklet describes some of the areas in which camping and sightseeing are particularly accessible.

Where Turning Wheels Stop, prepared by the Paralyzed Veterans of America Inc., 3636 16th Street NW, Washington, D.C. 20010. This booklet lists restaurants, hotel and motel information by state.

The Easter Seal Directory of Resident Camps for Persons with Special Health Needs, prepared by the National Easter Seal Society, 2023 W. Ogden Avenue, Chicago, Illinois 60612 ($1.00), lists camps by state, age groups, conditions, cost and sponsoring organization.

In addition, many of the local chapters of the Society for Crippled Children and Adults prepare guidebooks for the handicapped in certain cities. It would be worth calling the local chapter of this organization to see if such a book exists in your area or in the area of travel.

For the person traveling by car, it is helpful to know that as a general rule, Mobil Oil rest rooms are specially designed to be accessible to persons in wheelchairs. Look for the sticker portraying a person in a wheelchair.

RECREATION

Many recreational activities are accessible. Some are specially planned for disabled persons, but architectural barriers must be ascertained before arrival time. In some instances they can be avoided, and in other instances a different building will have to be used. For example, many movie theaters are accessible, but some are not. The disabled person may be able to see movies only when they come to the particular theater that is accessible.

It is always wise to inquire in advance about stairs inside and outside if a wheelchair is to be used. It is even wiser to go and look for yourself because in some cases persons who are unfamiliar with the problem provide partial or inadequate information.

Generally speaking, the disabled person can locate restaurants where the tables are not too close together to prohibit passage of a wheelchair. Many sports stadiums are accessible. Libraries, museums and so forth may be more difficult, since they are frequently housed in older buildings and, therefore, are more likely to be inaccessible. Newer theaters, such as the John F. Kennedy Center for the Performing Arts in Washington, D.C., are built to accommodate both the able-bodied and the disabled. This complex has elevators, ramps and special parking areas, and fountains and telephones at wheelchair height. Rest rooms have wide doors and grab bars. Features for the blind include knurled doorknobs to indicate danger areas. Some of the resources listed under travel also provides information on recreation.

The Smithsonian Air and Space Museum in Washington, D.C., is outstanding in its attention to disabled persons. For instance, the Apollo 11 capsule is set on its side so people in wheelchairs can look into it. The blind can learn about man's ascent into air by following the story on special paper that has three-dimensional images to be read with the fingertips. Deaf persons receive written scripts of movies and other audiovisuals. The book shop sells braille books and tapes on aerospace. Some guides are even trained in sign language.

In addition to public recreational facilities, there are special disabled sports groups. Disabled persons play basketball and table tennis and are involved in track and field events, archery, swimming and bowling. These activities are particularly important for the person who has always enjoyed participating in sports. In most instances, a medical social worker is familiar with these resources. The first issue of the *Wheelchair Competitor,* a magazine, was published in the winter of 1971. This magazine helps the individual to learn about various sports and recreational groups. The address is 30396 Stellamar Drive, Birmingham, Michigan 48010.

In addition, there are groups which focus mainly on socialization. These may emphasize social action, hobbies or purely friendship. Some are "condition" oriented, such as the Stroke Club in Galveston, Texas.

PUBLIC ATTITUDES

Certain countries attend to the needs of the disabled far better than others. Sweden may well do the best job. There, the government is committed to the importance of the key triad: mobility, housing and jobs. The United States is far behind. However, these issues are beginning to surface with greater visibility as the era of consumerism unfolds. Certainly the issue of jobs is a human rights issue, and the states of New York and Minnesota have work discrimination laws that now include the disabled.

Unfortunately, disabled persons are still too often treated as a minority group. While there are approximately 30 million of them, they are often overlooked. They are usually unable to be as independent as possible because of physical barriers. They are kept at a social distance and face segregation by virtue of people's personal attitudes and the indifference with which we build our schools, houses, sports arenas and other structures. Depersonalized charity, such as buying Easter Seals, may ease our conscience but does not solve the daily problems of disabled persons in their interactions with the rest of the community.

At the present time, the issue of whether disabled persons should be segregated or integrated in terms of housing has not been settled. Many facilities are actually built to isolate the disabled from the able-bodied. The question arises—Is this what the disabled want or is this what the able-bodied want? A few studies indicate that this is more the wish of the able-bodied than of the disabled person.

In many instances, the disabled also suffer from an unfair vocational disadvantage. The attitude and awareness of the public has been slow to change. The nurse and other professional health workers can truly assist disabled persons. By virtue of their awareness of the problems of the disabled, additional spokesmen help to step up the pace of improved conditions in the community.

HEALTH MAINTENANCE IN THE COMMUNITY

Once an individual is "rehabilitated," has returned home and become re-integrated into family and community life, new physical and psychological needs may arise. Therefore, a regular follow-up program is desirable in order to ensure that the person maintains optimal function. Ideally, this follow-up is carried out by a team of rehabilitation professionals so that physical assessment is not the only area of concern. In some instances the follow-up program may involve a few days of hospitalization.

The Sister Kenny Institute has two programs that may serve as examples. One is called SCIF (spinal cord injury follow-up) and is usually done annually. It involves a complete re-evaluation of function by nursing, physical therapy, occupational therapy, social service and psychology staff. A complete physical examination is done, with special evaluation of the urinary tract. The patient is an integral part of all conferences and planning. The Institute's other program is called SEAF (stroke evaluation and follow-up). This is done after hospital discharge to see if further progress is possible and is similar to SCIF in terms of completeness of areas of assessment.

FURTHER RESOURCES

Throughout this book, resources have been suggested for each problem area. In addition, invaluable help can be obtained from publications of organizations devoted to specific diseases. The following resources will provide additional information on various major diseases and health problems. The national organization can inform you of any state or local chapters that may be nearby geographically.

Aging

National Dairy Council
111 N. Canal Street
Chicago, Illinois 60606

Administration on Aging
U.S. Department of Health,
   Education and Welfare
HEW South Building
Washington, D.C. 20201

Arthritis

The Arthritis Foundation
1212 Avenue of the Americas
New York, New York 10019

Birth Defects

National Foundation–
   March of Dimes
P.O. Box 2000
White Plains, New York 10602

National Genetics Foundation
250 W. 57th Street
New York, New York 10019

Cancer

American Cancer Society, Inc.
219 East 42nd Street
New York, New York 10017

Cerebral Palsy

United Cerebral Palsy Association,
    Inc.
66 East 34th Street
New York, New York 10016

National Easter Seal Society
2023 W. Ogden Ave.
Chicago, Illinois 60612

Deafness

Alexander Graham Bell
    Association for the Deaf
1537 35th Street N.W.
Washington, D.C. 20007

National Association of Hearing
    and Speech Agencies
919 18th Street N.W.
Washington, D.C. 20006

Diabetes

American Diabetes Association
18 East 48th Street
New York, New York 10017

*Heart Disease, Hypertension, and
Stroke*

American Heart Association
44 East 23rd Street
New York, New York 10010

Kidney Disease

National Kidney Foundation
116 E. 27th Street
New York, New York 10016

Multiple Sclerosis

National Multiple Sclerosis Society
257 Park Avenue South
New York, New York 10010

Muscular Dystrophy

Muscular Dystrophy Association
    of America, Inc.
1790 Broadway
New York, New York 10019

Ostomy

United Ostomy Association
111 Wilshire Boulevard
Los Angeles, California 90017

Paraplegia and Quadriplegia

National Paraplegia Foundation
333 North Michigan Avenue
Chicago, Illinois 60601

Paralyzed Veterans of America
3636 16th Street N.W.
Washington, D.C. 20010

Parkinson's Disease

American Parkinson's Disease
    Association, Inc.
147 East 50th Street
New York, New York 10022

Visual Problems

American Foundation for the Blind
15 W. 16th Street
New York, New York 10011

Division for the Blind and
    Physically Handicapped
Library of Congress
Washington, D.C. 20542

SUMMARY

Once an individual has been rehabilitated physically and has come to terms with his disability psychologically, he is discharged from the hospital or rehabilitation center. At this point, the person begins a new life. In order to make that life whole, meaningful and varied, he or she will need to participate in the same activities in which we all engage. The world of work, the use of public buildings, education, travel, recreation and pleasure are all open to the disabled person. If health professionals know this, they will be able to seek local resources that are in keeping with the patient's interests. Together, they will seek a life that is as normal and as well balanced as possible for the disabled person.

REFERENCES

Akamu, Tom: Facilities and services for handicapped students at colleges in Hawaii. *Rehabilitation Literature, 36*:134, May, 1975.

Adams, Ronald C.: Bowling for the physically handicapped. *Interclinic Information Bulletin, 10*:9, 1970.

Annand, Douglass R.: *The Wheelchair Travler.* P.O. Box 169, Woodland Hill, California 91364.

Design for all Americans. A Report of the National Commission on Architectural Barriers to Rehabilitation of the Handicapped. Social and Rehabilitation Service, U.S. Department of Health, Education and Welfare, Superintendent of Documents, Washington, D.C. 20402, 1968.

Goldsmith, Selwyn: *Designing for the Disabled.* New York, McGraw-Hill Book Co., 1967.

Granger, Ben: Developing community-based, small-group living programs in rehabilitation services. *Rehabilitation Literature, 36*:170, June, 1975.

Greenstein, D., et al: "No one at home"; a brief review of housing for handicapped persons in some European countries. *Rehabilitation Literature, 37*:2, January, 1976.

Hagle, Alfred D.: The large print revolution. *Library Journal,* September 15, 1967.

Housing Needs of the Handicapped. Research Division, Massachusetts Association of Paraplegics, Inc., Bedford, Massachusetts 01730, November, 1970.

How to Get Help If You Are Paralyzed. The National Paraplegic Foundation, 333 N. Michigan Avenue, Chicago, Illinois 60601.

Lauder, Ruth: *The Goal Is: Mobility!* Social and Rehabilitation Service, U.S. Department of Health, Education and Welfare, Washington, D.C. 20201, 1969.

Lowman, Edward, and Klinger, Judith: *Aids to Independent Living.* New York, McGraw-Hill Book Co., 1969.

Lynton, Edith: The physically handicapped citizen: a human rights issue. *In* Garrell, J., and Levine, E. (Eds.): *Rehabilitation Practices With the Physically Disabled.* New York, Columbia University Press, 1973.

McGaughey, Rita: From problem to solution: the new focus in fighting environmental barriers for the handicapped. *Rehabilitation Literature, 37*:10, January, 1976.

Making Buildings and Facilities Accessible to, and Usable by, the Physically Handicapped. American Standards Institute, Inc., 1430 Broadway, New York, New York 10018, 1961.

Nyquist, Roy H., and Bors, Ernest: Mortality and survival in traumatic myelopathy during nineteen years, from 1946 to 1965. *Paraplegia, 5*:22, 1967.

President's Committee on Employment of the Handicapped: *Guide to the National Parks and Monuments for Handicapped Tourists.* Washington, D.C., U.S. Government Printing Office, 1966.

Roeher, G. Allan: Significance of public attitudes in the rehabilitation of the disabled. *Rehabilitation Literature, 22*:66, 1961.

Rusk, Howard: *Rehabilitation Medicine.* 3rd Ed. St. Louis, C. V. Mosby Co., 1971.

Siller, Jerome: *Attitudes of the Nondisabled Toward the Physically Disabled.* New York, New York University, May, 1967.

State University Construction Fund of Albany, New York: *Architectural Checklist: Making Colleges and Universities Accessible to Handicapped Students.* Reprinted by the President's Committee on Employment of the Handicapped, Washington, D.C. 20210 (undated).

Stohl, Dora: Preserving home life for the disabled. *American Journal of Nursing, 72*:1645, September, 1972.

Strauss, Anselm: *Chronic Illness and the Quality of Life.* St. Louis, C. V. Mosby Co., 1975.

Talbot, Herbert: *The Working Life of a Paraplegic.* Washington, D.C., U.S. Government Printing Office, 1962.

Weaver, Robert C.: *Housing for the Physically Disabled; A Guide for Planning and Design,* U.S. Department of Housing and Urban Development, Superintendent of Documents, Washington, D.C. 20402, 1968.

Where Turning Wheels Stop. Paralyzed Veterans of America Inc., 3636 16th Street NW, Washington, D.C. 20010.

Chapter 19

THE ELDERLY IN THE COMMUNITY

The elderly have complex health needs, require multiple kinds of services, and are heavy users of health services. They comprise almost 11 per cent of our population, and 95 per cent of the elderly live in the community. While the foregoing chapters of this book contain information applicable to care of the elderly, it seems fitting that a rehabilitation nursing text end by addressing itself specifically to a population particularly suited to the preventive and maintenance aspects of this field. Hospitalization and institutionalization of the elderly can be prevented or at least delayed by (1) monitoring their chronic conditions, (2) promoting a healthy social environment and (3) intervening with appropriate community services.

Rehabilitation of the elderly has special implications. It means that one views aging as a stage of development. It also means that one views aging as a *process* rather than as a disease or a chronicle of inevitable losses. There are a great many losses, granted, but there are ways of adapting to these losses. For instance, with experimentation, a balance between activity and rest can reduce the effects of loss of energy. Intellectual stimulation is available from tuition-free college courses, community lectures, public television and radio. Music and art can be found in most communities. Social centers, political activist groups (Gray Panthers, Senior Federations, political parties) and churches all provide opportunities for socializing and making contributions to society. In other words, unless an elderly person is severely incapacitated physically, psychologically or mentally (and this is not usual), quality of life, not just quantity, can be attained. It is up to society and the health professions to put the elderly in touch with the necessary resources.

To maintain and rehabilitate the elderly optimally, our society and present health care system require several changes. There is an urgent need for a greater number of physicians who are educated in geriatrics and who find care of the elderly rewarding. There is a need for more nurses who are educated in geriatrics and who will place greater emphasis on helping their patients socially and psychologically. Finally, our society needs to be more willing to release dollars to enable the elderly to live in the mainstream of life as long as possible.

PHYSICAL AND MENTAL CHANGES ASSOCIATED WITH THE AGING PROCESS

The aging process actually begins at birth and continues throughout the total life span. The rate of the process varies not only in the body systems of each individual but also between individuals. Individual variations are largely attributable to differences in genetic durability, general health habits, mental attitudes and general activity. Recognizing that there are individual differences in degree and timing, the following findings capsulize common changes.

PHYSICAL CHANGES

Both vision and hearing are affected by the aging process. Vision is affected by increasing farsightedness after the age of 45, diminishing visual acuity, poor night vision, difficulty in distinguishing blue and green light, and falling off of lateral vision. Hearing ability gradually lessens after 50 years of age. Other rather common ear problems are tinnitus and vertigo. Nearly all of our social, esthetic and intellectual stimuli are received through our eyes and ears. Therefore, medical care in these areas is essential to prevent a compounding of any mental and psychological changes.

Gum difficulties and recession of jaws increase the likelihood of dental problems and loss of teeth, which may in turn affect nutritional intake. While there is a diminishing volume of gastric juices, there continues to be a fairly good ability to absorb foods for tissue building. General appetite is good but somewhat smaller, probably owing to lessened physical activity.

In spite of an increased blood pressure and increased pulse rate, there is a decline in total blood flow. Breathing rates are slower, and there is a decreased ability to transfer oxygen to the blood stream. When an older person says he is "slowing down," this is one of the phenomena he is describing.

Other changes are principally related to the musculoskeletal system. Muscle tissue shrinks and becomes dehydrated and more fibrous, causing diminished strength. Ligaments contract and harden, causing the bent posture of the elderly person. Bones become more fragile because of a decrease in calcium content. There is also somewhat less padding on the feet and less sensitivity to temperature variation, resulting in a greater tendency to bruises and calluses. Much of the physical discomfort of the aged is related to these changes rather than to any specific disease.

MENTAL CHANGES

Intelligence and Learning. Present knowledge indicates that once intelligence reaches its peak, it is maintained if the individual is active and free of any physical or neurological changes. While a few areas of intelligence, such as arithmetic ability, may be diminished, most areas continue to be the same. The ability to learn is retained, although it may take a little longer—an important point for the nurse to remember while teaching an older person. Fear of failure or ridicule may also interfere with learning. Practice will help to assure retention of most skills. Brain and nervous system changes may be evidenced by an overall slowness in reaction time and loss of short-range memory, but these changes should not be confused with loss of intelligence or learning ability.

Sensation and Perception.   Loss of hearing and visual acuity have already been mentioned. These losses, along with diminished tactile sensation, decrease the individual's sensory intake. Because lack of sensory stimuli adversely affects mental and emotional health, it is vital to assist the elderly by providing environmental stimuli and cues.

Personality.   Elderly persons may suffer from mental illness like anybody else and naturally require therapy when it occurs. Aside from this, they have problems specifically related to their age, such as death of spouse, death of friends, reduced income and reduced energy.

Erikson takes the view that growth occurs whenever a developmental crisis is resolved. Since aging is a part of the development of life, one's adjustment to it will be similar to and influenced by one's previous life style. Two rather common negative reactions to aging are overdependence on others and anger, which may be expressed by blaming others or oneself. In spite of infirmities, many elderly persons achieve a constructive adjustment by which they adapt to their living situation without loss of self-esteem. In many cases a more successful adjustment is possible if safety and security needs are first cared for.

There are two frequently discussed theories related to the adjustment to aging. The first is the theory of *disengagement*. This theory states that, in preparation for death, the aged person retreats from society and society retreats from the aged. The theory has been modified, as it does not account for the many older persons who do favor engagement in life. The second theory is known as *role flexibility*. As a person approaches 65 years of age, his or her roles of worker, spouse and parent will be either discontinued or reduced. If, however, a person enters new roles, with citizen groups, church groups, friends and so on, and engages in hobbies that are artistic, intellectual or creative, he is said to have role flexibility. This is the emphasis of retirement preparation groups, which explore possible new roles for the future. Together, these two theories cover both groups of elderly persons—those who tend to drop away from society upon retirement and those who do not.

INDEPENDENCE–DEPENDENCE CONCEPTS IN THE AGED

The application of rehabilitation philosophy, knowledge and skills to the elderly population is basic to geriatric care. Maintaining function, reducing the effects of the aging process and increasing physical and psychosocial capabilities are of course primary aims. Depending on the extent to which an elderly individual has (1) reduced strength, (2) physical limitations, (3) diminished vision or hearing, or both, (4) altered ego strength, (5) changed social performance, (6) reduced cognitive skill and (7) slower motor responses, some degree of dependency will be necessary.

This dependency refers to a state of being, not a state of mind. It does not refer to the older person with a lifelong history of being dependent on others. For most elderly persons, one must identify the areas of dependence so that support can be given in these areas to prevent further dependency on others. This concept of carefully prescribed support to prevent dependency can be understood best by example. A person with reduced strength may need to depend on a homemaker for cleaning in order to allow himself enough energy to continue doing his own cooking and maintain at least minimal social function. In other words, by attending to one dependency, other dependencies may be avoided or reduced.

Many dependency programs for the elderly are found under the rubric of alternatives to institutionalization. Basically such alternatives consist of ways of preventing premature or inappropriate institutionalization. It is certainly better to allow a person to be as independent as possible as long as possible. However, the time will come in some persons' lives when institutionalization is preferred, as it may be the best way to support the person physically, psychologically and socially. Once a person has been institutionalized, personnel must be careful to provide help only where help is needed, as unncessary dependency can be induced by staff who perform tasks that the person can do. Elderly persons often view such assistance as indicative of a hopeless attitude toward their capabilities. They may then accept this "professional" opinion and give up trying to do things for themselves altogether. Nursing home personnel need to be constantly on guard for overdependence that is created either by staff attitudes and actions or by institutional characteristics such as lack of programming, policies that take away individual decision making, depersonalized routines and so on.

SPECIAL AREAS OF ASSESSMENT FOR THE ELDERLY

In order to develop a successful plan of care for an elderly person, the following factors must be considered:

Religion.   For the elderly, active church affiliation may or may not be important. The important issue is whether the person has any internal conflict about his or her beliefs.

Cultural Background.   What needs and attitudes will affect the plan of care?

Marriage.   How many marriages? How long married? Is spouse living?

Family.   How many children, grandchildren, siblings? Do they live nearby? Does the person have close ties with them?

Friends.   Any close companions available?

Education, Work and Retirement.   How much education in the past? Any present educational activities? What kind of work was done in the past? At present? Retirement enjoyable?

Economic Security.   Do combined sources of income provide adequate food, clothing, housing, medical care and at least minimal pleasures? What health coverage is available?

Housing.   Where is the person currently living? Are living quarters appropriate to the person's physical and mental capabilities? Is there a difference of opinion about the appropriateness of living situation between the person, the family and the health care professional?

Mobility.   Is the person able to drive, use public transportation, find assistance on his own? Does he require special equipment? Is it possible to obtain food, medicine? Is it possible to visit the physician, friends, relatives?

Physical History and Findings.   In addition to a thorough history and physical examination, it is vital to assess what equipment or adaptations will be needed if there is visual loss, hearing loss, a urinary problem, gait problem, energy problem or memory problem. Obviously these things will affect or influence the areas of dependence and independence.

Psychological History and Findings.   Besides taking a physical and social history, it is important to know of any emotional problems the person might have had in the past. It is also vital to know what recent losses have occurred and what recent feelings of anxiety, depression or loneliness exist, as well as the person's previous personality traits, sleep patterns and feelings about aging and death.

Once information about the foregoing areas is gathered, personal support systems can be planned around the special needs that emerge.

CONCERNS OF THE COMMUNITY HEALTH NURSE

It is essential that nursing services be available to the elderly person living at home. Although the nurse may enter the home because of a specific condition, she must be aware of the total needs of the elderly. Home health aides and homemakers, persons trained to perform housekeeping tasks, are available in most communities through the local health department, visiting nurse service or other agency. While an elderly person may be cared for by these persons regularly, it is the responsibility of the community health nurse to assess the needs of each patient and to develop a nursing plan for these persons to follow. In most cases, the nurse will monitor needs, follow up, and modify care plans at intervals. In addition to the primary purpose of home care, the nurse will need to assist in other matters.

SAFETY

Accidents rank as the sixth leading cause of death in those over 65 years of age. In addition, thousands of disabling injuries occur among those in this age group each year. Therefore, a primary nursing responsibility to the elderly is accident prevention.

Because elderly persons may have a tendency toward dizziness, weakness and numbness, they must learn to make allowances for it. Older persons should not get up from a bed or chair suddenly without support. Such movements should be done slowly and while holding onto something or someone. Older persons should get help if they need to climb on ladders or carry heavy loads. There should be good lighting and handrails at stairways, and night lights should be placed at the floor level of bedrooms and bathrooms. If dizzy spells are common, properly installed grab bars are essential in the bathroom for the tub, shower and toilet. Small scatter rugs should either be removed or secured to the floor. Well-fitting shoes should always be worn rather than loose slippers. Control knobs on stoves need to be carefully marked so that "on" and "off" positions can easily be seen. The older person should be cautioned against cooking while wearing full sleeves or long trailing robes, especially with a gas stove.

In addition, it is important to see that medicines and household cleaning agents are not stored near one another. The National Safety Council advises that internal and external medicines be stored separately and that cleaning agents and solvents be kept away from seasonings and cooking items. A large red ✕ or a piece of sandpaper should be placed on all items in the medicine chest that are for external use only. The elderly person should also be cautioned to turn on a light, put on eyeglasses and read both the label and the directions before taking any medicine. If pills are kept at the night stand, only one night's supply should be kept there, to prevent an overdose in a state of confusion.

MOBILITY

If a person wishes to participate in senior citizens' groups, go to church, go shopping, or see a physician, it is important for the nurse to know if the patient has transportation or is able to use public transportation. The person may not be able to afford the bus, or he may be unable to get on and off a bus or subway safely. He may not be able to make the trip without getting lost or confused. Many a social venture or clinic appointment is omitted for such reasons. A local community resource or relative may be able to assist if the problems are known. Activity is vital in overcoming loneliness and isolation as well as maintaining adequate physical health.

HEARING ABILITY

One of the most important social isolators is loss of hearing. Besides actual deterioration, tinnitus may occur and further interfere with hearing. Some hearing conditions may be surgically corrected, some may be helped by the use of a hearing aid and a few may require the learning of lip reading, more accurately called speech reading. The latter is, of course, impossible if the patient also has a serious visual problem.

Any person who has a hearing problem should be evaluated by a physician and an audiologist, if one is available, to establish which treatment may or may not help. If a physician or audiologist recommends a hearing aid, the most suitable requirements are prescribed for the particular problem. The patient is then able to ask the hearing aid salesman to demonstrate the aids that fulfill these requirements. Once the hearing aid has been prescribed, selected and purchased, it is important that the person understand how to operate and adjust it to a comfortable volume. If the aid has an ear mold, it must be washed frequently. It is vital that batteries in all aids be replaced regularly. Many an older person sets aside a hearing aid, saying it does not help, when in reality it needs volume adjustment, a new battery or removal of wax from the ear mold. The patient should always be referred back to the hearing aid sales representative, as this is the person who can be most helpful in showing how to use and maintain an aid. For communicating with the hearing-impaired person, review Chapter 7.

NUTRITION

The older person may not eat properly for a variety of reasons, including poverty, mental depression, loneliness, mental impairment, medications that impair appetite or utilization of food intake, and some physical conditions. Once physical reasons have been treated or ruled out, the nurse can assist the person with other problems related to nutrition. Adequate fluid intake can usually be attained by using thirst as a guide to quantity. As part of a nutritionally balanced diet, it is essential that the older person receive at least 1 gram of protein per kilogram of body weight in order to assure optimum tissue repair.

Consistency of food should be considered. Dental problems may require the use of puréed and soft foods. Because of discomfort from dentures, some persons choose to wear them only for eating. In many instances, it may be necessary to assist the person in securing dental care.

An older person's appetite may be normal, but he or she may overeat out of boredom (often snack foods that are not nutritious) or undereat for the reasons cited above. For the latter, small, more frequent meals may be beneficial. A little wine or beer may be used to stimulate the appetite, provided there is no tendency toward chemical dependency on alcoholic beverages. If a person lives alone or has low energy, cooking adequate meals may become a severe problem. In some communities, Meals on Wheels, a portable meal service that brings at least one hot meal a day to the home, is available. Some apartment residences provide one meal a day in a central dining room, leaving cooking of other meals up to the individual. The nurse must, therefore, assess both the elderly person's nutritional state and nutritional intake in order to make appropriate recommendations.

DRUG REACTIONS

The older patient reacts differently to drug therapy for several reasons. Biologic changes alter the absorption, metabolism, distribution, excretion and drug action. These changes result in a decreased absorption in the intestinal mucosa, more free drug in the plasma, decreased activation of the drug in the liver and less efficient excretion of the drug from the urinary tract. In addition, the target organ may be damaged, so that the usual dose of a drug may be excessive. In essence, this means that an elderly person's medications may have greater impact with any given dosage, may accumulate more readily and will have a longer lasting effect. These factors, along with the fact that the Federal Drug Administration's recommended doses are based on persons under 65 years of age, make it necessary to start any medication at a lower dose in order to observe the individual's response.

One other factor influences the prescription and administration of drugs to the elderly; namely, because of multiple physical problems, an older person may be taking as many as 15 drugs (polypharmacy), and this will cause drug-drug interactions. Knowing all of this, the nurse must be particularly cognizant of possible symptoms of drug accumulation, drug interaction and overdosing. Bizarre physical and mental symptoms may develop, unfortunately sometimes causing further drug prescription. The nurse should be particularly aware of a person's response to sedatives, mental confusion being a very common reaction.

There are special problems when the aged person administers his or her drugs at home. Self-medication without approval from a physician is frequent, as is improper taking of prescribed medications. Omission of a drug, taking incorrect dosage and improper sequencing are very common. The major causes of such problems are (1) lack of money to see a physician or to purchase drugs, (2) lack of understanding of or inability to hear the physician's reasons and instructions, (3) inability to get to the pharmacy, (4) inability to carry out the regimen because of physical or mental impairment and (5) dislike of the effects of the drug.

To prevent these problems, certain precautions are necessary. First, the person must have the ability to obtain and administer medications to himself. Second, the person must fully understand instructions for self-administration of drugs. If not, a spouse, a child or a nurse must be informed and available to give them. Third, all drug bottles must be clearly labelled with large print. They should be placed in clear (not brown) bottles, and safety caps for children should not be used. A periodic review of all medications should be done by the nurse, pharmacist or physician.

It would seem logical that if an older person were in a hospital or nursing home, the problems with drugs would be better managed. Unfortunately, that is not always the case, and many institutions make a practice of administering drugs for the purpose of keeping patients quiet rather than for strictly medical reasons. Dr. Ivor Felstein says that drugs should "never be a treatment based purely on the needs of the old person's attendants, be they relatives or nurses." The necessity for such a statement comes from what many physicians consider an overuse by institutions of sedatives and tranquilizers for noisy patients. Noisiness may be a sign of pain, frustration in making one's wants known, a full bladder, or a number of other discomforts. If the nurse spends a little time with a patient to try to discover the cause for the noisiness, the unnecessary use of medication can be reduced or even eliminated. An unfortunate part of such wrongly prescribed therapy is that it may mask an environmental situation that needs correcting, or actually worsen a physical problem.

HOUSING

The older person may be able to stay at home with the help of family, friends and minimal community services. If not, the person may require a living arrangement that maintains independent living but provides one or more daily meals, cleaning services, transportation services, emergency health services and possibly daily surveillance. These services may be available in special apartments, licensed board and care homes, multilevel geriatric centers and other innovative housing for the elderly.

Whether the elderly should be isolated in special housing or in housing where there is a variety of age groups is debatable. Some elderly persons actually prefer isolation, and some communities prefer that they be isolated. The best of both worlds can perhaps be accomplished by integrated areas with a segregated building for the elderly but one that is an integral part of the community.

Some elderly will naturally be housed in a nursing home. The rehabilitative nursing knowledge and skills discussed throughout this book are all applicable to nursing home residents. In addition, nursing homes are beginning to provide outreach services to the community, and hospitals are beginning to share services with nursing homes. As this trend grows, nursing homes, hospitals and community health services can provide a broad range of services to the elderly in a variety of living facilities.

SUMMARY

Rehabilitation of the elderly is basically a matter of prevention and maintenance. It most frequently begins in the home and may be unassociated with either trauma or a specific disease process, although multiple diseases are common. With appropriate assessment of elderly persons, rehabilitative approaches in the nursing home, hospital and community can bring about an improved quality of life. Institutionalization can then be selected for those who need more intensive, round-the-clock professional services.

REFERENCES

Alfano, Genrose: There are no routine patients. *American Journal of Nursing, 75*:1804, October, 1975.

American Nurses' Association: *Standards for Geriatric Nursing Practice.* ANA, 2420 Pershing Road, Kansas City, Missouri 64108.

Anderson, Helen C.: *Newton's Geriatric Nursing.* St. Louis, C. V. Mosby Co., 1971.

Burnside, Irene M.: Listen to the aged. *American Journal of Nursing, 75*:180, October, 1975.

Burnside, Irene M.: *Nursing and the aged.* New York, McGraw-Hill Book Co., 1976.

Busse, Ewald, and Pfeiffer, Eric (Eds.): *Behavior and Adaptation in Late Life.* Boston, Little, Brown and Co., 1969.

Carlson, Sylvia: Selected sensory input and life satisfactions of immobilized geriatric female patients. *American Nurses' Association Clinical Session,* 1968.

Clark, Margaret, and Anderson, Barbara G: *Culture and Aging—An Anthropological Study of Older Americans.* Springfield, Illinois, Charles C Thomas, 1967.

Costa, F., and Sweet, N.: Barrier free environments for older Americans. *Gerontologist, 16*:404, October, 1976.

Erikson, Erik H.: *Childhood and Society.* 2nd Ed. New York, W. W. Norton and Co., 1963.

Fann, W. E., and Maddox, G. L., (Eds.): *Drug Issues in Gero-Psychiatry.* Baltimore, Williams and Wilkins, 1974.

Felstein, Ivor: Precautions and problems in drug therapy of the elderly. *Nursing Mirror,* April 9, 1965, p. 53.

Greenberg, Barbara: Reaction time in the elderly. *American Journal of Nursing, 73*:2056, December, 1973.

Garrahenhart, D. G.: The use of medications in the elderly population. Nursing Clinics of North America, *2*:135, March, 1976.

Irion, Lou Anne: What's the difference in the care of the elderly? *Nursing Homes.* Part 1—December, 1969, p. 12; Part II—January, 1970, p. 15.

Kalish, Richard A. (Ed.): *The Dependencies of Old People.* Ann Arbor, Institute of Gerontology, University of Michigan–Wayne State University, 1969.

Kee, Joyce: Fluid imbalance in elderly patients. *Nursing, 73, 3*:40, April, 1973.

Levine, Rhoda L.: Disengagement in the elderly—its causes and effects. *Nursing Outlook,* October, 1969, p. 28.

Lewis, Robert, and Lewis, Myrna: *Aging and Mental Health.* St. Louis, C. V. Mosby Co., 1973.

Liederman, Herbert, et al.: Sensory deprivation. *Archives of Internal Medicine,* February, 1958, p. 389.

Long, Janet: Caring For and Caring About Elderly People—A Guide to the Rehabilitative Approach. Philadelphia, J. B. Lippincott Co., 1972.

Neugarten, Bernice: *Middle Age and Aging.* Chicago, University of Chicago Press, 1968.

Schwab, Sister Marilyn: Caring for the Aged. *American Journal of Nursing, 73*:2049, December, 1973.

Schwartz, Doris: Safe self-medication for elderly outpatients. *American Journal of Nursing, 75*:1808, October, 1975.

Schwartz, Doris, Henley, Barbara, and Zeitz, Leonard: *The Elderly Ambulatory Patient.* New York, Macmillan, 1964.

Stone, Virginia: Give the older person time. *American Journal of Nursing,* October, 1969, p. 2124.

Symposium: The special rehabilitation needs of the elderly. *Geriatrics, 31*:51–103, May, 1976.

Tobin, Sheldon: Social and health services for the future aged. *The Gerontologist,* February, 1975, p. 32 (Supplement).

INDEX

Note: Page numbers set in *italics* refer to illustrations; those followed by the letter t refer to tables.